T0247605

# Psychedelic
# Outlaws

# Psychedelic Outlaws

## THE MOVEMENT REVOLUTIONIZING MODERN MEDICINE

by Joanna Kempner, PhD

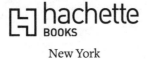

hachette
BOOKS

New York

Hachette Books

Hachette Book Group

1290 Avenue of the Americas

New York, NY 10104

HachetteBooks.com

Twitter.com/HachetteBooks

Instagram.com/HachetteBooks

First Edition: June 2024

Published by Hachette Books, an imprint of Hachette Book Group, Inc. The Hachette Books name and logo is a trademark of the Hachette Book Group.

The Hachette Speakers Bureau provides a wide range of authors for speaking events. To find out more, go to hachettespeakersbureau.com or email HachetteSpeakers@hbgusa.com.

Books by Hachette Books may be purchased in bulk for business, educational, or promotional use. For information, please contact your local bookseller or Hachette Book Group Special Markets Department at special.markets@hbgusa.com.

The publisher is not responsible for websites (or their content) that are not owned by the publisher.

Print book interior design by Amy Quinn.

Library of Congress Cataloging-in-Publication Data

Names: Kempner, Joanna, author.

Title: Psychedelic outlaws : the movement revolutionizing modern medicine / by Joanna Kempner, PhD.

Description: First edition. | New York : Hachette Books, 2024. | Includes
  bibliographical references and index.

Identifiers: LCCN 2024001704 | ISBN 9780306828942 (hardcover) | ISBN 9780306828966 (ebook)

Subjects: LCSH: Mushrooms, Hallucinogenic—Therapeutic use. | Mushrooms,
  Hallucinogenic—Research—History—20th century. | Mushrooms,
  Hallucinogenic—Research—History—21st century. | Drug development.

Classification: LCC RM324.8 .K46 2024 | DDC 615.7/883—dc23/eng/20240207

LC record available at https://lccn.loc.gov/2024001704

ISBNs: 978-0-306-82894-2 (hardcover); 978-0-306-82896-6 (ebook)

Printed in the United States of America

LSC-H

Printing 1, 2024

Tessa, Noah, and Joe. This book is dedicated to my family.

# AUTHOR'S NOTE

THIS BOOK IS AS MUCH ABOUT JUSTICE AS IT IS ABOUT PAIN. THE STORIES might sometimes read like fiction, but the book is grounded in years of research and lived experience that question the very norms of medicine and the justice—or lack thereof—embedded in our systems of care.

Between 2013 and 2023, I followed Clusterbusters, a patient community, wherever their search for pain relief took me. I often met people at community gatherings. I sometimes traveled to their homes and offices. But they usually met online in discussion groups, forums, and emails. Immersing myself in this digital landscape taught me about their daily struggles and helped me learn how they developed this movement. Tracking their journey introduced me to a range of new worlds, from the psychedelic underground network of spore dealers and clandestine chemists to the prestigious, credentialed aboveground scientists working at Ivy League universities in an epic story of survival at the edge of medicine.

Quotations within these pages are copied from digital recordings or historical records, apart from minor modifications to enhance readability and, when necessary, adjustments to identifying information. Pseudonyms are marked with an asterisk. More details about this research and its limitations can be found in the notes.[1]

**If you or someone you love needs help, please seek it.**
We offer the following resources as a starting point.

In the United States and Canada, you can call the National Suicide Prevention Lifeline for free and confidential support 24/7: **988**.

Outside the United States, the following websites provide information on accessing free and confidential support:
Find a Helpline: **https://findahelpline.com/i/iasp**
Befrienders Worldwide: **https://befrienders.org**

# CONTENTS

# TIMELINE

— 8000 BCE: Evidence suggests that humans across the globe are using psychoactive drugs, including hallucinogens.

— 1799: The *London Medical and Physical Journal* publishes the first medical description of a psychedelic mushroom experience, which it characterizes as a poisoning.

— 1887: Quanah Parker, chief of the Comanche tribe, gives fifty pounds of dried peyote to Smithsonian Institute archaeologist James Mooney.

— 1888: Anna Nickels, a cactus dealer, informs Parke-Davis, the pharmaceutical company, that local Mexicans use peyote to treat headaches.

— 1894: María Sabina born (approximate).

— 1896: D. Webster Prentiss and Francis P. Morgan publish a study suggesting peyote buttons can treat "nervous headache."

— 1897: Dr. Arthur Heffter isolates mescaline and demonstrates via self-experimentation that it is the psychoactive component in peyote.

— 1906: *Psilocybe cubensis*, a psychoactive mushroom, is formally identified and described by American mycologist Franklin Sumner Earle in Cuba, marking a crucial early step in the scientific documentation of psychoactive fungi.

— 1912: 4-Methylenedioxymethamphetamine (MDMA) is first synthesized by Merck Pharmaceuticals in Germany.

— 1914: US Harrison Narcotics Tax Act is passed. First attempt to regulate and control the production and distribution of opiates and coca products.

1918: James Mooney, the Smithsonian Institute archaeologist who obtained peyote from the Comanche tribe, writes a charter to protect Native American rights to worship with peyote, which serves as the basis for the Native American Church.

1937: Marihuana Tax Act places an excise tax on cannabis, marking a significant shift in US drug policy by laying the groundwork for the eventual criminalization of the substance.

1938: Albert Hofmann first synthesizes lysergic acid diethylamide (LSD) at Sandoz Laboratories in Basel, Switzerland.

1943: Albert Hofmann synthesizes dihydroergotamine (DHE), a vital headache medicine.

1943: Albert Hofmann resynthesizes LSD and discovers its psychoactive potential.

1953–1963: Central Intelligence Agency sponsors Project MKUltra, which involved the administration of high doses of LSD to experimental subjects.

1953: Aldous Huxley publishes *The Doors of Perception* detailing his experiences with mescaline.

1957: *Life* magazine publishes R. Gordon Wasson's travelogue "Seeking the Magic Mushroom."

1960: Timothy Leary initiates the Harvard Psilocybin Project.

1962: Congress passes the US Kefauver-Harris Drug Amendments.

1963: Sandoz allows its patent on LSD to expire.

1963: Federigo Sicuteri publishes a landmark study testing LSD and methysergide as a preventative for migraine and cluster headache.

1965: Congress passes the US Drug Abuse Control Amendments.

1965: Sandoz Pharmaceuticals abandons its production of LSD.

1966: California criminalizes the recreational use of LSD.

1966: National Institutes of Mental Health takes over the LSD stock from Sandoz.

1967: The Summer of Love, a significant cultural phenomenon, centers on the explosion of the counterculture and the widespread use of psychedelics.

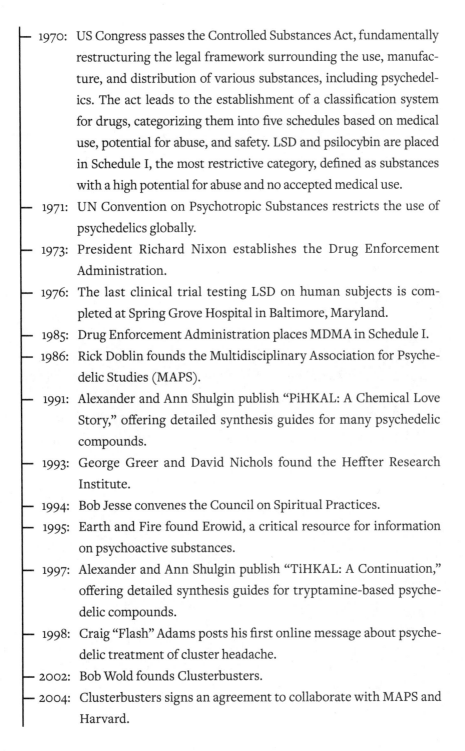

1970: US Congress passes the Controlled Substances Act, fundamentally restructuring the legal framework surrounding the use, manufacture, and distribution of various substances, including psychedelics. The act leads to the establishment of a classification system for drugs, categorizing them into five schedules based on medical use, potential for abuse, and safety. LSD and psilocybin are placed in Schedule I, the most restrictive category, defined as substances with a high potential for abuse and no accepted medical use.

1971: UN Convention on Psychotropic Substances restricts the use of psychedelics globally.

1973: President Richard Nixon establishes the Drug Enforcement Administration.

1976: The last clinical trial testing LSD on human subjects is completed at Spring Grove Hospital in Baltimore, Maryland.

1985: Drug Enforcement Administration places MDMA in Schedule I.

1986: Rick Doblin founds the Multidisciplinary Association for Psychedelic Studies (MAPS).

1991: Alexander and Ann Shulgin publish "PiHKAL: A Chemical Love Story," offering detailed synthesis guides for many psychedelic compounds.

1993: George Greer and David Nichols found the Heffter Research Institute.

1994: Bob Jesse convenes the Council on Spiritual Practices.

1995: Earth and Fire found Erowid, a critical resource for information on psychoactive substances.

1997: Alexander and Ann Shulgin publish "TiHKAL: A Continuation," offering detailed synthesis guides for tryptamine-based psychedelic compounds.

1998: Craig "Flash" Adams posts his first online message about psychedelic treatment of cluster headache.

2002: Bob Wold founds Clusterbusters.

2004: Clusterbusters signs an agreement to collaborate with MAPS and Harvard.

— 2006: Roland Griffiths publishes a landmark study in *Psychopharmacology*, documenting psilocybin's ability to occasion a meaningful spiritual experience.

— 2006: R. Andrew Sewell, John H. Halpern, and Harrison G. Pope publish a landmark case study series in *Neurology* documenting that people use psychedelics as a treatment for cluster headache.

— 2010: Matthias Karst, John Halpern, Michael Bernateck, and Torsten Passie publish a case series about BOL-148 as a preventive treatment for cluster headache.

— 2017: Food and Drug Administration (FDA) grants "breakthrough therapy" designation to MDMA-assisted therapy for treatment of posttraumatic stress disorder.

— 2018: FDA grants "breakthrough therapy" designation to psilocybin therapy for treatment-resistant depression.

— 2020: Oregon becomes the first state to legalize a psychedelic-assisted therapy, via Ballot Measure 109, allowing the "manufacture, delivery and administration" of psilocybin, a naturally occurring psychedelic prodrug.

— 2023: MAPS Public Benefit Corporation (now called Lykos Therapeutics) submits a new drug application for MDMA-assisted therapy to the FDA.

# Psychedelic
# Outlaws

# INTRODUCTION

MAGIC MUSHROOMS SAVED SEAN SLATTERY'S* LIFE.

Slattery has cluster headache, an almost comically banal name given the cruelty of the disease. Its signature symptom, the so-called headache, is widely considered the most painful phenomenon a human can experience. Attacks, which last between fifteen minutes and three hours, ignite the nerves behind one eye, turning it red and drowning it in tears. The eyelid droops, heavy with sorrow, the nose runs a relentless stream, and the body, caught in the storm's eye, shakes and shudders in fear.

Slattery once had one of those dream jobs, making people laugh at nightclubs and on cruise ships. Then cluster headache turned him into a recluse. He spent years in self-imposed exile, hiding away in the semifinished basement of his own home to protect his family from witnessing his violent attacks.

Six times a day, Slattery would be gripped with an attack that made him pace in circles till he dropped to his knees, buried his head in the cushion of the recliner where he slept, and screamed. Sometimes, in his desperation, he would hurl his head against the cold concrete floor, a futile attempt to knock himself unconscious. But there would be no mercy, not even in oblivion.

"That's when I would pray to God, 'Why are you doing this to me?'"

Something in him shattered the day he overheard his child pleading for someone, somewhere to do something. "Why won't anyone help Daddy?"

1

But he had no one left to ask for help. He'd already exhausted all his medical options.

"At those points you think, I'd be better off dead." Slattery's voice breaks as he recounts the darkest moments. His broad frame hunches over the small cafe table, leaning in so that I can catch every word. He is far from alone in his desperation. Cluster headache is called "suicide headache" for a reason.

Slattery's luck changed after reading about a clinical study at Yale University's medical school testing whether psilocybin, the active chemical in magic mushrooms, might work as a treatment for cluster headache. He called to volunteer as a participant, only to discover that the study hadn't yet begun enrolling. Dr. Emmanuelle Schindler, the physician running the trial, suggested that in the meantime he attend a patient advocacy meeting in Chicago run by Clusterbusters. "I think you'll find they can be helpful." (When I asked, she clarified that referrals to patient groups are "not specifically for any direction on psychedelics" but because they offer lifesaving personal support, family support, and important medical information.)

Clusterbusters proclaims its mission is "supporting research for better treatments and a cure, while advocating to improve the lives of those struggling with cluster headaches."[1] Their real purpose, so far as I can tell, is helping people with cluster headache survive a medical system that too often fails to provide adequate care. Psychedelic mushrooms are one of their key tools for patching the yawning gaps in the system.

Slattery took Schindler's advice. The gamble worked. People at the conference taught him how to obtain magic mushrooms and use them to treat his condition as safely as possible. Most found relief using a low dose, which they described as the psychedelic equivalent of drinking a few beers. The world around them got a little more vivid. Colors turned richer, walls gently swayed, and the sky deepened to a more intense blue. Emotions, the good and the tough ones, came to the surface with more ease.

Schindler was at the conference too, giving her annual update on the clinical trial at Yale. Volunteers for the study received three doses of pharmaceutical-grade psilocybin that replicated what Clusterbusters had already developed as a treatment. The study, she has said, would show that "patients know a lot more about their condition and how to treat it than they're usually given credit for."[2]

Slattery was glad he didn't wait for the trial to start. A low dose of mushrooms, which felt to him more like a strong cup of coffee, could suppress his attacks for nearly a week. The treatment wasn't perfect, especially since supply was a problem. But we were having a coffee in a city three hours from the basement he never used to leave.

Psychedelic drugs, once demonized, are now hailed as a new transformative medicine, hype that's fueled by a burst of scientific research.[3] As I write, the US Food and Drug Administration (FDA) is reviewing a submission to market MDMA-assisted therapy as a treatment for post-traumatic stress disorder (PTSD). If all goes as planned, American doctors will be able to prescribe MDMA-assisted therapy in the year 2024. FDA approval for psilocybin-assisted therapy may come as soon as 2025, given progress made on clinical trials testing this treatment for depression and end-of-life anxiety.

Other countries are already reforming their laws. In 2023, Australia chose to approve psilocybin- and MDMA-assisted psychedelic therapy on a limited basis for certain mental health disorders. Switzerland, Canada, and Israel allow the compassionate use of psychedelics in limited circumstances. Countries like Jamaica and Brazil, with more lenient laws, have become attractive locations for wellness retreats, drug developers, and research scientists.[4]

Outspoken figures across business, wellness, sports, and entertainment embrace psychedelics. Blake Mycoskie, founder of the shoe company TOMS, announced his commitment to fund $100 million of psychedelic research over the next eighteen years.[5] Tim Ferriss, Silicon Valley's productivity guru, is already one of the biggest investors and philanthropists in the field.[6] NFL player Aaron Rodgers attributes his best season to an ayahuasca experience that taught him to "unconditionally love myself."[7] Mike Tyson "smokes the toad"—a reference to a controversial practice involving secretions "milked" from a species native to the southwestern United

States and northern Mexico.[8] Will Smith and Prince Harry both speak about how the soul-searching invoked by psychedelic ceremonies helped them process the trauma and grief of their childhoods, while Gwyneth Paltrow has praised the trend as a wellness aid.[9] All this hype is reflected in a mad rush to patent psychedelic molecules.[10]

Public opinion about psychedelics is shifting too.[11] Voters in states unwilling to wait for the federal government have already legalized certain forms of psychedelic-assisted therapy. Oregon and Colorado were the first to do so. California, Massachusetts, and Washington seem primed to follow. Even conservative states like Texas are passing laws that expand psychedelic research and access, especially for veterans and first responders.

But even as everyone from tech bros to politicos have been touting the potential healing power of psychedelic medicine for mental health and addiction, the most innovative psychedelic research on pain is happening almost entirely underground—so far from the spotlight that scientists are only just catching up to the idea.

●  ●  ●●●●●●●●●●●●●●●●●●●●●  ●  ●

I've met hundreds of people like Sean Slattery experimenting with psychedelic drugs to relieve their pain. Their experiences, now documented in peer-reviewed articles, offer hope of relief amid a relentless opioid epidemic. Their story explains the vital—and mostly unacknowledged—role that citizen science in underground networks has played in nurturing psychedelic therapy over the last fifty years.[12]

It was half a century ago when US President Richard Nixon signed the 1970 Controlled Substances Act into law, a pivotal piece of legislation redefining federal drug policy. This act, which categorized drugs based on their potential for abuse, listed lysergic acid diethylamide (LSD) and psilocybin under Schedule I, its most restrictive label. Scientists must obtain government permission to research Schedule I substances—a requirement that led to a de facto prohibition on the study of psychedelic substances.

Or so the story goes. In truth, prohibition only pushed experimentation with psychedelics underground and out of sight, where it would be kept alive by a motley collection of clandestine chemists and curious psychonauts; community elders and a guild of guides; ethnomycologists and mushroom growers; shamanic healers and indigenous leaders; writers and musicians; cyberpunks and technovisionaries; Deadheads and Phish fans and counter cultural spiritual seekers.

Psychedelic medicine is back at universities thanks to these resistance movements. But from the perspective of the underground, renewed interest in psychedelic medicine looks less like a renaissance and more like a reckoning. The science we now see popping up at prestigious universities like Yale is better understood as a product of years of resistance, forged by outlaws and academics, working together, sometimes in partnership, sometimes in tension.

This is where I come into the story.

I study the politics of science and medicine. Pain, drugs, and the pharmaceutical industry are my bread and butter. I spend my time thinking about how ideological divides, funding sources, and scandals—let's say, a marketing scheme that foists highly addictive opioids on a population— shape our collective approach to health and illness.

The problem of pain is no small issue. According to a 2023 Centers for Disease Control and Prevention report, 20 percent of American adults live with chronic pain. Within this group, a jarring 7 percent endure what's known as "high-impact chronic pain," a condition that substantially limits daily activities.[13] That number seems like a wildly high estimate until we consider everything that makes us ache: arthritis, sickle cell anemia, diabetic neuropathies, kidney disease, endometriosis, peripheral artery disease, and vascular disorders. Migraine alone affects over forty million American adults and accounts for about four million emergency department visits each year.[14]

It's a challenging problem for medicine, a profession that much prefers symptoms that can be measured, standardized, and verified. Pain stubbornly refuses to be anything more than a private experience. You, and you alone, can feel your pain.

As a result, getting pain treatment relies on patients' ability to convince others that their pain is genuine and that they deserve help. Asking for care means navigating a broader set of moral quandaries, political issues, and social assumptions involving trust, blame, and responsibility. That opioids induce pleasurable sensations complicates these moral evaluations further. Ask any pain patient and they'll tell you that dodging the label "drug-seeker" and "malingerer" is a never-ending concern. In the cruelest, if most predictable, of ironies, the populations who bear the greatest burden of chronic pain—women, people of color, and the poor—are the ones who receive the least care and empathy for their conditions. Imagine how much more complicated these moral calculations become with psychedelics, a treatment that some people fear could inspire acts of political rebellion and transgression.

Dealing with pain is never easy, but it helps to have access to doctors who believe their patients. So here's a thought: if it's already a struggle for medical professionals to trust patients' reports of pain, how big a leap would it be to expect them to accept these same patients as partners in research? It's a significant jump forward, asking the field of medicine not only to acknowledge patients' experiences but also to value their contributions to medical knowledge.

People have learned they can organize and fight for recognition.

This book tells one such story from the clandestine world of psychedelic research: people with cluster headache, united only by pain and the internet, developed their very own treatment from homegrown magic mushrooms and have been trying to turn it into a legal medicine ever since. But the path from one world to the other has been fraught with conflict, mistrust, and misunderstanding. Even the strongest alliances with aboveground scientists face extraordinary barriers.

Their work is paying off. It's early days, but researchers are now looking at whether psychedelics might treat a wide spectrum of pain disorders, including migraine, fibromyalgia, arthritis, back and joint pain, complex regional pain syndrome, phantom limb syndrome, pelvic pain, and irritable bowel syndrome.[15] Even the excruciating pain associated with PTSD and cancer might relent when treated with this innovative approach.[16]

There's hope in this story. But it also raises so many questions: How much knowledge have we lost over the last fifty years? What political obstacles remain in the way? How will drug reform policies under discussion affect the people who might benefit from a drug's use? Who gets a seat at the table? What is the best way to incorporate patient knowledge into the development of medical therapies?

The members of Clusterbusters—a group of patients focused on treating physical pain rather than seeking spiritual enlightenment—have always been outsiders in the psychedelic world. But then again, for all the talk in psychedelia about the capacity of these molecules for creating a shared humanity, I've learned that the use of the word *community* to refer to those who use these drugs disguises how fragmented and contentious this world can be.

Indigenous communities, who have long struggled to gain access to good Western medical care, must now grapple with the reality of corporate entities patenting their ancestral knowledge. Meanwhile there's fear that these efforts have created an ideology of "psychedelic exceptionalism" that allows middle-class white people to talk openly about spiritual journeys and "plant medicines" while ignoring a punitive and racist approach to other forms of substance use. Psychedelic therapy might be a potent treatment for the racial trauma perpetuated by mass incarceration and medical racism, but most clinical trials have systematically excluded Black subjects, and there are real worries about how accessible legalized psychedelic therapy will be.[17] While these substances offer tremendous potential for healing, they also expose profound inequalities, ethical challenges, and cultural blind spots. The very systems that might benefit from psychedelic therapies are often the ones that have perpetuated the injustices that make these therapies necessary.

*Psychedelic Outlaws* offers just one slice of this story—patients forced to do extraordinary research by a healthcare system that remains woefully indifferent to their experiences. Understanding the twists and turns of the Clusterbusters' journey is a step toward disentangling these relationships, perhaps even beginning to realign drug policy to become more equitable, compassionate, and patient centered.

Part I

# Set and Setting

## Chapter One

# WHO ARE THE OUTLAWS?

Bob Wold always struck me as a most unlikely leader of an underground psychedelic network. Everything about him, from the baseball caps that he almost never takes off to his understated midwestern modesty, is unassuming. Even his signature bushy gray mustache is a testament more to a man whose aesthetic sensibilities stopped evolving in the 1970s than to a countercultural statement. Everything else, the button-down shirt that he wears when he's got to make himself look presentable and the comfortable pants, says "norm-core Grandpa" more than "revolutionary."

But it's not his mainstream looks that throw me off. Nor is it his aw-shucks, blue-collar, married-to-his-high-school-sweetheart, raised-four-kids, coached-the-Little-League-team-long-after-his-own-children-were-grown vibe. It's the general sense that he'd rather be talking about his grandkids and baseball than most anything else.

He didn't choose to be a psychedelic outlaw. The job sort of chose him. In fact, while I might describe him as the leader of an underground movement, Wold has always been open about his use of psychedelics, making sure that everyone, from his family and friends to the police officers in his small town, know what he is doing and why he does it. As he's argued many times, there's no shame in taking psychedelics for survival.

Wold is nothing short of evangelical about the healing power of magic mushrooms. They saved his life, and he's used them to save many more. Which is why, several years ago, I found him inside a crowded airport hotel suite, promising the four dozen people assembled there that he had found a way to treat their cluster headache cycles.

Everyone was already in good spirits—they always were when they got together. But a hush came over the room when Wold began unloading a cardboard box and setting its contents onto a table before him.

"It will cost $100 and take forty-five days, but you can produce all the medicine you need to treat yourself for a year."

He held up an empty canning jar and gestured toward a bag of vermiculite. Most of the materials necessary for growing magic mushrooms, he explained, can be easily obtained at a local hardware shop. It's legal to purchase mushroom spores, the "seeds" used to grow magic mushrooms, in almost all US states because of a loophole: spores don't contain any of the hallucinogenic compounds subject to legal penalties. Cultivating the spores at home, he emphasized, *is illegal*, but he assured the people gathered there that the process was both easy to do and easy to hide.

"I mean, honestly, it's very simple. It only takes you an hour in the kitchen. If you can bake a cake, you can grow mushrooms."

As proof, Wold held up a clear, vacuum-sealed plastic bag containing about a pound of mushrooms.

I would learn, over time, that growing mushrooms is not quite as simple as baking a cake. Nor are the legal consequences minimal. Wold understands both complications, but he'd rather not dwell on the challenges. After all, lives are at stake.

●  ●  ●●●●●●●●●●●●●●●●●●  ●  ●

The United States has a drug problem, perhaps best illustrated by the ancient Greek word *pharmakon*, which captures the idea that all substances contain the potential to be a cure or poison, capable of healing or harming, depending on dosage. But perhaps even ancient Greeks found this ambiguity challenging; the word *pharmakon* also translates to "scapegoat."

The complex and often contradictory ways we think about, interact with, and create rules for the use of drugs have a certain "pharmakologic." They reveal our worst fears more than they reflect any objective assessment of harms. How else can we explain America's simultaneous love affair with and revulsion for psychoactive drugs? Our adoration for substances that alter our minds is so deeply ingrained in everyday routines, it's taken for granted. But that morning coffee that helps us face the day, that bit of chocolate that brings us cheer, that beer after work—all are acceptable chemical pick-me-ups. Even sugar, which we arbitrarily consider a food rather than a drug, affects the mind, capable of releasing dopamine that makes us happy in the short term but ultimately irritable, unfocused, and— if we eat enough—depressed. Which is why we watch what we eat. Food is medicine, remember? There's that puritan impulse to temper indulgences and repress pleasures!

The cultural and regulatory logics dictating the contents of our medicine cabinets, where we tuck away little gems that can calm anxiety, uplift mood, focus attention, or gently lull us to sleep, are even more complicated. Consider the mix of suspicion and disdain cast upon those who rely on a pill to function—especially if there's any hint of nonmedical use. People in pain bear the weight of this scrutiny, especially now, amid an opioid crisis.

While the Food and Drug Administration allowed pharmaceutical companies to market opioids with abandon, the Drug Enforcement Agency (DEA) lists LSD, psilocybin, and marijuana as Schedule I drugs, despite evidence that all three drugs have pain-relieving qualities and low toxicity. Objective measures, like safety and efficacy, don't explain these discrepancies. And the implementation of these laws reflects deep racial inequities. Research consistently finds that white Americans use and sell illicit drugs at the same (or very similar) rates as Black Americans, but they are far less likely to be punished for doing so.[1]

Take marijuana, for example. According to the 2022 US National Survey on Drug Use and Health, as many as 22 percent of Americans over the age of twelve admitted to using marijuana at least once in the previous year, despite federal laws prohibiting the sale and use of the drug.[2] While some of these people will have used marijuana legally according to the laws of their state (to the tune of an estimated $14 billion in sales), marijuana remains a primary target of law enforcement agents. According to a recent report published by the American Civil Liberties Union, as many as 6.1 million arrests made between 2010 and 2018 were marijuana related. An astounding 90 percent of these arrests were for possession as opposed to trafficking.[3]

The fact that a Black person is 3.64 times more likely to be arrested for marijuana possession than a white person reveals a troubling fact: US drug law and its implementation have always reflected *whom* we fear more than *what* we fear. America's first drug laws were implemented in response to xenophobic fears about opiate use among Chinese immigrants and racist claims that "cocaine sniffing" among Black people increased their criminality. Never mind that white people already had a long history of using both drugs.[4]

As David Herzberg, a leading historian of medicine and the author of *White Market Drugs: Big Pharma and the Hidden History of Addiction in America*, wryly observed, we've built a regulatory system that's somehow too weak to contain greedy pharmaceutical companies poisoning our citizens, while simultaneously so strong, its harsh drug sentencing has fueled the largest carceral state in the world. Failing to understand the inequities built into drug policy requires a remarkable tolerance for cognitive dissonance.[5]

● ●  ●●●●●●●●●●●●●●●●●●  ● ●

Cluster headache affects people across the racial spectrum, but almost everyone I met at Clusterbusters' conferences was white. While they may not have wished to break the law, their ability to appear in a public space and talk about using (or potentially using) psychedelics must be understood against the backdrop of a racist justice system that imposes cruel punishments on Black and Brown citizens for their use of drugs while letting white compatriots go. Fear drives much of what we consider to be criminal. The rapid medicalization of psychedelics can't be separated from its whiteness.

According to surveys conducted by the National Institute on Drug Abuse, psychedelic drug use has become much more common since Bob Wold first experimented with magic mushrooms in 2001. In 2022, 8 percent of young adults reported that they'd used a hallucinogen in the previous year—a sharp increase from the 4.5 percent who had reportedly used a psychedelic twenty years prior. But the trend line isn't smooth: reported use ticked up sharply in 2020 and remained high for the next two years.[6]

It's not hard to imagine what might have changed. A global pandemic placed an unprecedented strain on healthcare systems, limiting access to conventional mental and physical health services, at the same time that people were experiencing an extraordinary level of economic disruption and isolation. Opioid overdoses increased by 30 percent during this period, despite well-funded efforts by public health and law enforcement.[7] Inject media hype about the miraculous benefits of "plant medicine" amid this chaos, and it's surprising that more people didn't use psychedelics.

● ● ●○●○●○●○●○●○●○●○●○●○● ● ●

Breaking a law is no small thing. But I can't tell Clusterbusters' story without wondering whether their actions make them "criminal."

Bob Wold doesn't consider himself or the other Clusterheads criminals—not when their survival is on the line. Nor do any of the physicians or advocates who work with them.

As I dug deeper into the racial overtones of the history of criminalized drug use, I found it fascinating, and more than a touch disturbing, that the Central Intelligence Agency (CIA) was the largest funder of LSD research in the 1950s. Its now infamous covert operation, MKUltra, sought to weaponize mind-altering drugs like LSD to control human behavior. Unknowing subjects underwent psychological torture in these experiments, offering a clear example of the role that power plays in determining criminality.

The authority granted to figures like Sidney Gottlieb, MKUltra's project head, allowed the requisition of human subjects for any form of abuse, including fatal experiments.[8] MKUltra even went so far as to hire Nazi doctors with experience in conducting mescaline experiments on concentration camp prisoners. CIA-operated secret detention centers in Europe and East Asia captured enemy agents and others deemed "expendable," subjecting them to abusive experiments. And a CIA-funded brothel in San Francisco served as a setting where agents secretly observed sex workers giving clients LSD without consent, before attempting to extract information from them after sex.

But nobody who worked at MKUltra was deemed a criminal. Not even Sidney Gottlieb, the mastermind behind the operation. At least not according to the United States.

Power and fear determine who and what make a person a criminal.[9] Wold, like other activists combatting the War on Drugs, must often break the law to do the work they feel is important. But if he's not a criminal, then what is he? "What do you think about the word 'outlaw'?" I asked him one day. Wold let out a laugh. "An outlaw? I could live with that."

Here, in a country founded by people suspicious of authority, we have a soft spot for outlaws—whether it's Billy the Kid as an irreverent rascal, Bonnie and Clyde as romantic killers, or Timothy Leary as spiritual leader of the counterculture. Outlaws don't just live by their own rules; they protect the populace from power. And so we admire their behavior, even if it's begrudgingly. The established social order doesn't register acts associated with whiteness as presenting nearly so great a threat as those linked to marginalized identities, allowing a double standard to persist in the narratives we tell ourselves about rebels and outlaws. This selective embrace of an archetype shapes, at times even dictates, the frameworks through which we interpret transgressive actions.

Writing this book while our country engaged, once again, in a national reckoning on race brought these issues right to the surface. Underground networks have been an especially important lifeline for Black Americans, who escaped enslavement by means of a clandestine Underground Railroad. A breach of silence could easily result in the loss of life or liberty.

The psychedelic underground described in this book is perhaps more accurately called a "subculture"—a visible space capable of taking up room in the public consciousness with minimal fear of punishment. That the narrative that unfolds in these pages is dominated by white men reflects their ability to speak openly and seize space in the spotlight without bearing as much risk of repercussion. Power has granted them both a stage and the ability to direct public attention, philanthropic dollars, and now public policy. In contrast, women elders of the underground have had a far quieter presence. Only now, as these medicines go mainstream, are we starting to see people speak openly about their use of psychedelics as treatments for racial trauma.[10]

Power, in all its forms, will be a steady thread in this book, guiding how I interpret the psychedelic world and its impact on the world around us.

## Chapter Two

SURVIVING MEDICINE

A INSLIE COURSE, A DETERMINEDLY CHEERFUL SCOT, LIVED HER LIFE according to the rules.

"I was the sensible one, always offering to be the driver to make sure everyone got home safely. The thought of trying anything . . . I was scared. I was always scared I'd be the one person to have an adverse effect, or worse, get caught."

Even a parking ticket felt too transgressive, let alone a joint. She thought it was ludicrous when someone suggested that a man all the way across the ocean in Chicago could help her use magic mushrooms to treat the cluster headache attacks that she no longer felt she could bear. But the doctors had never been any help. She'd given them nearly fifteen years, and they'd only made things worse.

The headaches began at age nineteen, when Course awoke to a pain so fierce and immediate, she thought she was dying. She leapt out of bed and paced the room in a frenzied attempt to escape the agony. The heel of her hand dug deep into her eye socket, until her fingers curled into a fist and began to pound her head. And then the pain disappeared.

Course, who was then a nursing student, carried out a quick triage to determine whether she had a stroke. Everything, so far as she could tell, seemed to be in working order. At least, nothing was paralyzed. Maybe a brain tumor, but nothing urgent. No need, she decided, to wake up her parents down the hall. Nobody at the National Health Service would be operating an MRI at 2:00 a.m. So she stiffened her upper lip and returned to sleep.

The pain returned two days later. This time, it brought her to her knees in broad daylight. Still nothing to worry about, she decided. She white-knuckled through daily attacks for several more weeks before seeing a doctor.

"I was in for all of about three minutes, and he said, 'Yeah, you have migraine. Here's some tablets. Off you go. If it doesn't get any better, come back.'" But the tablets didn't work. And that's how things went for years.

Course believed in medicine—she worked in a hospital—so she didn't give up. She returned again and again, seeking advice from a variety of doctors, hoping that the next one might provide, at minimum, a fresh perspective. "I think I trialed somewhere between fifty and sixty different meds, because I always had hope. And I thought that I should always try the next medicine because what if this was the one that made a difference?"

But doctors, she explained, began treating her like *she* was the problem. "I was very quickly labeled a time waster and an attention seeker. It was suggested to me on more than one occasion that my problems may be more psychological than neurological," she told me. She often felt like they saw her optimistic determination to find an effective medicine as a symptom of a psychiatric problem. She might never forgive the doctor who told her that her best course of treatment was a straitjacket.

A diagnosis would take fifteen years, a trip to London, and a costly consultation with a renowned headache specialist. He had an answer in under five minutes. She had a classic case of episodic cluster headache. The diagnosis had evaded her previous doctors due to a strange but once widely accepted medical theory positing that cluster headache primarily affected white men with hazel eyes and pitted, leathery skin. The specialist dismissed this as a myth, assuring Course that women were not immune.

Course burst into tears of joy when he gave her the news. The diagnosis came as a relief after years of uncertainty and self doubt. She explained, "[Cluster headache] has affected my family, my career, friendships. People say, 'Shit, she's got one of her headaches,' and I started to almost question myself. 'Am I weak? Can I not cope with this pain?'"

What Course didn't yet know was that a cluster headache diagnosis didn't guarantee that effective treatments would follow. Her doctor prescribed a standard course of treatment, which included sumatriptan, a treatment developed for migraine that has earned expanded approval for use with cluster headache from the US Food and Drug Administration and the UK National Institute for Health and Care Excellence.

Sumatriptan, when delivered as a subcutaneous injection, could stop an attack within fifteen minutes. But Course found it difficult to stick to her doctor's stern warning to limit her use of the medicine to two attacks per day, lest the treatment make the attacks longer and more severe.

Making choices about which of her daily attacks to medicate proved much easier said than done. She could do without the medication for mild attacks, but anything more intense was difficult to bear. Over time, she points out, "you become detached from the safety aspect . . . you know? You just want to treat what's going on."

Course's doctor's warning had been prescient. "If I could have used one for every attack, then it would have been fine, but what I did find was the more sumatriptan I used, the more I needed it. The more intense my cycles became, the more intense my attacks became." She'd entered what cluster patients sometimes call an "Imitrex death cycle," referring to sumatriptan's brand name in the United States.

Rock bottom occurred in 2002, seventeen years into her living with cluster headache. "I had a double-sided attack, well beyond my standard 'screamer.' I've only ever had four of them in, you know, thirty odd years."

Course had always had predominantly right-sided attacks, but during this attack, the pain started to hit on the left side as well. "I went into my shower, and I wet myself, I vomited, and I defecated on the floor of my shower room. The volume of pain was just off the charts. I remember looking through from my bathroom door into my bedroom, looking up at the light fixture and thinking, 'Will this lovely crystal chandelier, so delicate, take my weight?' And I thought, this is it."

But she wasn't beaten yet. "I sort of pull myself together, I clean myself up, and I thought I have to find another way."

Six months later, after quite a bit of hesitation, multiple email exchanges with Bob Wold, and careful research and consideration, Course again found herself looking at the ceiling. This time she was staring at Jesus, wondering how he'd gotten up there. She'd been careful to take a tiny dose of mushrooms, but it turned out that she's sensitive to psilocybin's effects. But the weird trip was worth it.

"All the pressure drained from my head. The only way I can describe it is like a boiled egg. Take off the top and put a pressure washer in there and clean all the shit out. Then put the top back again and seal it up."

"Bob Wold told me what to do, when to do it, how to do it, how often to do it. He saved my life."

● ● ●●●●●●●●●●●●●●●●●●●● ● ●

When doctors told Course that she had migraine, she thought, "Oh, my goodness, these poor people with migraine, you know this is awful." Did people really hurt this much when they had a migraine attack? Each one made her feel like she might die. "In fact, I [wished it] would kill me right now, because it was just so horrific."

It's natural to compare migraine to cluster headache and wonder, as I had, if having experienced one of the diseases might offer some insight into the other. It's far more common to have experience with migraine, a disease that affects 12 percent of American adults and 7 percent of children. That's a lot of people: there are more people living with migraine than there are people living in California. Cluster headache is *much* less common.

Depending on the study, cluster headache affects between one and three in one thousand people, or .124 percent to .381 percent of the population. To offer a comparison, Crohn's disease affects one in five hundred people.[1]

I've had a rough time of it, so far as migraine is concerned. My headaches began when I was five years old. As an adult, I'd become accustomed to living with two to three migraine attacks per week (each migraine attack, as per diagnostic criteria, usually includes a moderate to severe one-sided headache, alongside nausea, vomiting, and hypersensitivity to light or sound, but bone-tired fatigue and bodily pain are often more disabling features of the disease).

By the time I turned thirty, I had joined the 1 to 2 percent of the population with *chronic migraine*—that is, more than fifteen days of headache per month, of which nine must qualify as "migraine."[2] Managing life with only a few pain-free days per month is exhausting, so I figured I might relate to people with cluster headache. I should say, for the record, that I'm not a huge fan of comparing intensity of pain experiences, but I'm making an exception in this case.

Cluster headache is far more excruciating than anything I could ever imagine.

Each cluster attack is so intense, it might as well be considered a medical emergency. It's also accompanied by quite strange-seeming behavior. In much the same way one tries to shake off the sharp sting of a thumb slammed in a door jam, a person with cluster headache will rock, pace, and sometimes even repeatedly slam a hard object against the offending temple. Then, once it's done, it can seem like nothing has happened.

The term *cluster headache* refers to the distinctive timing of the attacks. Attacks occur in "cycles" or "bouts" that can last between a week and a year. Most resolve within six to eight weeks.[3] But about 15 to 20 percent of those with cluster headache have a "chronic" form of the disease, which means they never get a true break from the pain; if the bout persists without remission for over a year, as in the case with Sean Slattery, it is referred to as chronic cluster headache.[4]

Cluster headache cycles tend to have a circannual rhythm that syncs with the changing seasons—about half of the cluster headache patient population can predict the time of year their cycle will occur. Attacks also follow a circadian rhythm. As many as 70 percent of people with cluster headache can predict the exact time of day an attack will strike.[5] The clocklike regularity of cluster attacks points to the potential involvement of the hypothalamus, an almond-sized part of the brain that regulates our biological clock—a hypothesis supported by brain imaging studies.[6]

While medical terminology can be exacting, it often fails to capture the human experience of pain. To bridge this gap, Clusterbusters funded a groundbreaking study—the largest that had ever been conducted on the disease.[7] Researchers asked 1,604 individuals to rate the severity of their headache attacks on a scale of one to ten and indicate whether they had encountered other forms of pain. Those who said yes were asked to rate those as well. Ratings on this scale included

Stab wounds: 4.6
Migraine: 5.4
Gunshot wounds: 6.0
Kidney stones: 6.9
Pancreatitis: 7.0
Unmedicated labor: 7.2
Cluster headache: 9.7

(Yes, this survey included twenty-five people with cluster headache who had survived a gunshot wound and another sixty-seven with cluster headache who'd been stabbed.)

This is what is meant by "most painful phenomenon a human can experience."[8]

It's therefore unsurprising that cluster headache patients have found it necessary to develop a separate pain scale that suits a level of anguish most of us will never experience. The Kip Scale, named after its creator, Bob Kipple, a longtime member of the online cluster headache community, is adapted from the more familiar ten-point scales found in most doctors' offices. It ranges from a Kip 0 ("No pain, life is beautiful") to a Kip 10 ("Major pain, screaming, head banging, ER trip. Depressed. Suicidal"). Intermediate scores are likewise adapted to the realities of a cluster attack: while a 5 on a typical pain scale refers to "Can't be ignored for more than 30 minutes," a Kip 5 refers to "Still not a pacer, but need space."[9]

Time and time again, I have read and listened to testimonies from people with cluster headache about a level of pain so unbearable that they would do anything to make it stop, even at the price of their own lives.[10] Most of this compulsion is a desire for relief. If applying pressure to the temple provides relief, the next step might be tightening a belt around one's head. A step further might involve jamming a hard item into the source of the pain. Sometimes that's a telephone. But it might be a hammer. Or the head might be slammed directly against the hardest surface in the house with unconsciousness being a hoped-for but never-achieved outcome. One medical report documents a patient who tried to shoot the pain out of his eye with a bullet (he lived, but the effort failed to stop the pain).[11]

Despite the onslaught of such unfathomable pain, many cluster headache patients do not immediately rush to the doctor after their first attack. Larry Schor, professor emeritus of psychology at the University of West Georgia and a psychotherapist who has had cluster headache since 1983, tells people at Clusterbusters meetings that he initially found the experience too strange to explain to others. "The pain was so indescribably intense that I was afraid if I spoke it, I would breathe more life into it. There was this level of almost hallucination or delusional quality that it felt like if I said anything to anyone it would be more real. And maybe it'll just go away if I pretend it doesn't exist. It was like an alien in my head."

Years of counseling people with cluster headache has led Schor to conclude that they *want to live*, but the pain can become too much to bear.[12] "It hurts so fucking bad that . . . many of us think I would be collateral damage. I just want to kill it."

But why is it so difficult for people with this form of pain to get help? It's hard to imagine a disease as intensely awful as cluster headache going unnoticed in medicine. I expected at least some interest—if not urgency—from the people who care about suffering. It didn't take long to learn what might be happening. Literally: my research didn't take long. There's just not that much medical research on the topic.

● ● ●●●●●●●●●●●●●●●●●●●● ● ●

Doctors began to describe a set of cluster headache–like symptoms in the eighteenth century. But medicine only began to recognize the diagnosis in 1939, when Dr. Bayard T. Horton of the Mayo Clinic reported the discovery of a new, excruciating syndrome characterized by intense one-sided head pain. Histamine provoked an attack, which led him to believe the cause must be allergic. The treatment seemed draconian: he'd administer small, subcutaneous doses of histamine in increasing dosages until the patient was desensitized, that is, they no longer triggered attacks.[13]

(I've since discovered this treatment is still in use in an inpatient setting. Bob Wold endured four cycles of histamine treatment. Andrew Cleminshaw, a chronic cluster headache patient and former board member of Clusterbusters, went through five or six cycles; he described it as the "theory that if we induce enough headaches, the body will eventually get used to it.")

Horton's colleagues lauded his discovery of cluster headache as "medical history in the making," but few followed his exhortations to study the disease. Three decades after Horton's original article, only six dozen or so English-language articles had been published about cluster headache in medical journals.[14] Horton authored at least a few of these, including the study that introduced oxygen as a treatment for the disease.[15] Not even Dr. Harold G. Wolff, known as the "father of modern headache medicine," took more than a passing glance at "Horton's headache."

But 1970 was a banner year for cluster headache research. Ten articles came out in the research literature! Unfortunately for patients with the disease, the most influential of these research articles created a completely false but extremely persistent stereotype about cluster headache patients.[16]

Dr. John R. Graham, the author of this classic article and founder of the first headache clinic in Boston, had observed that his cluster headache patients shared several quite masculine physical and psychological features. Given that the vast majority of his patients (he estimated 90 percent) were men, he wondered if this might offer a clue. The article proposed a biological link between the male sex and the disease.

His patients shared a "look" (sandy hair, hazel eyes) and "hyper masculine" features: a heavily wrinkled, "leonine" face, pockmarked *peau d'orange* skin, mesomorph bodies, and athletic prowess. Their personalities matched: they drank "heartily," smoked tobacco "without inhibition," tattooed their bodies, and took unnecessary risks at work and leisure. Women with cluster headache only proved the rule by looking or behaving in a masculine manner. One woman, for example, had strong muscles. Another had a determined personality. A third violated the norms of femininity with her *peau d'orange* skin.[17]

Readers: there's no pockmarked, wrinkled man-look that gives away people with this disease. Nor is there any rule that women can't be determined or have muscles or (gasp) bad skin. An experiment in the 1990s tested if headache specialists could diagnose people with cluster headache from pictures; they couldn't. Perhaps it's not surprising, then that recent research suggests that men may be only slightly more likely to have the disease than women.[18]

Women may find it easier to get a diagnosis now than ever before, but like Ainslie Course, they remain plagued by a myth that sounds as if it was ripped from the pages of a nineteenth-century phrenology textbook.

What went wrong?

Pain has a long history, but a few key moments in medicine might have gone better. For starters, medicine really struggles to cope with any phenomenon that blurs mind-body boundaries. So there's always this lingering idea that pain might operate the way seventeenth-century philosopher René Descartes had once proposed: as a sort of mechanical process, like a cord that connects our nerve endings to our brains. You hurt your toe, a string is pulled, an alarm bell rings in your brain, and a sharp sensation is registered.

It was during this period that the medical field began to prioritize physical evidence and empirical data over the subjective reports of patients' symptoms. Michel Foucault, the renowned French philosopher, high-lights this era as a critical juncture in the history of medicine. According to Foucault, this was the moment when modern clinical practices began to emphasize observation, examination, and the categorization of diseases based on visible signs rather than patient testimony. In other words, doc-tors stopped caring about what patients said, and instead began to care a lot more about finding visible signs of damage in the body—and that, ultimately—would make life more difficult for people in pain.[19]

Not that pain had ever been a popular specialty in medicine. Migraine might have gotten a boost in the mid-twentieth century after Harold G. Wolff produced experimental evidence that proved a biological mechanism "caused" the pain of migraine. (*Life* magazine even featured his experiment on a cover.[20]) However, Wolff believed that the mind caused the migraine itself. Every migraine patient he saw shared the same personality profile: ambitious, successful, perfectionist, and efficient. But that was just the men with migraine. His female patients, he argued, expressed their Type A per-sonalities via sexual repression.

Wolff's "migraine personality" hit a sweet spot, breathing scientific legiti-macy into stale ideas about repressed women. So it wasn't entirely surprising that his star student, Graham, had been looking for a similar set of personality traits in his cluster patients. But why did his idea last so long? By the 1990s, Course and most of her doctors would have raised an eyebrow at the overt sex-ism in the old headache research literature. But people hadn't yet tuned their ear to hear masculinity presented as a disease. I suppose it sounded plausible.

Headache patients are deeply stigmatized in medicine. Unfair as it may be, headache patients maintain a reputation for being "whiny," "difficult," "anxious," and "depressed." And apparently, this isn't the kind of person that doctors enjoy treating. As one headache specialist warned me, "Head-ache neurologists are kind of the . . . lowest caste of neurologists. To stand up and say that you are interested in headache is a chance for you to be stig-matized [among neurologists]. You should be aware of that."[21]

Cluster headache might affect more men than women, but it still falls under the aegis of headache medicine—a small, under-resourced field.

Migraine, a disease associated with women, is the big fish that gobbles up the little funding and attention the specialty gets.

Headache medicine attracts vanishingly few physicians. The United States has only around six hundred board certified headache specialists. And neither medical students nor residents learn much about headache treatment in training. This perhaps explains why it takes patients an average of five years to receive a correct diagnosis of cluster headache. Some wait more than ten. It's also difficult to find a doctor who understands how to treat cluster headache.[22]

A back-of-the-envelope calculation suggests that the average cluster headache patient will experience 168 unmedicated attacks every year while waiting for a correct diagnosis and effective treatment. This means that while the average patient is off consulting an average of two to five clinicians and receiving an average of 3.9 incorrect diagnoses, the healthcare system expects that same average patient to survive 840 attacks—each of which, as we know, feels worse than giving birth without medicine, a gunshot wound, or passing a kidney stone.

One of the kindest men I met at Clusterbusters lived in pain for forty-five years before learning that his so-called migraine attacks were cluster attacks. I never could quite reconcile his beatific Mr. Rogers demeanor with the fact that he'd spent nearly a half century going to sleep knowing he'd wake up ninety minutes later and spend an hour screaming, only to repeat the entire scenario once more before his workday began. Maybe optimism provided a measure of protection against what I estimate were 32,850 unmedicated attacks.

In the interim, people invariably undergo a series of invasive, painful, and ultimately useless interventions: brain scans, sinus surgeries, tooth extractions, nerve ablations, and a broad range of alternative therapies. The cost—not just in missed work but also in the search for care—is astronomical.[23]

· · ·············· · ·

Effective treatments for cluster headache exist, but the road to relief isn't straightforward. Providers rely on a "trial-and-error" approach "based on very few and small studies not fulfilling modern standards."[24] As a result physicians often rely on their collective clinical experience, rather than strong clinical trial data, when treating their cluster headache patients. It's a scenario that leaves patients feeling a bit like guinea pigs. Knowing a little about their treatment options makes it a little easier to understand why these particular patients might have been willing to experiment with psychedelics long before they surged back into public view.

Treatments come in three varieties: abortives or "acute" medicines, which stop an attack in progress; "bridge" or transitional medicines, which temporarily suppress attacks; and preventives, which keep a cycle from starting. Expert guidelines recommend two "first-line" acute treatments: sumatriptan (taken as an injectable) and high-flow oxygen.[25]

As Course learned, sumatriptan is easy to administer and can, for many people, deliver miraculous relief. But if taken too often, sumatriptan can paradoxically increase attacks. The dreaded "Imitrex death cycle" is all too real.

High-flow oxygen, in contrast, can be used to abort as many attacks as needed. It also has a safer side effect profile than most other medicines, but tanks are difficult to transport. (Traveling by plane can be especially harrowing.) Obtaining access has been an ongoing problem in the community. It's not FDA-approved, which makes insurance reimbursement more difficult. Doctors also often fail to prescribe this option, and even when they do, they neglect to teach their patients the correct way to use the treatment.

"Bridge," or transitional, medications offer a crucial respite from the brutal cycles of cluster headache. Often a short course of steroids or another strategy is deployed with the hope of suppressing attacks long enough for preventive medications to take effect or for the cycle to naturally conclude.

Clusterheads have a love/hate relationship with steroids. These medications act swiftly, but the relief is typically short-lived; attacks often resume

once the medication depletes. Prolonged use of steroids has grave consequences: weight gain, diabetes, cataracts, osteoporosis, and vascular necro-
sis of the hip or shoulder, a condition marked by bone tissue collapse due to
failed blood supply. Such necessary relief, but at a terrible cost.

So doctors dig deeper into their medicine bags, looking for anything that
might keep people from experiencing this extraordinary pain. But the overall picture is a patchwork of care that seems far more experimental than
one might hope.

Preventive options are limited. For now, I'll just mention that verapamil,
an FDA-approved drug for hypertension, is considered a first-line preventive treatment for cluster headache, despite mixed evidence supporting its
effectiveness. Clusterheads often worry that there are risks associated with
the high doses they've been prescribed. Constipation is a known side effect
of verapamil. "I had to go to the hospital after two weeks of not going to the
bathroom. It cost me $1,800 to take a shit," said one person. One man told
me that he couldn't "remember [his] dosage [of verapamil] but it was four
or five times what you would normally get." When he mentioned his pace-
maker at a cluster conference, "about five young men came up to me and
told me the heart issues they had around verapamil."

●  ●  ●●●●●●●●●●●●●●●●●●●  ●  ●

What happens when treatments fail?

Ethnographers talk about "saturation" to refer to the experience of
knowing we've learned everything we can on a topic because we keep hearing the same story on repeat. But what is it called when saturation can
never be reached because, even when the stories speak to the same malfea-
sance in medicine, there's no bottom to the horror they reveal?

One Clusterhead told me about the time when his doctor, probably frustrated that none of his prescribed treatments were working, had essentially
advised him to kill himself. "Well," the doctor had said, "you know the only
cure is a .357." The Clusterhead recounted, "I thought for a minute. And I
went, 'Jesus.' I looked at him and he looked away. And I said, 'Are you saying
the only way for me to find relief is to blow my brains out?' And he said, 'That's

the way it is.' And I said, 'You don't want me to come back, do you?' He said, 'Well, you know, you're not getting better. We like to see people get better.'"

The story took my breath away—I wanted to believe it couldn't be true. But then another Clusterhead told me his doctor—in a completely different part of the country—had said something very similar. How could it be possible that physicians, whose most basic oath is to refrain from doing harm, might suggest so devastating a course of "treatment" to a patient with a high risk of self-harm?

● ● ●●●●●●●●●●●●●●●●●●● ● ●

It can be puzzlingly difficult to get ahold of the therapy that most of the patients I met agreed was the safest, most effective, and most affordable of anything they'd tried and could be used as often as needed without any risk of arrest, addiction, or unwanted side effects: oxygen therapy.

Doctors have known that high-flow oxygen can abort cluster headache attacks since 1952, when Horton first proposed it as a treatment. But the challenges involved are multiple. For oxygen to work properly as an abortive, it must be inhaled at a high flow rate (between twelve and fifteen liters per minute) using a non-rebreather mask that seals around the mouth and nose, guaranteeing that 100 percent of all breaths are taken from the oxygen tank, excluding even small amounts of air from the surrounding room.

However, doctors rarely prescribe oxygen correctly if they prescribe it at all. Clusterheads were constantly commiserating over the challenges they faced in obtaining oxygen. Most people seemed to have had doctors who didn't understand that oxygen needed to be delivered by a non-rebreather mask and instead prescribed a nose cannula. "You might as well be told to take Extra-Strength Excedrin," a patient told me. "I used mine for my fish tank."

I once heard a doctor offering the following suggestion to Clusterheads whose doctors had prescribed them a cannula. "You get the cannula, snap it in two, and your first piece goes around the neck of the person prescribing it."

Then there are the doctors who refuse to prescribe oxygen for reasons that are not entirely clear. According to their patients, these doctors worry about the safety of high-flow oxygen, but it's hard to say what their precise concerns might be. High-flow oxygen is considered one of the safest interventions, especially since cluster headache patients only use oxygen for short periods.

Risks associated with the use of high-flow oxygen are easily mitigated with small interventions. For example, falling asleep with a non-rebreather mask is dangerous. Suffocation if the tank runs out of oxygen is a real danger; also, a long dose of pure oxygen can damage lungs. So Clusterheads advise one another to hold their masks to their faces rather than use its straps. That way, if they fall asleep, their mask will just slip off.

Oxygen therapy is a great example of what the network provides for its members because the rest of the world just doesn't get it. Clusterheads know they need oxygen, because they know how effective it is, and they have learned the hard way that it's far more difficult to access than it should be.

Clusterbusters' website coaches Clusterheads on obtaining a prescription for high-flow oxygen therapy and, importantly, how to use oxygen effectively. But unlike traditional advocacy groups, Clusterbusters offers an advice page providing a bunch of unconventional suggestions for obtaining oxygen. Fire stations, they suggest, usually have emergency medical technicians who might be friendlier than the doctors and nurses working in emergency rooms. The website also mentions that some people have been known to use welding-grade oxygen when they can't get their doctors to prescribe medical-grade oxygen for them. The two are identical, but the latter must be stored in sterile, certified tanks. Many are willing to take the risk of accidentally huffing a noxious chemical if the preferred alternative isn't available.

Regarding this industrial oxygen, Clusterbusters writes emphatically (in bold type), "DO NOT recommend using anything other than prescribed medical oxygen provided by an approved vendor." They know they shouldn't recommend that anyone do something so dangerous. But they also know how desperate their fellow Clusterheads are. "Yes, that is the disclaimer."

When all else fails, Clusterheads activate their network. Someone, somewhere, will have an oxygen tank to lend to a person in need, even if this means driving several hours to reach salvation. They spend a good percentage of time teaching one another hacks to make the oxygen therapy more effective: Swap out the short tubing that the oxygen supply company provides with something longer to enable pacing. Chug an energy drink containing caffeine and taurine to amplify the beneficial effects. Use breathing techniques akin to hyperventilation to make oxygen work even faster. Cover the holes of the non-rebreather mask to increase the flow of oxygen, or better yet, invest in an on-demand regulator.

Oxygen therapy, with its minimal side effects and proven high success rate, stands as an especially useful treatment for those who endure agonizing bouts of cluster headache attacks. So why is obtaining oxygen therapy so difficult? Why, despite the clear evidence and passionate advocacy from those who have experienced its benefits, is it so challenging to get the right equipment and clear instructions on its use? It's just one of many frustrations in the world of pain medicine, where patients' needs too often fall on deaf ears.

But patient advocacy is making things better. Many people with cluster headache are now finding hope in a new breakthrough treatment that owes much to the relentless advocacy of Bob Wold. Eli Lilly, the pharmaceutical company responsible for Emgality (galcanezumab)—a medication initially developed for migraine—expanded its focus to investigate the drug's potential application for cluster headache. The results offered enough promise that the FDA approved it for episodic cluster headache on June 4, 2019. The United Kingdom's National Institute for Health and Care Excellence and the European Union declined to do the same based on a lack of evidence.

Like all therapies, even a marvelous new medication has its limitations. Clusterbusters' website advises, "Treating Cluster Headache is done widely by way of trial and error." It's common for a medicine that once worked wonders to stop being effective. It's vital to remember the trial and error nature of treatment and to maintain hope that one of these therapies will work. And if conventional treatments fail? Clusterbusters and the community it represents offer a reservoir of alternative treatments and creative hacks. Wold, of course, is always willing to help talk someone through the psychedelic protocol. Other strategies, like chugging a coffee or an energy drink containing $B_{12}$ and taurine at the first sign of an attack, can boost the effectiveness of a regular abortive treatment. And plenty of people swear that the best preventive is an easy-to-follow high-dose vitamin D regimen.

● ● ●○●●○●●○●●○●●○●●○●● ● ●

Bob Wold didn't have much experience with psychedelics when Ainslie Course sent him an email in the fall of 2002 to ask for help. A few people had sent him direct messages on the internet forum where cluster headache patients were talking about the treatment, but nobody had ever reached out by email before—and from so far away! Scotland had always been on his bucket list.

Advising her, however, was a daunting prospect. Wold, a building contractor with no medical training, had only been treating his own cluster bouts with psychedelic mushrooms for a year. But nothing in his twenty-three-year experience with cluster headache had ever worked as well, or as quickly, and he'd tried dozens of therapies, including over sixty prescription medications and four in-patient hospitalizations.

"I felt a deep sense of responsibility [when Ainslie] reached out. . . . I can say, '[Mushrooms] don't help everyone' all I want, but in the case of someone on the brink of suicide, the most important thing I can offer is hope. I can downplay it all I want but can't make a response absent of hope."

The task wasn't easy then, and it's only getting harder. "I appreciate it when people come up to me and tell me that I saved their lives, but that just reinforces that same responsibility when the next person comes up and, without saying the words, is asking me to save their life."

It's wearying to patch up an entire medical system on your own. Wold, now seventy, wonders if, and how, he might ever retire. Who would take care of all the people who write and ask for help? People assist him—Ainslie Course is now one of his most dedicated volunteers. But he can't help worrying about the people still in need. He knows all too well what it's like to live on the brink. He thanks goodness for the stranger he met online who sent mushrooms to his house in the summer of 2001 in a UPS Priority box with a return address reading simply "Atlanta."

Chapter Three

● ● ●●●●●●●●●●●●●●●●●●● ● ●

# THE SOCIAL MYCELIUM

OUR CULTURE MAINTAINS AMBIVALENT ATTITUDES TOWARD FUNGI. The word *fungus* itself evokes disgust. Green, moldy leftovers. Itchy feet and dirty locker rooms. Black mold spreading behind damp walls. A deep-seated aversion fuels a thriving industry of remediation services, while wild mushrooms—though long a staple of human diets—are often regarded with caution because some are poisonous and deadly. Cultivated mushrooms seem much safer but come with a downside: agricultural workers who grow mushrooms risk developing a lung disease called hypersensitivity pneumonitis because of overexposure to so many spores.

But fungi also provide pleasure, joy, nourishment, and healing. Traditional medicine around the world has always drawn on the therapeutic properties of molds and mushrooms, a practice mirrored in Western "allopathic" medicine, which derives many of its most potent pharmaceuticals from these same natural elements. Penicillin is derived from a bread mold; lovastatin, a cholesterol drug, from oyster mushrooms; and cyclosporine, an immunosuppressant, from a fungal parasite. Scientists are now studying fungi in their search for new antiviral medications capable of defeating flu, smallpox, and SARS.

And now a wellness scene flush with cash is embracing the "shroom boom." Various kinds of mushrooms are said to boost the immune system, improve cognitive capabilities, support gut health, decrease cancer risks, and lower cholesterol levels. Consumers seeking to supplement their diets with medicinal mushrooms may purchase tinctures containing their extracts or, if they prefer, replace their morning coffee with a healthful mushroom drink. And, of course, any of us may also eat the mushrooms as food.

Mushrooms may contain the medicine, but they are hardly the most interesting or important component of the fungal organism. Mushrooms are just the fruit of a much larger fungal body, albeit one that we humans rarely see or notice. These fruits are important for reproduction; they produce and disperse spores—essentially microscopic seeds. With the correct moisture, temperature, and nutrients, some of those spores germinate into threads of cells called *hyphae*, the basic building blocks of fungi.

The real magic happens when hyphae gather and form *mycelium*, thin, white filaments that branch like a network, absorbing nutrients from decay and in the process creating layers of rich soil that nourish entire ecosystems. The fine threads of hyphae may be too small to see, but once knitted together into mycelial mats, these fungal forms make much of the matter holding together the earth beneath our feet. A single square inch of healthy soil can contain enough mycelium to stretch for eight miles. And yet, even as mycelium forms the bulk of the planet's forests, its foundational role in our ecosystems has, until recent decades, escaped scientific notice.

Paul Stamets, perhaps the best-known champion of fungal networks, has argued that fungi are the "keystone species" that sustain all ecosystems, flora, and fauna.[1] Fungi can't photosynthesize like plants can, which means they must consume food for energy—a feat they accomplish by extracting nutrients from dead trees, plants, and animals. The process creates fertile soil, filled with nutrients that plants need, like nitrogen and phosphorus. Scientists are now looking into how we might harness fungi's ability to break down complex organic molecules like toxic chemicals and plastics to solve challenging environmental problems. In a world threatened by human-made climate change, fungi may be our savior.[2]

Stamets makes the compelling case that mycelia, with their branching weblike threads, function as nature's neurological network. This metaphorical comparison underscores how mycelium serve as a mode of communication that connects ecosystems. Just as the internet connects communities, mycelium forms a "Wood Wide Web" enabling plants—even of different species—to share information and resources. For instance, should a maple tree lack certain nutrients, mycelium can collaborate across species to transport the necessary sustenance. Similarly, when a fruit tree is besieged by ants, a mycelial network can alert other plants in the area while delivering immunotherapy to the affected tree.

Learning more about this underground network has transformed how I understand my landscape. My house sits on a city street lined with towering oaks and maples, interspersed with odiferous ginkgo and a glorious magnolia. I had always seen each tree as an individual, each bringing its own personality to the block. But now I think their real lives take place underground, where an entire subterranean world of mycelium and its tangled skeins share messages along mycelial routes. Now I wonder, *Is the oak in front of my house talking to the rose bush in the back garden? Are they sharing nutrients alongside neighborly gossip? Are they in cahoots with the wisteria crawling up the side of my house? What secrets do they spread beneath Philadelphia's sidewalks and potholes?*

To the untrained eye, each oak tree on my block looks like a mighty individual that grew strong from a tiny acorn. Humans, with a partial view, might believe that a mushroom on an oak's roots is parasitic, there only because the oak provides the fungus with essential nutrients. But most fungi offer trees far more food and water than they consume. Fungal networks are not just necessary to the oak's survival but an essential precondition of its existence.

Mycology speaks to me more as a sociologist than as a nature lover. The concept of sociological imagination prompts us to see individual behavior as interconnected with and nurtured by broader structural and societal influences, often hidden from our view. At their best, fungi offer a model of symbiotic living in which everyone benefits. By embracing a sociological imagination, we can develop a worldview recognizing the interplay between individual behavior and the larger social and structural forces that shape our existence.

This lens of interconnectedness, reflected in mycelial networks, emphasizes the significance of recognizing the subtle but powerful forces shaping our lives. This perspective is pertinent in the United States, where the prevailing belief in meritocracy often overshadows the influence of government policies in determining access to resources such as healthcare. By adopting this sociological mind-set, we gain a clearer understanding of the complex interplay between individual actions and the larger forces that govern our existence.

People, like trees, require a broad network of support for survival.

● ● ●●∶●●∶●●∶●●∶●●∶●●∶●●∶● ● ●

Clusterbusters offers this kind of support by providing education, building community, offering peer support, and advocating on behalf of patients' interests. They've been building a parallel set of offerings through MigraineBusters. Both websites offer information on how *to bust*—their term for using psychedelics to treat headache disorders.

Migraine and cluster headache, according to Clusterbusters' research, can be treated with classic psychedelics, a category that includes psilocybin (the psychoactive compound in magic mushrooms), lysergic acid amide (LSA), which can be derived from morning glory seeds, and lysergic acid diethylamide (LSD).[3] Each of these substances has a chemical structure called an *indole ring* that's similar in shape to a neurotransmitter called serotonin (5-hydroxytryptamine, or 5-HT).

Serotonin influences some of our most important bodily functions, including sleep, memory and learning, mood and emotions, sexual behavior, hunger, and perceptions. Many commonly prescribed antidepressants and headache medications target serotonin receptors, each of which regulates distinct physiological responses, from gastrointestinal functions to complex cognitive processes.

Classic psychedelics cause their signature altered states of consciousness because they have a strong affinity with the serotonin 2A receptor (5-HT2A). This interaction is key to their potential therapeutic effects in treating conditions like migraine and cluster headache, as well as their more widely recognized psychoactive properties. In high enough doses, these substances trigger a cascade of chemical and electrical signals that produce hallucinations and perceptual shifts, but subperceptual doses (sometimes called "microdoses") may also affect how this receptor does its job.

Clusterbusters offers education and peer support for several classical psychedelic substances. But most of the information on the site is specific to psilocybin mushrooms since it is possible (albeit often illegal) to forage or cultivate a psychoactive fungus. Even still, this leaves a lot of choice for Busters, given that there are over 180 species in the *Psilocybe* genus of mushroom.

Foragers depend on whichever psilocybin-containing mushroom grows near them. In the United Kingdom, this is *Psilocybe semilanceata* (Liberty Caps), a teeny, ugly, brown mushroom that might not attract much attention at all but for its ability to induce psychedelic states. Foragers in the Pacific Northwest have more choices, including potent *Psilocybe azurescens*. But foraging requires confidence in one's ability to distinguish the correct species from a toxic look-alike.

Most people rely on *Psilocybe cubensis*, an easy-to-cultivate fungus with a reliable psilocybin content. Even limiting oneself to *P. cubensis* can be confusing, given that it comes in a broad range of strains. A "Golden Teacher" can look so different from "Penis Envy" that it's easy to assume they belong to different species. It's a bit like how a tomato can be large and savory, like a Brandywine, or small and sweet, like a cherry tomato.

Cultivation usually begins by injecting spores that were purchased online into canning jars holding a sterile, moist substrate, then incubated in a dark, warm space for several weeks. Successfully incubated jars will soon be packed with mycelium—the root structure of mushrooms—at which point they will be emptied into a "birthing chamber." Under the right conditions, the mycelium soon fruit mushrooms. Instructions for growing psychedelic mushrooms are easy to locate online, and the required materials can be purchased anywhere. The substrate can be made from brown rice and vermiculite; a birthing chamber can be fashioned from a large Rubbermaid container; moisture can be supplied with a simple spray bottle; and the temperature of the whole setup can be maintained with a cheap aquarium heater sold at any pet store.

Those who value convenience or, like me, doubt their ability to create a sterile environment anywhere in their house might be relieved to learn they can purchase preassembled, sterilized grow kits online.

Clusterbusters' website provides guidelines on how to bust effectively while minimizing risk of harm. Busting, according to their guidelines, is an all-purpose tool. It can end a cluster headache cycle, prevent a cycle, and/or abort a single attack.

Most individuals find relief through a regimen of three "low-dose" psychedelics administered five days apart. Unlike a microdose, which is sub-hallucinogenic and shouldn't cause noticeable effects, a low dose induces a mild euphoria. Bob Wold likens this sensation to the relaxed feeling of a "two-beer buzz." "Expect very blue, blue skies. Your favorite music will sound better than ever, [and expect a] smile on your face for 4–5 hours."[4]

The potency of mushrooms can vary, their website warns. Some people are more or less sensitive to the effects, so Clusterbusters recommends starting with a low quarter-gram dose that usually doesn't cause perceptual effects and titrate up slowly. Most people, in their experience, feel better with a one to two gram dose, which might lead to more euphoric sensations and a sense of connection to something greater, blurring the sense of self and causing feelings of oneness with the universe. As the dose increases, hallucinations can include alterations in colors and shapes or synesthetic experiences like "hearing" colors and "seeing" sounds. The self might dissolve entirely. The experience may be sociable and uplifting for some and overwhelming for others.

Classic psychedelics are not considered addictive, and they present little risk of toxicity to the body. They can, however, cause some people to experience physical distress while they are intoxicated. LSD and psilocybin can raise blood pressure, heart rate, and body temperature, as well as dilate pupils. Psilocybin can also cause nausea and even vomiting.[5]

Psychological risks are a bigger concern. Fear, anxiety, grief, confusion, and even feelings of insanity, isolation, or paranoia can make for a "challenging" experience. (The term *bad trip* is out of fashion.) A trip can also cause a dissociative reaction, a feeling that nothing is real. While many derive value or insight from a challenging experience—Wold believes that psychedelic medicine can heal the trauma of living with cluster headache—problems can occasionally take a long time to resolve.

Preparation can go a long way in minimizing risk. Psychedelics amplify one's mind-set, so busting just after a terrible breakup or while grieving can be especially difficult. Psychedelic experiences can occasionally have long-term consequences. There's a small risk of so-called flashbacks, known more formally as *hallucinogen-persisting perception disorder*, when perceptual disturbances persist well after the experience is over. Some people don't mind, but others find this distressing. An online survey asking people about their challenging experiences with psychedelics found that 24 percent experienced negative psychological symptoms, like fear, anxiety, or depression, for a week or more after their dose; 10 percent experienced negative symptoms for over a year. Intriguingly, the degree of difficulty experienced corresponded with how personally meaningful the psychedelic experience had been. A safe setting that promotes a sense of security is a must. Taking the medicine alone is not recommended. It's far better to be with someone trusted and, preferably, sober. Psychedelics amplify one's mind-set, so busting just after a terrible breakup or while grieving can be especially difficult.

There have been reports of sexual abuse in clinical trials testing psychedelic therapy and in the psychedelic underground. Underground drug markets, of course, increase risk. Ensuring the safety and quality of substances is difficult without regulation, and encouraging people to hide their activity makes it so much harder for people to reach out and get the help they need.

Clusterbusters offers education and peer support to reduce the risk of harm but can't make it disappear. No matter what happens, Clusterbusters urges people to be patient. They're just a small team of people trying to patch a broken system.

● ● ●●●●●●●●●●●●●●●●●●●● ● ●

The social mycelium offers an important corrective to the romanticized notion of scientific progress: the idea of a lone genius, standing on the shoulders of giants, reaching ever upward like a tree toward the sun, all the while drawing from an embedded network of roots pulling knowledge from the earth. It's a powerful narrative—but it comes at a cost.

Lauding the genius who runs the laboratory renders invisible the collaborative nature of science, as well as the historical contribution of countless scientists who have added to our collective knowledge. Sometimes this means ignoring the input of a junior colleague, a research assistant, a graduate student, or a spouse. Often it means women, people of color, and other marginalized groups are robbed of recognition for their role in making important discoveries.

Mycelial networks also provide a model for how science gets made. Picture science not as an ivory tower from which knowledge is broadcasted downward but instead as an interwoven mycelial network. In this network, each thread—each hypha—represents a different scientific field or even an individual within that field. Like a mycelium network where nutrients and information are constantly exchanged, science also involves a dynamic interchange of ideas across a vast network.

The ivory tower metaphor suggests that wisdom emerges from a singular, all-knowing source, but the reality of science is far more communal and interconnected. It's a system of constant growth and exploration where each participant—from credentialed scientists with MDs and PhDs to people in desperate need of relief—contributes expertise and insight, helping the entire network thrive, adapt, and expand our collective understanding.[6]

• • •••••••••••••••••••• • •

Much like the mushrooms it often studies, modern psychedelic research operates within a complex ecosystem. Most of us know about the "aboveground"—this is psychedelic research on and advocacy for psychedelic substances that occur legally within well-regulated, well-respected institutions, like universities, pharmaceutical companies, philanthropic organizations, and nonprofit entities. But the truth is that the psychedelic aboveground consists of a rarefied group, mainly because governmental regulations have made this kind of science extraordinarily difficult to pursue. As a result, the work of the aboveground relies on an extensive underground network.

The "underground" includes all contributors to psychedelic research who lack the legal and institutional authority to do such work. (Some people argue that the phrase *psychedelic underground* refers to a distinct subculture of psychonauts interested in exploring consciousness. This book uses a more capacious and inclusive definition that includes indigenous communities who have long used these substances, clandestine chemists whose laboratories produce consciousness-altering research chemicals, traditional healers trained as shamans, psychologists and psychiatrists offering guidance with "integration," Silicon Valley tech executives microdosing to increase their productivity, creatives seeking a shift in perspective, couples seeking the intimacy offered by an MDMA session, parents desperate for a holiday from their children, and, of course, an increasingly large group of sick, depressed, and anxious people desperate to find a better way to treat their health.)

Like any vibrant subculture, the underground has its own superstars and ne'er-do-wells, and is rife with drama and subtext that occasionally consume too much of its own oxygen. There's also an almost religious devotion to leaders who provide a sacramental experience believed to offer divine connection. But the underground does not fetishize credentials and authority in quite the same way as aboveground institutions. Instead, it supports a wide range of expertise, from scientists and physicians with multiple advanced academic degrees and years of laboratory and clinical experience to those with no formal education whatsoever who contribute vital data and produce valuable knowledge about psychedelic experiences.

Underground researchers must do so, however, without the same sorts of institutional support, let alone protection, that aboveground researchers enjoy. Nevertheless, the underground has developed sophisticated ways to create and distribute its research over time. At first, print and word of mouth operated as the primary modes for communicating underground knowledge. In the 1970s and 1980s, bookstores that carried underground books and magazines, like *The Anarchist Cookbook* and *High Times*, were significant sites for distributing psychedelic knowledge.

During the 1990s, the internet became a powerful worldwide platform for creating and sharing information about psychoactive substances. Early sources of such knowledge included Usenet groups frequented by drug aficionados. In 1995, an American couple going by the names Earth and Fire created a website called Erowid, where they post information about psychoactive drugs, including their history, dosage, legality, and safety, as well as "experience reports" written by people who have taken them. A screening process helps ensure that information is "objective, accurate, and non-judgmental."[7] By the new millennium, Erowid's curated "trip reports" had become a vital resource for those seeking to understand the effects, risks, and advantages of different substances, be they "drug geeks" seeking a novel way to explore their consciousness or physicians hoping to learn more about how these drugs affected their patients.

Erowid, however, was only one of many websites offering information about psychoactive drugs.[8] Online forums, like the Shroomery and Mycotopia, offered detailed advice on growing, identifying, and using psychedelic mushrooms. The Shroomery's detailed instructions on growing mushrooms, combined with its vibrant community, helped develop the underground network while offering mushrooms a vital new way to spread their mycelial networks. Eventually, forums like Clusterbusters were created. The neighborhood mycelium had vastly expanded its range, and the aboveground would soon benefit hugely from the growing reach of the World Wide Web.

● ● ●●●●●●●●●●●●●●●●●●● ● ●

It's not surprising that drug prohibition fostered the growth of clandestine networks. Indigenous people in the Americas continued using psychedelic substances as sacraments, albeit covertly, despite Spanish prohibition of the substances. Mafia-controlled speakeasies and moonshine kept Americans sloshed during the United States' brief flirtation with alcohol prohibition. Criminalizing marijuana, heroin, and cocaine spawned a lucrative underground economy.

Prior to the 1960s, psychedelic use was uncommon in Western culture, with experimentation largely limited to scientists, physicians, and a few notable intellectuals. Not until the rise of influential advocates and cultural figures did psychedelics begin to gain popularity in the United States and Europe. Pioneers such as Allen Ginsberg, Ken Kesey, and former Harvard professors Timothy Leary and Ram Dass (born Richard Alpert) played significant roles in popularizing LSD within youth culture. Key figures like clandestine chemists Augustus Owsley Stanley and Melissa Cargill supplied Deadheads with quality acid while Nick Sand and Tim Scully produced the famous "Orange Sunshine" LSD, distributed by the Brotherhood of Eternal Love. Alexander "Sasha" Shulgin's extensive contributions to the field further broadened the scope and acceptance of these substances.

The psychedelic underground networks inspired and sometimes led by these iconic figures created "safe spaces" where the exploration, development, and promotion of psychedelics could continue even in the face of legal restrictions and cultural stigma. These networks, much like the resilient mycelium in the natural world, could slow down or go into a state of dormancy when faced with unfavorable conditions, preserving their structure and potential for future growth. Sociologist Verta Taylor argued that social movements can survive challenging and even oppressive political environments if they can find a safe space—an "abeyance structure"—to regroup while waiting for a more supportive environment.[9] In the case of the psychedelic movement, this mycelium-like ability to endure and adapt allowed the ideals and practices to persist, ready to flourish again when societal acceptance and legal landscapes shifted.

While we often consider these psychedelic networks as a single, unified counterculture, they consisted of diverse threads, each pursuing distinct interests, philosophies, and practices. Spiritual seekers saw LSD as a sacrament for communing with the sacred. Technologists viewed the drug as a cognitive enhancer that could spark innovation. Artists turned to LSD to unlock creativity while fans of the Grateful Dead use it to deepen their musical appreciation. Even at "The Farm," a utopian community in Tennessee, midwives administered LSD to assist women in labor.

Not every mycelial thread flourished into an enduring network, and some, like Charles Manson's notorious cult, inflicted lasting damage on the reputation of psychedelic drugs. Yet these collective efforts not only preserved the knowledge and techniques of psychedelic use during a time of widespread prohibition but also laid the groundwork for the resurgence of interest and acceptance in modern times.

One locale played a crucial part in shielding the psychedelic movement during the heated days of the War on Drugs—a place so verdant that those who congregated in this newfound sanctuary might occasionally lose sight of the fact that their movement was lying in wait, dormant and unnoticed.

Established in 1962, the Esalen Institute in Big Sur, California, a veritable Eden perched on a cliff overlooking the Pacific, is a breathtaking New Age retreat center focused on the cultivation of human potential. Its cofounders, Richard "Dick" Price and Michael Murphy, drew inspiration from one of their earliest visitors, British writer Aldous Huxley. Huxley's exploration of consciousness, enriched by psychedelic substances, resonated with the burgeoning counterculture's interest in transcendent experiences. This laid a blueprint for Price and Murphy's Esalen, guiding them to foster a multifaceted approach to personal growth centered on introspection and the exploration of altered states of consciousness as avenues for self-discovery.

Huxley did not witness the lasting influence of Esalen on Western spirituality; he passed away before he could see the full scope of its impact. However, his vision and philosophy did not perish with him; it found a champion in his widow, Laura Huxley. She supported the institute, molding its ethos and steering its journey in a direction that aligned with her late husband's commitment to exploring and enhancing human potential, an ethos that maintained Huxley's advocacy for the therapeutic use of LSD.

It may have helped that *Island*, Huxley's last novel, envisions a utopian society where a drug quite like LSD plays a pivotal role in fostering a community grounded in awareness, empathy, and self-realization.[10] One can't help but draw parallels between the utopia envisioned in *Island* and the very real, physical space of Esalen, a haven of exploration and spiritual growth sprouting in the same timeline, as if bearing testimony to the possible realization of Huxley's dream.

Over the decades, Esalen has hosted the most recognizable names in New Age spirituality *and* the superstars of the psychedelic world, including Alan Watts, Ram Dass, Timothy Leary, Andrew Weil, and Stanislav Grof. Their workshops on plant medicine, spirituality, consciousness, and alternative therapeutic modalities attracted both psychedelic elders and newcomers to the field. The campus became a refuge where scientists, psychotherapists, intellectuals, and seekers could find refuge and communion while preserving the integrity and continuity of psychedelic exploration. Over time, small networks of people debated the best way to return important work on psychedelic medicine to the aboveground.

At least three significant initiatives emerged from these networks: Rick Doblin's Multidisciplinary Association for Psychedelic Studies (MAPS), George Greer and David Nichols's Heffter Research Institute, and Robert "Bob" Jesse's Council on Spiritual Practices (CSP). Each of these organizations offers the vital support that underground psychedelic networks need to bear fruit in aboveground settings. But they've each employed quite different strategies.[11]

●  ●  ●●●●●●●●●●●●●●●●●●●  ●  ●

Rick Doblin formed MAPS in 1986 as a response to the decision of the US Drug Enforcement Administration (DEA) to permanently class 4-methylenedioxymethamphetamine (MDMA) as a Schedule I drug. Most people today still know MDMA as an illegal street drug called Ecstasy (when sold as a tablet) or Molly (when sold as a crystal). Less known, however, is that people had been using MDMA legally for at least fifteen years before the DEA decided to criminalize its use.

MDMA, a drug first synthetized by the pharmaceutical company Merck in 1912, is a stimulant that produces a euphoric sensation, along with a profound feeling of empathy and closeness with others. In the 1970s, a network of underground psychedelic therapists, many of whom met one another at Esalen, began using MDMA, which they called Adam, in their psychotherapy practices. When used along with psychotherapy, Adam allowed their clients to approach even their most traumatic and frightening memories with gentle love and kindness.[12]

Therapists who used MDMA insisted that the practice be kept secret, since they worried that the US government would criminalize the substance if it learned of its use. Their fears materialized when officials noticed a huge amount of the stuff being sold at dance clubs and bars in Texas. The DEA announced its intention to place MDMA on Schedule I of the Controlled Substances Act.[13]

Esalen, naturally, became the headquarters where the underground could mobilize against this new injustice. Dick Price immediately organized a meeting at the Pacific paradise so that the psychedelic elders could brainstorm a way to stop the DEA. Rick Doblin, who was just twenty-eight years old at the time, had no real business being there, but his innovative advocacy on behalf of MDMA had reached none other than Laura Huxley. She was so impressed that she'd made sure he was invited.[14]

Doblin wasn't shy about expressing his opinions or taking charge despite being the junior member of the group. Taking on the DEA was no joke, and he lacked confidence that the elders' newly formed Association for the Responsible Use of Psychedelic Agents had the gumption for the job. So Doblin took action.

He began by taking over a friend's inactive nonprofit called Earth Metabolic Design Laboratories, which would serve as a base from which he could coordinate a response to the DEA.[15] He then sued the agency in the most public manner possible.[16] The courts agreed with Doblin—twice. But the DEA wasn't mandated to accept either ruling. They placed MDMA in Schedule I on a permanent basis anyway.

Rick Doblin embraced his leadership position as a public psychedelic outlaw with evangelical fervor. He believes—truly believes—that MDMA can provide the spiritual awakening that can bring humanity more peace. And true believers need to testify.

Like the best evangelicals, Doblin is an optimist—so much so that in 1986, smack dab in the middle of a decade marked by fearmongering about illegal drugs, including psychedelics, he founded MAPS, a "research and educational organization that develops medical, legal, and cultural contexts for people to benefit from the careful uses of psychedelics and marijuana."[17] Public service announcements warning that drugs fry brains be damned.

Doblin hasn't changed his evangelical style, and he also projects a remarkable amount of authenticity. One gets the sense that what you see is what you get with Doblin. So while MAPS exists to fund the kind of research that will lead to the legalization of MDMA and other psychoactive drugs, it does not shy away from embracing recreational use of psychoactive drugs or advocating for drug decriminalization.

It's an unusual strategy with a psychedelic community on high alert for government interference. Even now that the underground movement has come so far toward legitimacy, the entire community still feels precariously balanced on the knife-edge of potential regulatory clampdown.

The Heffter Research Institute, the second major psychedelic philanthropy that emerged from Esalen's networks, implemented a far more cautious strategy. Professor David Nichols, a stalwart from the aboveground
world of academia, spearheaded Heffter's meticulous approach. His
position as a professor of pharmacology at Purdue University (prior to
retirement he held the prestigious Robert C. and Charlotte P. Anderson
Distinguished Chair) afforded him a perspective that straddled the realms
of the forbidden and the conventional in drug research.

Nichols is one of the few academic researchers who have managed to
study psychedelic substances for an entire career. His interest in these compounds reaches back to the late 1960s when he studied mescaline as a PhD
student. He was able to continue this work at Purdue because laboratory
researchers didn't experience nearly as many restrictive obstacles to studying Schedule I drugs as those conducting clinical research in humans. He
even obtained a license from the DEA that permitted him to synthesize
Schedule I drugs. Most of the psychedelic substances tested in contemporary clinical trials were created in his laboratory.

But Nichols worried about the lack of clinical research on psychedelics.
Laboratory experiments had a limited ability to reveal how these drugs
affected human consciousness. But he didn't know many physicians who
wanted to do this research until autumn 1984 when he traveled to Esalen
to join Dick Price's resistance movement. Rick Doblin, of course, was there,
along with a great many legends in the field whom he'd long admired but
never met.[18]

In recollections of these meetings, Nichols described how impressed
he'd been by everyone's conviction that psychedelic substances had the
capacity to heal. So he was dismayed to learn how few of the scientists in
attendance truly believed that the government would ever again allow their
use. Maybe Nichols felt differently because of his experience as a laboratory scientist, but he thought they were being overly pessimistic. An aboveground scientist at a prestigious institution ought to be able to gain the
necessary approvals. So far as he could tell, the biggest challenge would be

funding. A philanthropy dedicated to providing grants and financial support for this research would make a big difference.

In 1993 Nichols cofounded the Heffter Research Institute with psychiatrist George Greer to serve this mission. The institute bore the name of Dr. Arthur Heffter, a German chemist and physician with the distinction of isolating mescaline from peyote. Aligning the institute with Heffter—a figure synonymous with "outstanding scientific work"—would symbolize a commitment to excellence and the pioneering spirit of exploration in the scientific study of psychedelics.[19]

But aligning themselves with aboveground science also meant keeping the underground and the counterculture at arm's length. To do so, they established a clear, focused vision: back the highest quality of scientific research carried out in renowned institutions and passing through rigorous checks by other experts in the field. Getting this science done would mean a concerted effort to prevent controversy. LSD and MDMA might have therapeutic benefits but carried too much cultural baggage. So Heffter chose to concentrate on psilocybin, since most people in the public hadn't yet heard of the chemical. Obtaining financial backing from Bob Wallace, a key figure from the early days of Microsoft and a passionate supporter of psychedelic research, allowed Heffter to forge a path dedicated to careful, serious, and safe exploration of the potentials housed in psilocybin.

Esalen's network of psychedelic elders proved indispensable to Bob Jesse when he began organizing the Council on Spiritual Practices (CSP), which is now one of the most influential organizations in the movement to use psychedelic substances to transform modern medicine. Jesse, who was then a vice president of business development at Oracle, was interested in psychedelics more as a means to invoke spiritual transformation than as a medical treatment. But he found the old scientific research on LSD fascinating.

Jesse, like most tech executives, lived in the Bay Area, a hub for psychedelic enthusiasts. He'd been washing dishes in the Shulgins' kitchen, according to Michael Pollan, when he learned that, in January 1994, Esalen would be hosting a meeting of elders who were plotting a comeback of psychedelic science.[20] Meetings like this were small, exclusive events, but Jesse found a way to attend.

The meeting was useful. In addition to solidifying his relationships with a network of elders, he learned that the political situation was a lot more optimistic at the federal level. The Food and Drug Administration (FDA) had decided that it would evaluate applications to study psychedelic substances using the same set of criteria as proposals for any other drug. And it didn't seem to be all talk, either. The FDA gave the go-ahead for a clinical trial testing the effects of dimethyltryptamine (DMT), a potent hallucinogen, on healthy human subjects at the University of Mexico.[21]

Hearing so much enthusiasm for the restoration of research on psychedelic medicine inspired Jesse to create the CSP to help develop scientific research on the use of psychedelics for more spiritual purposes. By 1996, Jesse was hosting his own meeting at Esalen under the aegis of the CSP.

Jesse is always described as a meticulous person, so I have no doubt that he'd thought carefully about the fifteen people in attendance. Most were psychedelic elders, like Brother David Steindl-Rast, Huston Smith, and Jeffrey Bronfman, then head of the US branch of the União do Vegetal, a religious society that considers ayahuasca a sacrament. But Jesse also invited at least two people who very much inhabited the "aboveground" worlds: Harvard Kennedy School professor Mark Kleiman, an influential drug policy scholar known for his interest in well-regulated, legal markets for marijuana, and Charles "Bob" Schuster, former director of the National Institute on Drug Abuse under both Ronald Reagan and George H. W. Bush.

Schuster, a relative outsider to the group, found the conversation sufficiently captivating to introduce Jesse to his colleague, Roland Griffiths of the Johns Hopkins University School of Medicine. Griffiths, despite a career centered on studying the addictive traits of psychoactive substances, had been harboring a growing interest in spirituality, fueled by a personal meditation practice.

Jesse saw in Griffiths a potential ally and persuaded him of the potent research avenue that psilocybin offered in examining altered states of consciousness in clinical research. In 1999, Griffiths began his research into the therapeutic potential of psilocybin. Their collaboration has been fruitful. In 2006, Griffiths and Jesse coauthored a landmark study documenting that psilocybin could "occasion" mystical states of consciousness. Jesse is now described as the "quiet force" steering the research that's been pouring out of Johns Hopkins ever since. Jesse's influence can be seen right there in the name of Hopkins's new center dedicated to this work, the Center for Psychedelic and Consciousness Research.

One more initiative, crucial to the resurgence of psychedelic research albeit not originating from Esalen, is firmly anchored in the underground scene. The Beckley Foundation, established in 1996 as the Foundation to Further Consciousness before a name change in 1998, funds scientific research on psychedelic substances and collaborates with political leaders and researchers on drug policy reform. Its founder, Lady Amanda Feilding, a powerhouse in Europe's psychedelic movement, runs the Beckley Foundation from her childhood home, a stately Tudor hunting lodge in the lush green hills of Oxfordshire. Like Doblin, Feilding is open about her own experiences with psychedelic drugs in her advocacy for reform. Since the mid-1960s, she's been impressed with the ability of LSD to occasion mystical states of consciousness and heighten creativity.

The Beckley Foundation has long been a visible force funneling money from the psychedelic underground to European universities. Its support has enabled much of the foundational neuroimaging research on psychedelics produced at Imperial College London, Britain's premier science and engineering university.

• • •••••••••••••••••••• • •

What is the relationship between these vast underground networks and the aboveground researchers now flourishing in the current psychedelic renaissance? Those involved in rehabilitating psychedelic medicine have worked hard to distance themselves from the moral and legal stigmas that smothered the entire enterprise in the 1960s. Funders of psychedelic research far prefer collaborating with the most prestigious universities; psychedelic researchers dress in suits and ties to curry respect and emanate authority; some in the field even refuse to discuss whether they have ever used psychedelics themselves.

Few mainstream news reports connect the illegal use of psychedelic drugs to this movement, despite how obvious this is to anybody paying attention.[22] I suspect the lack of media coverage has something to do with the fear of government backlash: at least, that's what many of the leaders in psychedelic medicine told me off the record. Anything that might threaten the eventual medicalization of psychedelics has to be hush-hush.

Hiding the origins of the knowledge that scientists now produce has its own ethical problems—whether it comes from generations of indigenous wisdom or underground patient populations. And as it happens, the relationship between these worlds is much closer to the mycorrhizal relationship shared between fungi and oaks: the aboveground psychedelic renaissance bears the fruit of a much deeper movement happening underground. In fact, not only are underground networks producing some of the best knowledge we have on the therapeutic uses of Schedule I drugs, but the aboveground scientists depend on these underground efforts to organize, design, and legitimate their clinical trials. In the meantime, the underground offers essential resources for people who have hit a dead end with their regular doctors.

Clusterbusters is far from the only patient group that has formed an underground network to develop new psychedelic therapies. These movements span various medical challenges. In the 1980s, Howard Lotsof pioneered a patient-led effort to use iboga for addiction treatment, following his personal discovery at age nineteen that it eliminated his heroin addiction. Within professional sports, the healing potential of psychedelics for concussions has led many athletes to explore these treatments. Recognizing this trend, former professional hockey player Daniel Carcillo founded Wesana, a company focused on developing such treatments. Internet forums have become meeting points for people with autism, sharing ways to use MDMA to mitigate social anxiety. (A recent clinical trial testing whether MDMA might reduce social anxiety supported the claims made by patients online.[23])

Patients form underground networks for all sorts of other treatments too. Transgender people have created secret networks for hormone treatments since the 1960s, often driven by societal misunderstandings and legal barriers. The 1970s saw Jane's Collective aiding women in accessing safe abortions during a time of stringent legal restrictions. In the world of pediatric epilepsy, parents have united to develop high-CBD tinctures on their own before these were available for purchase. Perhaps most famously, the AIDS crisis gave rise to underground "buyers clubs" to import and share experimental drugs the FDA hadn't yet allowed.[24] These collective efforts reflect a common human drive to find hope and healing, even in the face of institutional shortcomings and legal constraints.

It is funny, isn't it, that depending on our political orientation, our sympathies for outlaws can shift one way or the other. The governmental—and social—policing of illicit drug use has always been uneven. The FDA knew that AIDS patients were importing illegal drugs, but they looked the other way. Not only did police leave parents of children with epilepsy alone, but their plight conjured so much sympathy that medical marijuana advocates made them the poster children for their medical marijuana campaigns. And while people can and do get imprisoned for psychedelic-related offenses, the justice system doesn't seem interested in pursuing outlaws like Rick Doblin or Bob Wold.

In other contexts, policing turns certain forms of banal DIY medicine into criminal behavior. For example, an alarming number of poor people are incarcerated simply because they had a prescription medicine that didn't belong to them.[25] And there's no doubt that people use opioids—at least in the beginning—because they lift mood and reduce pain. But how many of us consider open-air opioid drug markets a form of DIY medicine?

Who gets to draw the line?

Mapping out the "pharmakologic" of a psychedelic ecosystem reveals a complex underground network feeding into a regulated, bureaucratic system of universities, biotech start-ups, pharmaceutical companies, private philanthropies, government agencies, nonprofit organizations, legislators, indigenous communities, religious belief systems, a media market hungry for news to hype, and the US War on Drugs and its bloated and racist carceral system.

If I wanted to understand Clusterbusters and its path from the underground world of online psychedelic dosing advice to the halls of Harvard, I would simply need to pick up and follow each connective thread and see where it took me.

But as I would quickly discover, every thread selected uncovered a network denser and more matted than I could have ever anticipated. I needed a heuristic to pick and choose investigative leads. What better place to start than the knotted strands of mycelium that have led hundreds of people in pain on a pilgrimage to a rotating set of airport hotels each September.

# Part II

# Incarnations

Chapter Four

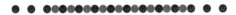

# COMMUNITY

I SPUTTERED AND STUMBLED MORE THAN USUAL WHEN I PITCHED THIS study to Bob Wold. We had met in 2012 at an annual advocacy event called Headache on the Hill, which brought advocates to Washington, DC, to meet their congressional representatives for a day. I had been attending as part of my research for a book that I'd been writing about migraine and stigma, and had grown accustomed to seeing the same staid faces. In those days, the event was small, just a few dozen headache specialists—mostly a staid group of neurologists dressed in business casual, who greeted each other with hearty handshakes before retreating into their screens during downtime. I knew that the organizers wanted more participation from patient advocates, but it had taken them some time to figure out how to connect with patient-led groups. Truth be told, there weren't many patient-led communities back then.

So I noticed when Bob Wold and a crew of Clusterheads appeared at the Capitol. First off, just by dint of participation, Headache on the Hill suddenly felt like a bigger, more substantial advocacy effort. But they also changed the feel of the event. The Clusterbusters didn't look or act like the other participants. Their dress leaned far more toward casual than business. And unlike the doctors, they seemed to genuinely enjoy one another's company. They embraced each other when they said hello, they hung out together, telling stories and jokes, and they would let out the loudest, most raucous laughs.

They also suffered, sometimes visibly. Large oxygen tanks—a necessity for those in cycle—accompanied the group wherever they went. I noticed at least one advocate managing a cluster attack during advocacy training—I could tell by the way she gripped her temple and used her hand to shake her head repeatedly that she wasn't having a run-of-the mill migraine. Another, who had been paired with me the next day on Capitol Hill, told me that he spent the night having multiple cluster attacks in his hotel room. Like most people with cluster headache, REM sleep triggered his attacks. I worried about how he would get through the day, but he assured me that he was used to it. He had chronic cluster headache, so not only had he not gone a night without cluster attacks for decades, sleep itself terrified him.

I decided to ask Wold if he might meet me for lunch the following year. He'd been public about his use of psychedelics, but this was 2013—before the shroom boom made psychedelics the latest wellness fad, and it seemed a bit much for me to just *ask* him about it, point-blank.

My explanations grew longer each time he pushed his chicken Caesar from one side of the plate to the other. Wold, I would learn, likes to listen.

I needn't have worried. As it turns out, Wold wasn't remotely interested in hiding. He viewed my interest in Clusterbusters as an opportunity to increase awareness.

By the end of our first lunch together, Wold had offered me access to whatever materials I would need for my research. Five months later, while I was attending my first Clusterbusters annual meeting, the entire community was just as welcoming. So much so, that when I introduced myself, the attendees burst into applause, nearly drowning me in a chorus of thank-yous. Their gratitude overwhelmed me. I had done nothing at all aside from show up.

Their gratitude, I eventually learned, was borne of the devastation wrought by their disease, combined with the certainty that nobody else cared, nobody else understood, and except for one another, they were completely alone. "Suffering," observes author Kate Bowler, "is a lonely place. . . . But when there is a witness to that suffering, someone who sees you in it—will be *with* you in it—you are not alone anymore with that choking vulnerability, and it is bearable."[1]

● ● ●●●●●●●●●●●●●●●●●● ● ●

I hadn't been at all sure what to expect when I showed up to that Clusterbusters conference. Would people be wearing business casual or psychedelic chic? Would the airport hotel approach the magical serenity of soaking in the Esalen Institute's hot springs on a clear dark night? Would we be opening chakras or tapping into previous lives?

What would the people be like? Would I be greeted by a salacious counterculture filled with patchouli-scented nudists? Or would it be more of a futuristic aesthetic, like the kind of psychedelic experimentation rampant at Burning Man, an annual festival in the Nevada desert that celebrates art, community, self-expression, and self-reliance, where interested participants can attend talks on "orgasmic meditation," "shamanic auto-asphyxiation," and "ecosexuality" as a prelude to a sunrise cuddle puddle?[2]

Or maybe the Clusterheads I'd be meeting would fit the increasingly common version of psychedelic enthusiasts seen in wellness circles—more like the attendees of the luxury retreats that Gwyneth Paltrow features in goop: healing spaces where each "sitting" is "integrated" with "experiences" of "yoga, breathwork, journaling, creative expression, [and] floral baths" in a setting that is somehow both verdant and always within earshot of the ocean.

But that was just my imagination on overdrive. Come to Clusterbusters in search of a lush retreat and you'll be disappointed. They meet in a plain hotel. The people there would blend in at any suburban mall. There's not a hint of spirituality to be found. No yoga offered during rest breaks. No drum circles. Not a single *namaste*.

Instead, I found a large gathering of people in front of the hotel, huddled over coffee, cigarettes, and cans of Red Bull, trading jokes and stories, just passing time while waiting for asylum from their pain.[3]

Replace the Black Rock Playa with a beige, bland hotel conference room, swap out personalized nutritional protocols for bottomless urns of luke-warm coffee, and don't expect lectures on "femtheogens and the tantra of our menses."[4] You're more likely to be signed up for a detailed workshop on the medical use of high-flow oxygen and inexpensive mushroom growth techniques.

I soon discovered that each three-day conference looks more like a mutual-aid group meeting than a psychonaut scene. Organizers place cans of Red Bull and dozens of giant oxygen tanks in an empty "comfort room." Additional needs are taken care of by a volunteer brigade tasked with tend-ing to anyone in cycle having an attack.

There is, to be fair, a touch of counterculture. Plenty of people are wear-ing tie-dyes, and there are drugs to be had. Weed is everywhere. Psyche-delics are also available for anyone who knows how to have the coded conversations that end in handshakes in which drugs were transferred.

But as I started to meet the group, it became obvious that these events are rare pleasures in the lives of those with cluster headache—a three-day reunion with their tribe. While each day is spent attending sessions marked by the sort of pent-up emotional release one might find in a twelve-step program, the nights are filled with an immersive joy that comes from spending time with people who completely get it. These people have all experienced repeated, lonely, excruciating pain, stared down the tempta-tion of suicide, and somehow made it back to this conference for another year. The drugs on the scene don't create these feelings, but they certainly amplify them. In a nondescript airport hotel, I see the most emotional bac-chanale I've ever witnessed.

Imagine sitting poolside at the O'Hare Hilton experiencing deep psyche-delic awe with a friend you've met at previous conferences who a few years ago was a newfound acquaintance but is now someone you consider more important than people you've known your entire life. In the next moment, you feel a tap on your shoulder. It is a first-time conference goer, gathering the courage to tell you about the last seven years of her life, in which she has lived in excruciating, suicidal, and largely undiagnosed pain. She's been sipping the same cocktail all night. She doesn't enjoy the feeling of being out of control, so the idea of using a psychedelic frightens her but not as much as the thought of her next cycle. The conference has taught her about so many other treatment options. She tells you that she's never felt more connected in her life than she does to the people she's met today. What might feel like an awkward interruption in another context feels perfect in the current moment. A blue aura pulses from her head as you hug her. You both cry for a long time. She's part of your family now, you tell her. You are safe now. She squeezes you tighter because she knows that what you say is true.

● ● ●●●●●●●●●●●●●●●●●●●●●● ● ●

After hearing enough heart-wrenching stories, I finally began to understand why people come to Clusterbusters. They're refugees. They aren't here to *find* alternatives to medical care so much as they have arrived only after just managing to narrowly *survive* medical care.

It would be wrong to think of Clusterbusters as a psychedelic organization. It can't afford to be—its constituency has so many pressing needs, many of which take precedence over treatment.

Bob Wold seemed to have an intuitive understanding that people needed to be in the same room as one another. I'd later learn that he'd met several Clusterheads in the 1990s while an in-patient at Chicago's Diamond Headache Clinic, one of the rare facilities with a floor devoted to headache patients. That encounter transformed him.

"Everybody I met was my instant friend because every time you mentioned anything, it'd be like, yeah, that's right, me too. It was just a really big deal to have somebody that knew what you were talking about. You didn't have to explain anything at all. And up until that point, all I wanted was to talk to somebody that understood what I was going through," he told me.

Conferences offered a similarly transformative experience to those who attended. Days might be spent listening to talks in a cold, partitioned conference room, but the annual event always felt joyful. Lots of people return year after year—after all, Clusterbusters is basically family. The vibe is open and friendly. Stick around long enough and there's gossip and an occasional undercurrent of resentment too. Like I said: family.

Every three-day conference began with a Thursday evening reception, where people could register and then have a drink and a bite to eat. Informational talks would begin the next morning at 9:00 a.m. "These conferences are just amazing," said a man sitting in the row in front of me, eyes wide with appreciation. "I'm hooked. Can you believe I just met a guy who has had cluster headache for six years, and I was the first person he's met who had the same disease?" He shook his head. "People don't understand how amazing it is to meet someone else with cluster headache."

Conferences always have a charismatic emcee. At this conference Dan Ervin, a silver-haired Clusterhead with a wide grin, took the stage. Ervin has an easy way with the crowd, a personality that's equal parts warmth and bombast.

"Welcome, everyone," he called out, his voice reverberated off the walls. "If you could state your name, where you're from, and whether you're episodic or chronic?" A roomful of eyes awaited further instruction. Ervin might own a liquor store in real life, but he's a minor celebrity in this room, having starred in a National Geographic TV episode featuring his use of homegrown psilocybin mushrooms as medicine. He flashed another grin and kick-started the process: "I'm from Abilene, Texas, and I've had a lifetime being a chronic, then went to episodic, and then back to being chronic."

Mary, Bob Wold's wife, took the microphone and handed it to a man sitting in the room's front row for the next introduction. And so, it went down the line, as they introduced themselves.

Some attendees explain in their introduction that they are in pain and are looking for information about new treatments. Others say that they "bust" the pain away but that they're "here to help people." Several introduce themselves as caregivers to people with cluster headache. Attendance didn't seem to be a solo affair. Although people didn't bring children, a few younger attendees had brought parents. Many were married couples, in which one person introduced themselves as a patient and the other as their caregiver.

Nearly half the attendees described themselves as "supporters"—people there to care for a loved one. This group, especially "cluster moms" or "cluster dads," occasionally come by themselves, searching for useful information they can bring home. Supporters, I noticed, always got lots of applause from everyone in the audience. As one attendee told them during his time with the microphone, "Nobody here is just support. I don't know what I would do without my mom."

It was as if AA attendees brought all their Al-Anon people with them to their annual meeting to find fellow sympathizers, though I suspect it was also something of a practical necessity as well. If an attack hit at an event like this, far from home, people would need help managing the excruciating onset of symptoms.

For a disease that causes so much pain, both physical and psychic, these get-togethers overflow with joy. I have met so many Clusterheads over the years who have tried to explain to me the profound emotional pull of these meetings. Aaron*, a longtime attendee, likened the experience to landing on a planet where you finally find your people.

Ashley Hattle, a professional writer and author of a popular self-help guide to living with cluster headache, spent most of her first conference in tears, releasing the emotions she'd saved up over seven years of brutal interactions with doctors who refused to believe how much pain she experienced.[5] Three years later, she married Andrew Cleminshaw, a chronic Clusterhead she met at that first conference. They timed their wedding, officiated by a fellow member, to coincide with a Clusterbusters conference to make it easier for other attendees—their adopted family—to attend. Bear hugs, tears, and affirmative nods of what Ashley described as "profound legitimation" replaced the usual small talk.

Over time, I learned that it's not uncommon for those who have cluster headache to hide their diagnosis from others. People hide during cycles for a variety of reasons. Some of the things they do are so strange, they wonder if they might be going insane. They worry—often from experience—that others won't understand how a headache could hurt so badly. They hide to protect others from the trauma of witnessing an attack. But they also hide to protect themselves. Strangers, they worry, might misinterpret an attack's odd and sometimes frightening behavior as a psychotic break.

Marginalized populations might have more to fear, especially Black men, who are already frightened about police brutality. "People might think you're on drugs or you're crazy," explained Andy Berry,* a frequent conference attendee. "As a Black man, if they call the police, it's even worse. I don't want anybody else's hands on me."

The secrecy surrounding cluster headache not only serves as a shield against misunderstanding but also erects barriers to empathy and support. Silence, a profound consequence of stigma, amplifies the fear of solitude in one's suffering, reinforcing a solipsistic nightmare. The breakthrough comes with the moment of connection—discovering another who bears the same invisible burden. It acts as a revelation, akin to a mirror reflecting one's own experiences, shattering the walls of solitude with the recognition of a shared reality.

Connecting this deeply also creates room for sharing a far messier, more transgressive emotion: the desire to end one's life. For some, this is the first time they've been in a room filled with people who might understand how a headache made them want to kill themselves or, worse, inspired an actual suicide attempt.

● ● ●●●●●●●●●●●●●●●●●●● ● ●

The courage on display at these conferences is palpable, with individuals sharing experiences that, in any other context, would remain shrouded in secrecy. Conversations this personal are built upon mutual trust and understanding. This trust extends beyond personal stories; it shapes the very fabric of the community, dictating who is invited into these spaces. Clusterbusters curates its events, welcoming only those doctors and professionals who support their cause, while pharmaceutical representatives, if present, remain silent observers. The absence of a police presence, except for the occasional noise complaint, underscores a sense of safety and autonomy.

However, this embrace of openness and safety raises questions about who remains absent from these gatherings. The stark racial homogeneity within the room mirrors a larger issue that extends beyond the confines of these conferences, reflecting a serious equity problem pervading both psychedelic medicine and the treatment of pain.

Pain invites doubt, leaving the wounded on trial to defend their moral integrity. In the absence of proof that pain is "real," people are vulnerable to labels like "malingerer," "drug seeker," "neurotic," "hypochondriac," and "sensitive." The opioid epidemic has only increased the stakes. Everybody at this conference understands all too well what it means when others invalidate their lived experience.

Not every patient is viewed as a reliable narrator of their own symptoms. Women are more likely than men to be dismissed as weak, sensitive, and demanding. Poverty increases people's chances of being accused of drug seeking. Meanwhile Black patients, even now, continue to struggle getting doctors to recognize that they're capable of experiencing pain—a holdover from eighteenth- and nineteenth-century scientists who claimed that people of African descent could handle the inhumane conditions of their enslavement because of a biological inability to feel pain.[6]

I was relieved to find so many women with cluster headache at these conferences, even if it was troubling to hear that so many of them still found it difficult to obtain a cluster headache diagnosis because their doctors still believe old, debunked myths. Overcoming these stereotypes is even harder for Black women. Ask Bernice Clark,* whose doctor told her she couldn't possibly have cluster headache. "Number one, women don't get clusters. Number two, Blacks don't get clusters." Bernice's case, of course, proved him absolutely wrong.

● ● ●●●●●●●●●●●●●●●●●●●●● ● ●

Black people of course can get cluster headache. But if they're lucky enough to have been diagnosed, finding treatment or relief is yet another bridge they must cross.

Both Bob Wold and his right-hand woman, Eileen Brewer, president of the board, have often told me that they are disappointed that they've had so much difficulty creating a more inclusive environment. Brewer told me that she's contacted by people of color all the time. But only a few ever make it to the conference. The criminalization of psychedelics presents real risks to a lot of people. Black people with cluster headache, Brewer tells me, are especially afraid of the police. She says she's had at least three dozen conversations that end with folks telling her, "If I try these medications, and I get caught, I'm going to get shot. I'm going to wind up dead."

She takes their concerns seriously. "We've had people threaten to call the cops over the years, but it's never happened. A lot of people wouldn't come to the conference if they thought that their place of employment found out that they were there. So, we just try to be sensitive to that," Eileen told me. "But honestly, if the cops showed up and arrested me, I would be thrilled. I would call every news station in the country."

When I asked if she might change her mind if the conference wasn't so white, she said, "Absolutely."

Risk of arrest and imprisonment isn't theoretical—it happens. One Clusterhead I spoke to faced serious repercussions after police discovered a small amount of mushrooms in his car during a traffic stop. He was charged with a fifth-degree felony, a sentence that carried mandatory rehab, attendance at twelve-step meetings, and probation.

Brewer has friends in prison on drug charges (not linked to medicinal use). She's had her run-ins with the law too. But she's a white woman who has never feared police brutality. "They really are trying to balance the 'Am

I going to wind up dead from cluster headache' with the 'Am I going to get shot by a police officer.'"

Immigrants face similar dilemmas. "I have talked to some people who are citizens of countries where this is, like, absolutely illegal. And the penalty is not going to a horrible prison for a few years, but a death sentence for using these substances. So, they have to consider whether they're going to leave their family and their heritage and their culture in order to seek treatment more safely." Talking to people about having to choose between life and freedom breaks her heart, and like me, she finds much of the color-blind conversation about psychedelic treatment tone-deaf. Consider, for example, the generic kind of advice typically offered on how to have a "good trip." Finding a "safe and familiar space" to be "undisturbed" for five to seven hours, ideally "a home with an enclosed yard or other outdoor space," during a day without "obligations to work or care for others, including children" is a high bar for most every family I know in the city. Crowded housing, a lack of safe, green space, fear of police, and the reality of work and caregiving make some of these recommendations a pipe dream for many people. Brewer isn't sure how to make Clusterbusters an inclusive organization, but she's doing her best to advocate for legislative policies that promote equity and access.

• • •••••••••••••••••• • •

Receiving so many emails and phone calls from people who have been told that Bob Wold is their last hope is a heavy burden. He answers every single one, no matter how burned out he feels. Too many Clusterheads he knows have already lost their lives. He knows how that particular rock bottom feels. And he knows he can help them.

Wold's celebrity at Clusterbusters meetings is, at least, partly driven by the countless people who attribute their survival to his interventions, many of whom thank him for saving their lives. Wold is always happy to hear when someone feels better. But he brushes off their effusive expressions of gratitude in much the same way another person might nod in reaction to being thanked for holding a door open.

He feels compelled to help. People are in danger, and he can see no other way forward. One gets the impression that this moral imperative to prevent every single potential suicide is so strong that he would no sooner step away from his work with cluster headache than ignore a child running in front of a car.

Wold infuses this same ethos into everyone affiliated with Clusterbusters at their annual conferences. His effort to do so leaves a vivid impression. Science and medicine, he explains to attendees, are terrific, which is why Clusterbusters supports academic research. But he's learned the hard way that they can't afford to wait for scientists and doctors to save them. The ever-present threat of suicide means that cluster headache patients can and must step up and do this work for themselves if they want to get it done.

At this point in the meeting, the audience will begin to see slides of previous years' attendees who are no longer alive. "Yes, it's important to study and collect data. But while we are collecting data"—a woman's face appears on a screen—"Sarah's* family and friends are collecting pieces of their lives and trying to put them back together." And then the next slide. "Pierre* was here from the very beginning, but clusters became too much for him and he took his life."

I only had to attend two conferences before someone I recognized appeared on the screen: Walter Roberts*, a stocky, middle-aged Black man—one of the only people I ever met at the conference who wasn't white. I held my breath while Wold continued. "Mrs. Walter Roberts is collecting widow's benefits, and Walter was just here in 2013."

Wold's next slide shows a clipping of a news article describing Clusterbusters as a classic example of "citizen scientists" who "roped in scientists to validate what their experiences have shown and plan clinical trials and other research to take the treatments forward."[7] Wold points out that Clusterbusters can make these advances quickly *because* they're citizen scientists.

"One nice thing about Clusterbusters is we don't always follow the rules, and we're not always stuck with the same constraints that professionals have, so we are able to do things a little bit quicker." Wold leads by inspiration and by hard work. "We are making great progress," he tells the assembled Clusterheads. "But it's not good enough. We need to do good work at a better pace." They cannot wait for the system to catch up because they themselves are the most important part of the system. "We need all hands on deck. We need to continue to knock on every door. We need to not only ask, but demand attention."

Wold is sociable with a wry sense of humor, and he enjoys the boisterous parties that unfold each night after the conference winds down. But the man does not play around at the podium. "Take a look around," he says. "Look at the person sitting next to you. The person sitting in front of you. The person sitting behind you. You may save their life. They may save yours."

A lifetime of smoking has carved a dry rasp into Wold's voice, which now lingers in the air around us. I look around, then up and back over each row of attendees, as they too scan the room. Do they see themselves in Wold's dire prediction? Are they wondering who in this room will be the next to be memorialized? Or are they beginning to believe that they will be someone's salvation?

The community that emerged from this neglect is resourceful, inventive, and committed to creating a system that saves lives. Psychedelics, however, are never anyone's first treatment option. Clusterbusters begins by encouraging people to work with their physicians to find effective, legal treatments, and they provide a wide range of tools to help people advocate for themselves within the existing medical structure. Wold and his board of directors collaborate with physicians, professional headache advocacy organizations, and pharmaceutical companies to make all this easier for patients and their caregivers.

But eating a mushroom seems like a small transgression when survival is at stake.

## Chapter Five

THE HACKER

Bob Wold has never taken credit for inspiring Clusterheads' interest in psychedelic therapy. He traces the movement's origins along a mycelial thread to an online forum dedicated to cluster headache support, clusterheadaches.com (CH.com), established in April 1998.

Three months later, a message from Scotland made its way across the wire, posted by a stranger claiming he'd treated his cluster headache cycles with psychedelics. Years marred by misdiagnoses and botched treatments had made skepticism the community's currency. Wold's voice lowered when he remembered the dismissiveness, the doubt. But something about the post lingered, a faint trace of hope amid despair.

I traced the digital footprints back to their origin. As promised, there was a post, preserved like an ancient manuscript, dated July 28, 1998. A man named Craig Adams had been bold enough to write, "I use small doses of LSD to treat cluster headache."

A response came quickly, a warning, tinged with a knowing wariness: "Good luck," someone named James* fired back. "Hope you used an alias. Trust no one."

Craig Adams heeded those words. He vanished, swallowed by the virtual void, only to be followed, six months later, by a new voice, "Flash," extolling the therapeutic virtues of psychedelics.

●  ●  ●●●●●●●●●●●●●●●●●●●●●  ●  ●

*Why*, I wondered, *would anyone heed the advice of a stranger from the digital shadows, especially a person urging experimentation with an illicit substance?* The forum contained a patchwork of desperate efforts to find relief: extreme cardio exercise regimens, antifungal diets and medications, and a practice called "Water Water Water," a treatment involving so much hydration, it bordered on water poisoning.

I tried to find somebody who might have met Adams so I could learn a bit more about how the story unfolded. Veterans of the online boards remembered him as Flash. Their eyes would grow misty recalling how he had helped them through their most brutal attacks. Nobody seemed to know many details about the guy, but the longer version of his nickname, "Flash of Aberdeen," suggested his location: a small city in Scotland.

Thankfully, Bob Wold's meticulous files yielded a long-buried email address. It felt like a gamble when I reached out. To my astonishment, Adams replied, eager to share his story. A few months later, while packing my suitcase to visit him in Aberdeen, my son, age eight, squealed with delight when I told him I was off to meet a man who had discovered that a mushroom helped people in pain.

"Flash?" he said. "Sounds like a superhero."

●  ●  ●●●●●●●●●●●●●●●●●●●●●  ●  ●

We rendezvous in my hotel lobby, two figures connected by a digital thread now facing each other in the tangible world. Flash (his preferred nickname in real life) has a powerful costume for his superhero alter ego: a white Gen X hipster dad, wearing straight-cut jeans, retro sneakers, and a slim-cut T-shirt bearing the logo of Krakatoa, Aberdeen's "authentic Tiki dive bar and grassroots music venue."

Nevertheless, I soon discover that Flash has several qualities in common with the classic superhero archetype: a tireless energy that powers a compulsion to view even the most intractable problems as a puzzle that he can solve; a moral compass oriented toward the public good; and the resourcefulness, leadership, and courage to carry out his ideas—no matter how batshit they might seem to most people.

Luckily for me, Flash is much more comfortable talking about psychedelics now than he used to be. He hasn't had a cluster headache attack in years, so there's been no need to use psychedelic drugs. And it helps that he's financially secure. In the 1990s and early naughts, he worried that his use of an illicit drug would hurt the business he was trying to build. That business is now a multinational company that provides him with a passive income.

But he's quick to point out that he's far more of a rebel than the usual tech bro. He's a subversive, an anti-capitalist devoted to redistributing wealth using industrial unions and worker ownership.[1] His ideological orientation is built into the design of his IT company. Rather than replicating conventional hierarchical structures, Flash decided on a much flatter model, with share options being distributed among all workers. His belief in this model was so strong that he was taking it even further at Krakatoa, the venue he runs with the Black Cat Collective, a nonhierarchical, nonprofit worker cooperative. Free time is spent planning out how to replace Aberdeen's dying oil industry with a more sustainable and circular economy, one built on a network of worker cooperatives.

What about the Porsche he drives to work every day? Flash quipped, "Everyone should have one!"

Bread and roses, indeed.

Flash's principles might seem paradoxical, but this blend of innovation and equity made him exactly the right person to launch an underground research network.

● ● ●●●●●●●●●●●●●●●●●●●● ● ●

After a long conversation over coffee, we head back to Flash's home in the country, a beautiful stone dwelling that once housed the neighboring church's pastors. Flash had just recently completed a painstaking renovation of the rectory. The basement has been kitted out as a massive gym for his two parrots. When he's home, Flash allows the birds to fly freely over the emerald shire. Their care is one of the reasons he rarely leaves Aberdeen. Parrots require structure. But he's also intensely afraid of airplanes. (I'm starting to understand why he's more myth than man in the cluster community.)

His home renovations also reflect his overall approach to medicine. Most people use drywall, but Flash replastered the entire house using historically accurate sheep's wool insulation and old-fashioned paints to allow the house to breathe. Turning to his girlfriend, Dee, for confirmation, he said the cost and labor had been worth it, hadn't they? She nodded. They hadn't gotten so much as a cold since they'd lived there, he told me.

His experience with doctors over the years had eroded his trust in their expertise and made him wary of a "pharmaceutical industry, with its huge advertising budget, ties to the media, and lobbying power."

At times, he veers so close to debunked conspiracy theories in medicine . . . well, there's no avoiding it. Talk to Flash long enough and he'll begin to "ask questions" about settled scientific debates like vaccines and autism and the veracity of climate science. It's concerning but understandable. As he likes to say, "The medical orthodoxy failed people with cluster headache, yet it had transpired that there had been a way to treat it all along . . . and that this was likely known about. How many other conditions and diseases was this true of?"

●  ●  ●:●:●:●:●:●:●:●:●:●:●:●:●:●  ●  ●

At this stage in his life, Flash appears ready to settle down. He and Dee moved in together as single parents, each bringing a son from previous relationships. Their six-month-old, Archie, filled their kitchen with the most joyous, gummy smiles. Dee is just as delightful as Flash and cheerfully asks me polite questions over a dinner of Turkish takeout.

Dee, I am surprised to learn, knows very little about the reason for my visit and next to nothing about Flash's days with Clusterbusters. But after spending so much time with him that afternoon, I can imagine that Flash has so many ideas to discuss and problems to solve that, despite how long they've been together, it probably had never come up.

"Dee, did you know that Flash had cluster headache?"

She nods slowly. She knew he had terrible headaches. "But he doesn't seem to have it anymore," she added.

How is it possible that she doesn't know? It's after 9 p.m. when I ask her this, even as I wonder whether they might want to pause our conversation to put Archie to bed. But the sun is still high in that northern summer sky, so we press on. Flash puts on the kettle to make a pot of tea, and Dee leans back and settles in, eager to hear about the time that Flash hacked an entire patient community's worst health problem.

● ● ●●●●●●●●●●●●●●●●●●● ● ●

Flash was sixteen when he began having multiple, severe headaches every day. The doctor told him not to worry—teeth clenching was likely the culprit. Flash figured the doctor was right since the headaches disappeared after a few weeks. But seven months later, when the pain returned, he grew skeptical.[2]

A naturally curious person, Flash headed to his local library to do his own research. It didn't take long to figure out what was wrong with him: Flash instantly recognized himself in a description of cluster headache he found in a textbook about head pain. The illustration next to the diagnosis captured how he felt: a face with a dark patch over one eye, indicating where the pain of cluster headache is located. He could almost feel the ink searing through the man's eye socket.

He brought a copy of the description to his doctor, who agreed immediately. But as plenty of others with cluster headache know all too well, a proper diagnosis rarely translates into a helpful treatment. Everything the doctor prescribed was useless or, worse, caused terrifying side effects.

Flash felt great for ten months out of the year. But his attacks prevented him from sleeping, eating, or leaving his house for a month at a time, twice a year. His slim frame looked skeletal by the end of each cycle. Relationships seemed like an impossibility. He might start dating a girl, but he had no idea how he could explain this strange wasting disease to somebody he really liked, let alone subject her to the horror of going through his cycles alongside him.

By age twenty-one he could no longer keep up with his university courses. His cluster cycles occurred in the fall and spring, right when he ought to have been studying his hardest. His grades were dismal; his social life, in tatters; his mood, depressed.

His friends thought he was "having a laugh" when he told them he needed to drop out of university because of his headaches. They thought he was attention seeking or lazy or just very, very tired. It probably seemed odd to them that as far as they could tell, he looked and felt fine for most of the year, when suddenly he'd disappear for weeks at a time. They couldn't fathom that a headache could be so bad. His professors had just as little sympathy.

Life as a university dropout was grim. Flash felt he had no career prospects, and his attitude toward his future was becoming increasingly nihilistic. Unable to hold down a proper job, he was offered a small consignment of LSD on "sale or return" by a barroom acquaintance. Not being much of a drug user, other than some recreational pot smoking, he felt ethically obliged to try it out first. Plus, it might be fun. And he did need some fun.

● ● ●●●●●●●●●●●●●●●●●● ● ●

In hindsight, he said, with a mischievous grin, his first tab of acid must have been strong because "it was quite an experience. It was a whole level beyond anything I'd ever taken before. Time slowed down, like right down," until his own sense of self became indistinguishable from his surroundings.

At first, this started with the dots of a duvet cover pulsing with breath. Then it "felt like I had left my body and had zoomed back over toward the duvet, like flown over the top of it, and as I was flying over the top of the duvet in slow motion, I looked down, and all these LEDs were popping up, like circuits with dual legs coming out of the duvet. They were all lit up red and blue and green and yellow and everything."

Wonder struck again when he stepped outside. Walking up the hill from his flat made him feel diminutive against the city's tallest buildings. Walking down hills made him feel like a giant. He delighted in how the once familiar streets of the city of Aberdeen sparkled with lights as bright as the dance floor in *Saturday Night Fever*. What luck to live in a town so ancient and magical! In retrospect, he realized the disco effect had merely been slick granite streets reflecting the traffic lights.

Drug dealing, and the lifestyle that went with it, suited Flash for a while, especially when his anticipated cluster cycle failed to appear as expected the following month. The supplier would drop off a fresh batch on Thursday. He'd go on a four-day booze- and weed-fueled bender, with his customers treating him to food and drink. He'd sleep all day Monday, trip on Tuesday, sleep all Wednesday, then do it all over again. "'Highway to Hell' was the soundtrack of my life," he told me.

But Flash had never intended to be either a layabout or a criminal. In September 1993, after realizing he'd gone a year without a single headache, he returned to university to finish his degree.

School was easy now that he was feeling well. He graduated in 1994 with decent grades, a degree in computer science, and a steady girlfriend. He dropped one last remaining acid tab that summer, and then launched his IT business. Entrepreneurial purpose and idealistic vision replaced his former nihilism.

He tried not to worry when, in April 1995, he felt that dreaded but familiar creeping sensation tingle up the back side of his head. As usual, his doctor had little to offer in the way of either advice or help. The cycle only lasted a few weeks, but Flash was devastated. That September, Flash landed an essential contract for his business—a job that could make or break his company. How would he manage if his cycle returned?

He had until the coming November, when the next cycle was likely to hit, to figure out a treatment. It was one thing to have debilitating head pain as a precariously housed drug dealer in his early twenties, but now he had a toehold in a lucrative business. He had too much to lose to return to a life marked by multiple cycles of cluster headache a year.

He began to wonder if he'd been doing something in his pain-free years to keep his cycles from returning. "In desperation, I decided to make a list of everything I'd done differently between [August 1992 and April 1995]." It took hours of deliberating to come up with a "remarkably short list, consisting of just three letters: L.S.D." But how could LSD have made a difference?

Flash had once discovered a reasonable explanation for his head pain by doing some research in his local library. In 1995, people with access to the internet had a lot more potential information at their fingertips. Most Scots didn't yet have access to the web, but Flash ran an IT company. He could access the internet at work. So he loaded up Netscape on a work computer and typed "cluster headache && LSD." (In the early days of the internet, two ampersands indicated "and" in a search engine.) No hits.

The internet at that time, Flash reminded me, "was very small"—mostly tech information about Unix and, he joked, a "solitary nude photo of Sharon Stone."

He broadened his search. Maybe "cluster headache" by itself would produce some information. Still no hits.

"LSD," on the other hand, returned too much information. So, he tried limiting the search with "migraine && LSD."

That's when he first saw the name Albert Hofmann.

●  ●  ●●●●●●●●●●●●●●●●●●●●  ●  ●

Albert Hofmann's memoir, *LSD: My Problem Child*, dispelled all the misconceptions that Flash held about the street drug he used to sell. Hofmann, a research chemist who worked at Sandoz, a major Swiss pharmaceutical company, had no intention of creating a potent hallucinogen when he discovered LSD—the whole thing had been an accident in the everyday process of pharmaceutical drug development.

Hofmann's memoir described a time when scientists and physicians conducted legitimate, useful research on LSD. He'd enjoyed the success of LSD while it lasted, but alas, the "joy at having fathered LSD was tarnished after LSD was swept up in the huge wave of an inebriant mania that began to spread over the Western world, above all the United States, at the end of the 1950s."[3]

Even still, LSD did result in quite a few remarkable medical advances, one of which had been a major advance in headache medicine. Flash recognized the name of the medication—methysergide, marketed as Sansert—from a doctor's prescription he never filled. The list of side effects was far too frightening: anxiety, dizziness, significant gastrointestinal distress, edema, weight gain, and cramping; in rare cases, if used for an extended period, it could lead to a serious fibrotic condition affecting the heart. What his doctor *hadn't* mentioned was that methysergide was a modified version of LSD.

Flash didn't need any more details. He was desperate now, and the memoir offered all the encouragement he needed. If only he knew where to get LSD these days. Returning to the seedy bars he frequented as a youth was not an option.

"I didn't want to hook up with my former associates again." His shady former life as a drug dealer could not be allowed to compromise his future.

He tried to think of an acceptable workaround. Then he remembered: it was September. Magic mushroom season.

● ● ●●●●●●●●●●●●●●●●●● ● ●

Foraging is practically a lifestyle in Aberdeenshire, where the chilly, damp climate nurtures verdant grasslands and vibrant fungal life. Chanterelles, morels, seaweed, and berries dot the mountains, valleys, lochs, rivers, and shores. Land access in Scotland is largely democratized via the ancient statutory "right to roam." Everyone has access to almost everything with few restrictions, no matter where it is or who owns it. Anyone can make a foraged feast, so long as they know enough to distinguish the delicious from the deadly.

Flash, alas, did not know what he was doing, but over the years, he had picked up bits of information here and there about magic mushrooms that grew around his hometown. It would be hard not to, given how many people in the area enjoyed the occasional trip, including his girlfriend at the time.

Flash had been under the mistaken impression that these little fungi would provide the LSD he needed. But LSD is a synthetic chemical made in laboratories. Magic mushrooms contain the psychoactive compounds psilocybin and baeocystin.[4]

Foraging for psychedelic fungi, however, held an important advantage over LSD. Magic mushrooms were, technically, legal, due to a loophole in the otherwise stringent regulations of the British Misuse of Drugs Act of 1971, the UK counterpart of the US Controlled Substances Act. The law outlawed psilocybin and psilocin. But prior to 2005, when legislators amended the act, Brits could forage, possess, and even sell fresh psychedelic mushrooms, since the law only banned isolated chemicals.

The law, however, did place limitations on what people could do with these mushrooms. Preserving and/or eating a magic mushroom could get a person in trouble. But Flash could manage a few small transgressions; buying from drug dealers, on the other hand, was a risk he refused to take.

So, on an overcast September morning, Flash drove to a beach just north of the city where he and his friends had always enjoyed smoking grass. A mate once told him he'd seen Liberty Caps growing in a large cow pasture just behind the grassy dunes. Flash brought a local mushroom guidebook to help with identification, ignoring the description of Liberty Caps as inedible.

Tiny, conical Liberty Caps, *Psilocybe semilanceata*, thrive in the phosphorus- and potassium-rich soil of pastures and grasslands where sheep and cows graze. While some mushrooms are quite beautiful,

Liberty Caps are decidedly not. They are scrawny, brown things that, when wet (and it's always wet in Scotland), develop an unappetizing slimy, chestnut-brown membrane called a *pellicle*.

Flash would return to the same field many times in subsequent years, but never, he told me, his voice filling with a reverence for this unforgettable moment, would he ever see as many mushrooms as he did then. He wouldn't need the guidebook that day. The entire field was covered with tiny brown mushrooms, "like little toy soldiers all over the grass."

Flash hoped this ugly fungus that grew in piles of shit might offer a chance, however tiny, of freedom from nearly unendurable pain. Maybe their distinctive nipple-tipped, conical caps, named for the Phrygian caps worn by formerly enslaved people in ancient Rome to signify freedom, were a good omen.

● ● ●●●●●●●●●●●●●●●●●●● ● ●

Taking the mushrooms alone seemed depressing to Flash, so he invited some friends over to participate. He wouldn't mention the real reason for the party—his experience in university taught him that people didn't understand how devastating a "headache" could be. But nobody asked any deep questions. They were up for a fun night.

Flash brewed his harvest into a tea following instructions from a mate and portioned it out, but his friends worried that the infusion would not suffice. His mate had warned them not to eat the soggy mushroom bits at the bottom of each cup, but they figured it couldn't hurt. Fifteen minutes later, Flash's stomach cramped something awful. He retreated to the loo and tried to throw up. Nothing happened. He sat on the toilet, morose, and thought, "It's too late. I've poisoned myself and everyone else in the house. We're all going to die."

"And then, all of a sudden, I can hear through the house, everybody starts laughing, right? And everyone was farting like mental, which was making it even funnier."

The shrooms cast a mesmerizing spell. Flash, ever the DJ, could now make the walls pulsate in sync with the beat, each new song infusing the room with a kaleidoscope of vivid colors. Their laughter, now harmonized, could lift anyone's spirit.

Flash invited his friends back the next month to "work through his stash." His gambit worked. November came and went without so much as a single attack. When Hogmanay—the traditional Scottish celebration of the New Year—arrived, he shared his third dose, a massive two-liter bottle of tea. He and his friends reveled in the ancient, jewel-like fortress of Stonehaven, set majestically above the chilly waves of the North Sea, a night spent enraptured by music that fused the mossy green walls with a tempestuous sky and the spinning trails of family tartans.

Missing his fall cluster cycle offered strong evidence that the mushrooms worked as a preventative medicine. But continuing the experiment would require that Flash learn how to become a better psychedelic outlaw. The mushroom season was over, and the curious legal loophole in British law that allowed for the possession and sale of fresh *Psilocybe* mushrooms prior to 2005 strictly prohibited most preservation techniques. But he discovered yet another loophole: although drying and freezing Liberty Cap mushrooms was illegal, storing shrooms in honey was technically legal. Why? Honey somehow preserves fungus while keeping it fresh.

The downside: this storage method made it more challenging to calculate dosage since the honey absorbed psilocybin from the mushrooms. But the technique complied with the letter of the law, if not its spirit.

Flash also discovered in those intervening months that there were better and worse ways to take magic mushrooms. Fewer Liberty Caps produced a more leisurely, more relaxing trip than the higher doses he had taken at parties. And, as always with psychedelics, "set" and "setting" were vital. One's frame of mind (set) and the location's aesthetics and environment (setting) could make or break a trip.

But learning what he liked took experience. The music he might enjoy elsewhere put him on edge when he was high. "All the stuff that people think they want to listen to when they're tripping, stuff like Pink Floyd, you can't do it, it's too scary, it's too frightening. You have to listen to stuff like country and western, stuff that's nice and safe. That's all the excitement you can handle," he told me.

Flash eventually stopped enjoying recreational psychedelic trips. Perhaps he grew out of them once the novelty began to wear off. Or maybe the experience started to feel isolating. If psychedelic experiences amplify one's mind-set and the attendant physical and sociocultural settings, I suspect it might grow tiring to attempt to heal oneself on psychedelic trips when surrounded by others using the same drug for fun.

Flash's girlfriend was the only person he took mushrooms with who knew why he'd suddenly developed this interest in Liberty Caps. But he often felt she only cared about his pain insofar as it affected her life. And Flash continued to keep his health history to himself, having learned long ago that most people had no frame of reference for the existential terror unleashed at the onset of a cluster cycle.

The trick, he decided, would be to discover the lowest necessary therapeutic dose to prevent a cycle. To do so, he'd run experiments in which he served as both scientist and subject. Would his cycle return if he lowered his dose to a dozen mushrooms? What would happen if he dropped it to eight mushrooms? Did it continue to work if he used only six in his brew? How often did he need to consume mushrooms? Could he extend the time between doses to six months? To nine months? Could he go even longer? The predictable, seasonable onset of a cycle served as his control: his body served as the best barometer of success or failure.

Four mushrooms, the lowest dose he tried, cleared his head and made him giggle but worsened his attack. Eight mushrooms was the lowest dose that effectively aborted an attack, but twelve consistently prevented a cycle from forming. Each batch of mushrooms varied in strength, so he eventually settled on ten to twelve Liberty Caps, taken fresh, as a dose that consistently and effectively prevented his cycles with the fewest possible psychedelic effects. He described it as "tripping" only in that he'd "see some mild visuals." But if he took any less, he'd feel a slight twinge indicating the impending onset of a cycle.

Anyone who has managed to tame a chronic illness knows only a fool would mess with a medical regimen that works. But Flash mediates his adventurous curiosity with a hyperrational approach to problem-solving—an intuitive Popperian, willing to subject even his most cherished theories to the experiments designed to prove they are false. He knew he wouldn't be satisfied until he could prove that the mushrooms were indeed preventing his cluster headache cycles.

Flash decided the best way to see how long it took for the next cycle to emerge would be to sit out the fall 1996 mushroom harvest. That year, he managed to go just over twelve months without dosing before an attack hit. The following Christmas and New Year's Eve were a living hell.

A doctor prescribed him painkillers. Flash took the maximum dose and spent a week vomiting blood and not sleeping. "It got to the point where I was getting hit six times a day, three hours each hit . . . I didn't know where I was." He broke down in front of the doctor. The last time he had cried so hard, he told me, was in 1978, while watching Bambi after a trip to the dentist.

The doctor told him the cycle had got this bad because he was taking too many painkillers, which was true. Nobody told him the drugs had that effect. The doctor told him to quit the opioids immediately and prescribed propranolol, a beta-blocker, instead. But then Flash said something that made the situation even worse. He asked the doctor for his opinion.

"What do you think about LSD or mushrooms for treatment?"

The doctor threatened to throw him out of the office and accused Flash of being a "junkie" who just wanted "hard drugs."

Flash quit the painkillers. Nobody had told him they could be making the pain worse. The doctor was right: getting off those meds helped.

But nothing else about that medical interaction went well. Like most cluster headache treatments, propranolol is an old drug, developed for hypertension. Doctors use it "off-label" to treat migraine and cluster headache, but experimental evidence for these indications is weak, especially for the latter.

Flash did poorly on the drug. "My blood pressure must've dropped right down. My pulse went so low it was really scary, below fifty, and normally my pulse is quite rapid. It was frightening, and I really began to lose faith in the doctors."

So that was that. Western medicine must be trying to kill him.

Flash took me to the pasture where he had first collected Liberty Caps. He told me a little about his family as we neared the fields. His mother had such a profound fear of World War III that she couldn't handle any news. "If the news came on, we had to leave the room. All we had was, like, the *National Enquirer*."

We continued past the cows until we reached the top of the dunes, where we were met with a spectacular view of the North Sea. So stunning that Donald Trump, who was—at the time—the president of the United States, had built a golf course in that exact location.

"Should we walk through it?" Flash asked, gesturing at the edge of the course. He'd just told me a rather worrying story about a local retiree arrested for urinating in a dune close to the property—out of desperation or as a political stance, we could not speculate—but we forged ahead nonetheless.[5]

As we walked, Flash continued to tell me about his mother, laughing in anticipation of what came next. One day, his grammar schoolteacher asked everyone to bring in newspapers from home, which was how he learned that old unsolved murders and alien abductions didn't count as news.

Was this sudden awakening to reality the source of his skepticism of institutional knowledge? Maybe, but all his experiences with Western medicine thus far had undermined his trust in the entire institution. Now, he told me, he wasn't sure if the vaccines that the pediatrician wanted to give his son Archie were safe. He refused to accept a physician's advice without doing independent research.

Flash's experience with his doctor not only convinced him that psychedelic mushrooms were the only way he'd find relief but also compelled him to find a way—any way—to share what he'd learned with others like him who needed an effective treatment and had never found anyone or anything able to help.

● ● ●●●●●●●●●●●●●●●●●●● ● ●

Flash began his efforts at outreach by ringing a neurologist in London— one of the world's leading experts on cluster headache. The doctor listened until Flash stumbled over a bit of medical jargon. "Tell me in English what it is you're trying to say, and I'll be the doctor. Stop using words you don't understand." Flash understood when he was being patronized. Doctors, he later told me, believe they know better than patients, but they "can only go by what the patient tells them or what the blood test tells them." They "don't really know what it feels like inside."

Doctors just didn't try hard enough to be helpful. But Flash had never been one to stop at a dead end. In his world, problems were made to be hacked.

Although Flash doubted experts' commitment to solving problems, he felt sure people could effect change through direct action. He needed to take his message to the people. And he knew just how to do it: the internet.

That was how, during the summer of 1998, Flash found himself combing through all the posts on CH.com. Posting a message about psychedelics wasn't a casual decision. He thought people would excoriate him. Or worse, he might somehow post something that could get people in trouble.

He described himself in the post as a reasonable person. "I run a successful IT business, employing twelve people." He wanted everyone to know that he understood the moral implications of his behavior: "I'm going to do something horrible in an effort to prevent CH recurring for a while. I'm going to take a very low dose of LSD-type substance obtained from Liberty Cap mushrooms."

By then, Flash knew that Liberty Cap mushrooms contained psilocybin rather than LSD. But "LSD-type" might make more sense to people. He had only learned about psilocybin a few years back himself.

"These headaches are terrible things," he continued. But the mushrooms offered "periodic relief." He told the rest of his story straight, explaining how he discovered, and why he planned to continue taking, Liberty Caps "for the foreseeable future."

● ● ●●●○●●○●●○●●●○●●○●●●● ● ●

Memory is a funny thing. Everyone I spoke to about these early days of psychedelic experimentation described discussions around psychedelics as contentious. Flash remembered it the same way. But when I looked over the forums, I thought people tended to be receptive to the idea.

In fact, not only was Flash spared the moralizing he dreaded, but his earliest posts elicited support, cheers, and intrigue from those who remembered how fun LSD had been in college.

Still, there were concerns. Foraging for forbidden mushrooms came with serious risks: a psychedelic mushroom might be mistaken for something fatally poisonous. At least one Clusterhead on the board understood that LSD and legally prescribed methysergide had similar properties. He asked why Flash wasn't just asking a doctor to prescribe Sansert (methysergide). Given that this legal, nonhallucinogenic, and widely available drug "is real close on the ol' chemical tree," why was he going to all this trouble?

Flash knew this treatment would be a challenging sell.

Over the following months, Flash would return to the board with occasional updates regarding his treatment. Every message he posted received the same dutiful cheers and an occasional murmur of concern. *Wasn't he scared he might have a cluster attack during a psychedelic trip?* A psychedelic experience might be challenging on its own—how would Flash handle the terror of cluster headache while lost in the depths of his mind?

In October 1999, Flash embarked on a risky experiment, one that involved inducing a ferocious headache with a glass of Scotch. "It always triggers a headache, and it always triggers a bad one. . . It was scary because it could've gone awfully, awfully wrong, you know? But I'd had bad trips before by that point, so I was prepared for the worst."

The fear was real, but so was his resolve. Sure enough, the headache came on fast and furious, a maelstrom of pain that threatened to engulf him. But Flash was ready, armed with his unique remedy: a tea brewed from psychedelic mushrooms. With a mixture of hope and apprehension, he gulped down the tea as soon as the waves of pain started rolling in. His heart pounded as the seconds ticked by, each moment an eternity as he awaited the outcome of his daring experiment.

Fifteen minutes later, the cluster headache was gone. Vanquished.

Chapter Six

● ● ●●●●●●●●●●●●●●●●●●● ● ●

# TAKE TWO TABS AND CALL ME IN THE MORNING

Visiting Flash had given me some insight into the origin of Clusterbusters, but his story raised questions about the role that LSD had played in the development of headache medicine. And I couldn't stop thinking about the audacity of that whiskey experiment. It took true commitment to empirical inquiry to trigger an attack so painful just to see if an intervention might work.

Like Flash, I wanted to know how this simple brew could have achieved what years of medical treatment could not. And I couldn't help but wonder if the pharmaceutical industry, as Flash suspected, already knew the answer.

Uncovering this story would require that I trace the mycelial threads connecting Flash's psychedelic treatment back in time. Choosing the first stop on the journey seemed simple enough. I had to get my hands on Albert Hofmann's memoir.

● ● ●●●●●●●●●●●●●●●●●● ● ●

Albert Hofmann (1906–2008) holds an iconic status in the psyche-delic world, a standing made tangible by a thriving market for Hofmann memorabilia. T-shirts, hats, mugs, puzzles, belt buckles, boxer shorts, and, of course, blotter art are all adorned with the visage of a middle-aged man whose graying, receding hair and unruly eyebrows frame an intense, almost sage-like gaze. Among the various portrayals, a favorite rendition shows Hofmann in the act of juggling an oversized molecule of LSD while other images are crafted to convey a mind-bending aesthetic. Of course, his allure in the psychedelic community had to do far more with his outlook on life than with his looks. Unlike his contemporaries, who often erected rigid barriers between the worlds of science and spirituality, Hofmann imbued his work with a personal exploration of the interplay between nature and the human psyche's ability to tap into profound moments of awe, transformation, and a unifying connection with the cosmos.

Hofmann traced his spiritual inclinations to a childhood spent wandering the Swiss meadows and forests, immersed in the rhythm of the changing seasons. Those close to Hofmann, including his parents, found it peculiar that a child so enraptured by the arts, the humanities, and nature's beauty would gravitate toward the precision of research chemistry. But Hofmann's interest was much more specific to the chemistry of flora— those "deeply euphoric" connections with nature had made him curious to discover what else he might find hidden within the forest.[1] Pursuing a PhD in chemistry was also a pragmatic choice that offered the possibility of a career that married his passion with well-paying work. Basel, Switzerland, was home to a newly thriving pharmaceutical industry, where plants were the genesis of powerful medicines.

Consider the profound impact that plants with psychoactive properties had on shaping the colonial economies of Europe. Empires were built on the trade of tea, thanks to its caffeine content. Cacao, when transformed into chocolate, contributed to a general uplift in mood across the continent due to its mix of euphoria-inducing compounds. Europeans had a deep affection for wine, a beverage that produced feelings of joy through the fermentation of grape juice. Tobacco and sugarcane—both of which activate the brain's reward circuits—became two of the most lucrative imports from the New World.[2]

The pharmaceutical industry emerged in the nineteenth century, a time of unbridled exploration into the potential applications of substances derived from bioactive plants and fungi. Among the most notable derivatives came from the opium poppy. In the early nineteenth century, advancements in chemical processes led to the development of morphine, a drug hailed as an effective—and at first nonaddictive—salve for pain. Friedrich Sertürner, the German pharmacist credited with the discovery of morphine, marketed it as a treatment for addiction, even as it beguiled him into dependence. The drug itself could be purchased without a prescription at any apothecary (indeed, prescriptions didn't yet exist). The 1855 invention of the syringe made morphine even more addictive. Nevertheless, injecting morphine became very fashionable among the elite, so much so that many had their own personalized hypodermic syringes. Smoking morphine, on the other hand, became gauche—associated with poverty and Chinese immigrants. In 1898, the German pharmaceutical company Bayer marketed its new "heroin" as a nonaddictive replacement for morphine, safe enough to be sold as a cough suppressant and headache treatment. Heroin probably stopped coughs and headaches, but it caused much more addiction than morphine ever had. Bayer's marketing campaign did little to slow that century's opioid epidemic.[3]

Not every pharmaceutical that treated pain created huge public health problems. In fact, Bayer introduced aspirin, a veritable miracle drug extracted from willow bark, the same week it put heroin on the market. Cannabis, a relatively gentle medication, found favor among influential physicians like Sir William Osler, who extolled its virtues for treating migraine. A few investigations suggested mescal (peyote), a classic psychedelic, might treat some forms of headache.

Anna Nickels, a cactus nursery owner from Laredo, Texas, first brought peyote to the attention of the pharmaceutical company Parke-Davis in 1888, after witnessing indigenous people using it to treat headaches.[4] Her observation spurred scientific interest, leading to a groundbreaking study in 1896 by Drs. D. Webster Prentiss and Francis P. Morgan. They found potential in peyote for the treatment of nervousness, irritative cough, and "nervous headache," a term for migraine.[5] Self-experiments published by influential figures like neurologist Silas Weir Mitchell and British psychologist Havelock Ellis, however, cast doubt on the drug's therapeutic effects, but there were hundreds, maybe thousands, of other fascinating bioactive plants that an aspiring research chemist like Albert Hofmann might study in the hope of discovering the next great therapeutic miracle.[6]

● ● ●●●●●●●●●●●●●●●●●●●● ● ●

Albert Hofmann received his PhD in a privileged position, receiving job offers from all three pharmaceutical companies in Basel, Switzerland. Sandoz Pharmaceuticals, though offering the lowest salary and benefits, caught his attention and eventually won him over because they were focused on the chemistry of natural plants that were known to possess medicinal value but had been underutilized in therapeutic applications.

The challenge with these natural substances was twofold: they were often unstable, and getting their dosage correct when used in their natural form was fraught with difficulties. These challenges intrigued Hofmann. Here was an opportunity to apply his scientific expertise to bring stability and precision to medicines derived from nature. The lure was not monetary reward but intellectual pursuit, the chance to unlock the therapeutic potential of substances that had so far eluded conventional medicine.

Arthur Stoll, the biochemist who founded the pharmacology department and the man who would be Hofmann's boss, gained prominence for his work standardizing ergot, a parasitic fungus that attacks cereal grains and wild grasses, especially rye. Ergot was best known for causing massive poisonings across Europe that devastated entire villages. The symptoms included diarrhea, vomiting, convulsions, hallucinations, and a gangrenous condition that caused extremities to blacken. The excruciating pain, often described as a "holy fire," led to its being called St. Anthony's Fire, named for the saint tasked with caring for those afflicted. Some historians even speculate that ergot epidemics might have spurred witch-hunting panics, as the paranoid delusions it induced could lead to accusations of witchcraft.

Luckily, poisonings decreased dramatically once ergot was identified as the cause of these outbreaks.

Despite its reputation, ergot wasn't all bad news. Midwives and physicians had long recognized its medicinal properties. Its potential lay in its powerful ability to constrict blood vessels, including those in the uterus. This made it a tool for both abortive purposes and childbirth assistance. Ergot's capability to strengthen contractions helped in delivering babies, and its effectiveness in stopping hemorrhage during and after childbirth was vital at a time when excessive bleeding was a leading cause of maternal death. However, the potency of ergot was inconsistent and unpredictable. A therapeutic dose could easily turn damaging; too much could even lead to uterine rupture. However, the inherent risks often outweighed the potential benefits, particularly in cases where excessive bleeding might occur during and after childbirth.

The desire for a standardized and safer form of ergot made it a compelling fungus for a research chemist looking to discover a novel pharmaceutical. In 1918, Stoll synthesized ergotamine, a derivative of the sensitive, unstable fungus. This marked a significant achievement, transmuting a substance once fraught with risk and variability into a standardized, consistent form.

Sandoz originally marketed ergotamine in obstetrics because of its success in controlling hemorrhaging. In 1925, Stoll's colleague, Dr. Ernst Rothlin, a professor at the University of Basel, administered ergotamine to two of his migraine patients who weren't responding to any other treatments. The drug stopped their pain in its tracks.[7] Over the next fifteen years, ergotamine became a standard medical treatment in Europe and the United States. Unfortunately, side effects made it difficult to tolerate, especially in patients with cardiovascular problems. Stoll decided that the small research staff at Sandoz ought to redirect their attention to other, less toxic, easier-to-handle plant and fungi.

● ● ●●●●●●●●●●●●●●●●●●● ● ●

Ergot, however, continued to be a fungus of interest elsewhere in the world. In 1934, American scientists had successfully identified the chemical structure of lysergic acid, an essential component of ergot alkaloids. Recognizing the potential of this breakthrough, Hofmann, who had spent his first five years at the company working on other plant medicines, cautioned Sandoz that the company could forfeit its position in the market if it failed to fully investigate these prospects. The company, he argued, ought to redirect its attention back to ergot research—an effort that he would like to lead. Stoll obliged.

Hofmann thought he could quickly discover a medication derived from ergot. A competitor made a stimulant called Coramine from nicotinic acid diethylamide. Could he craft a similar compound using lysergic acid as a base?

His laboratory began creating new lysergic acid derivatives. As per protocol, he sent each version, including the twenty-fifth derivative, which he'd created in 1938, to the pharmacological department to screen for bioactivity. The pharmacology department had not been impressed with any of these efforts, although it did note that animals had become more restless than usual when administered lysergic diethylamide-25 (LSD-25). But the overall assessment: LSD was a dud.

The lysergic acid derivatives might not be working out, but that same year, 1938, was still a big one for Sandoz and ergot. American neurologist Harold G. Wolff and his mentee, John R. Graham, published a research paper about the use of ergotamine that used a clever experiment that revealed a biological mechanism responsible for migraine pain.[8]

Physicians had long theorized that migraine attacks had something to do with a cranial vascular system that expanded and/or contracted. Wolff and Graham's experiment tested what was really happening inside people's heads. Wolff had already shown that a histamine injection induced a migraine-like headache, and everyone knew that ergotamine could stop it. The innovation was a Rube Goldberg–esque machine that he'd invented to measure the expansion and constriction of cranial blood vessels.

Twenty volunteers agreed to have a histamine-induced migraine, which the investigators aborted with ergotamine. And voilà: the cranial vasculature did expand during the pain of a migraine attack. Ergotamine, a known vasoconstrictor, made the attack disappear. Wolff and Graham's 1938 study became an instant classic in headache medicine. Harold G. Wolff became a legend in the field.

And Hofmann? He convinced Arthur Stoll that they ought to work on ergotamine again. In 1943, they synthesized dihydroergotamine (DHE), a little-known drug that made an enormous impact in headache medicine.[9] But as we know, neither ergotamine nor dihydroergotamine was the drug that caught Flash's attention in Hofmann's memoir. Instead, another discovery that Hofmann made with that shelved drug in his laboratory would change Flash's world.

* * ●●●●●●●●●●●●●●●●●●●● * *

Once Sandoz's pharmacology department decided to shelve a substance that a chemist had synthesized, additional testing was discontinued. But Hofmann had never agreed with his colleagues' assessment of his twenty-fifth derivative, lysergic acid diethylamide-25. He couldn't quite say why—perhaps it was his spiritual side—but something about LSD-25 "called out" to him.[10]

Hofmann resynthesized LSD-25 five years later. His report to Arthur Stoll, dated Friday, April 16, 1943, described a problem with the experiment. After producing the chemical, he began feeling odd symptoms. "A remarkable restlessness, combined with a slight dizziness . . . a not unpleasant intoxicated-like condition, characterized by an extremely stimulated imagination. In a dreamlike state, with eyes closed (I found the daylight to be unpleasantly glaring), I perceived an uninterrupted stream of fantastic pictures, extraordinary shapes with intense, kaleidoscopic play of colors. After some two hours this condition faded away."[11]

Hofmann thought he might have been poisoned by the substance he'd made that day. But he couldn't figure out how since any contamination would have been too small to have such a dramatic effect. The logical step would be a self-experiment on Monday when he returned to the office. (If only all our Mondays in the office held such promise.)

Albert Hofmann's trip with LSD-25 on April 19, 1943 is so well-known in psychedelic circles that it's celebrated around the world as Bicycle Day. Hofmann, opting for prudence, ingested the smallest dose that he anticipated might induce a reaction: .25 mg (250 µg).

A mere forty minutes later, Hofmann started to feel dizzy, anxious, and giddy. His vision was distorted, and some parts of his body felt paralyzed. Writing, let alone speaking, became too difficult. He asked his laboratory assistant to accompany him home.

Hofmann usually enjoyed his bicycle commute home from work. The historic streets of Basel, Switzerland, felt like an illuminated fairy tale, even in 1943 when much of Europe was under Nazi occupation. The war made the streets quieter. A fuel shortage meant fewer motors and more bird song. Jasmine, lilac, lavender, and honeysuckle infused the air, still crisp from winter's final thaw. He would have heard the rhythm of his wheels over the cobblestone roads, while noting the new leaves gently unfurling in search of the warming sun.

But these ordinarily charming details took on a darker shade on Bicycle Day. Although his assistant insisted they were moving quickly, Hofmann felt paralyzed, as though trapped in a mirrored fun house. Arriving home solved nothing. A doctor, called to check on him, found nothing wrong with Hofmann's vitals. But the patient's inner self had somehow disintegrated, leading him to worry that he'd fallen into madness. Worst of all, he thought he might die, leaving his wife and children behind. "I had not even taken leave of my family (my wife, with our three children had traveled that day to visit her parents, in Lucerne). Would they ever understand that I had not experimented thoughtlessly, irresponsibly, but rather with the utmost caution, and that such a result was in no way foreseeable?"[12]

Once the visions and mania passed, Hofmann emerged to find that he had not only survived the experiment but could also find solace and beauty in the changed perceptions he experienced as the drug wore off. Despite the "bad trip," he woke up the next day alive and enlivened.

Hofmann knew he had stumbled onto something powerful. No other drug could produce such an extraordinary shift in consciousness with so tiny a dose. Even his colleagues were skeptical. In science, the precept has always been "seeing is believing," but the powerful effects that Hofmann described could only be observed through experience. His colleagues would only believe once they experimented with LSD themselves.

Nobody, however, knew how LSD-25 ought to be used in medicine. One possibility emerged from the demonic visions the drug created. Similar experimentation with mescaline, the psychoactive chemical in peyote, had already inspired interest among psychiatrists in *psychotomimetics*—drugs that could mimic the symptoms of mental illness. The first clinical trial in humans, conducted by Dr. Werner Stoll—Arthur Stoll's son—supported the theory that LSD could produce a model psychosis and suggested that low doses might help resurface repressed memories.

Sandoz extended this research by offering a free supply of LSD (under the brand name Delysid) to a wide range of researchers, loosely defined. All they required was a written promise that those who requested samples of Delysid would supervise studies and document their observations. Choice of topic and research method were left to the individual researcher. This may sound astonishing today, but such open-ended distribution was a hallmark of pharmaceutical research during that era, and reflected a vastly different regulatory and scientific landscape.

Sandoz did, however, include an insert with a basic overview of the drug and guidelines for its use in every package of Delysid it shipped. Emphasized, for example, was the need for medical supervision, especially for those with suicidal tendencies or those nearing a psychotic episode, and the use of chlorpromazine as an antidote in case of adverse reactions.

But it was the company's recommended uses that caught my eye. Sandoz offered two possibilities: Delysid might be employed as an adjunct to psychotherapy, as it could "elicit the release of repressed material and provide mental relaxation, particularly in anxiety states and obsessional neuroses." Or those curious about the minds of mental patients could consider using Delysid as a psychomimetic to simulate the experience of mental illness. Some might choose to self-administer the drug "to gain an insight into the world of ideas and sensations of mental patients." But those with more scientific ambitions might consider administering Delysid to "normal subjects" to induce (and therefore study) psychosis in the laboratory.[13]

In other words, the suggested uses included treatment for mental illness or the simulation of insanity. But these were just suggestions.

● ● ●●●●●●●●●●●●●●●●●●●● ● ●

LSD was released into a world teetering on the edge of discovery and paranoia, optimism, and fear. Though the West had triumphed over Nazi Germany, the postwar period was far from tranquil. World War II brought heightened attention to psychiatric conditions, including a misplaced concern that the United States was experiencing an epidemic of schizophrenia. (Historians have since shown this "crisis" was caused by looser diagnostic standards, professional rivalries, and racial and gender discrimination.[14]) In 1949, the US Congress founded the National Institutes of Mental Health to develop better mental health treatments.

The pharmaceutical industry had already demonstrated the power of medicine to tackle a wide range of ailments. Insulin, sulfa, penicillin, cortisone, and vaccines had transformed healthcare, strengthening the conviction that even mental illnesses were conquerable through discernible biological pathways. A novel compound from Sandoz that could simulate insanity? This offered an enticing prospect. If LSD could act as a psychotomimetic, inducing symptoms like schizophrenia, it might reveal a tangible biochemical target, which meant that a "magic bullet" drug could be developed to cure it.

Meanwhile, a shifting geopolitical landscape had created a new powerful enemy of the United States. The Cold War had begun, and the threat from the Soviet Union was all too real. The Central Intelligence Agency sought potent tools for mind control, truth extraction, and even incapacitation of enemies. The Department of Defense saw in LSD the potential for a chemical weapon that could stun entire populations, allowing occupation without a single shot fired.

This convergence of interests meant that funding flowed for LSD research across universities, hospitals, and prisons in the United States.

The sources of this support were sometimes shadowy, funneled through newly created foundations, but the money was there, and scientists were ready to explore the potential of this unique and potent drug.

The emergence of LSD was a product of its time—a mixture of scientific curiosity, medical optimism, and political maneuvering.

● ● ●●●●●●●●●●●●●●●●●● ● ●

Even though many scientists, including Albert Hofmann, had enjoyed their self-experiments with LSD, research on LSD-assisted therapy didn't gain prominence until the mid-1950s.[15] The shift toward the therapeutic potential of LSD occurred due to the influence of an unexpected advocate: the British novelist Aldous Huxley.

Huxley, already a figurehead for his progressive and intellectual pursuits, harbored a keen interest in psychoactive drugs. His opportunity to experiment with a psychedelic substance came in May 1953, when he invited Dr. Humphry Osmond, a British psychiatrist based at Weyburn Hospital in Saskatchewan, Canada, to travel to his home in Los Angeles to administer mescaline to him and his wife. Osmond agreed, despite concerns he might ruin a national treasure.[16]

The session transformed Huxley. Mescaline, he explained in his 1954 best seller *The Doors of Perception*, hadn't induced psychosis but had instead showed him "how things really are." There were benefits to shaking oneself "out of the ruts of ordinary perception."[17]

Huxley's account inspired a new generation of psychedelic scientists, including Osmond and his collaborator, Albert Hoffer, to experiment with LSD and mescaline as conduits for profound personal transformations rather than as simple chemicals that interacted with neurotransmitters. They developed new methodologies that integrated the profound experiences elicited by high doses of psychedelics with psychotherapeutic interventions to treat a broad range of psychiatric and behavioral problems, including alcohol addiction, schizophrenia, depression, anxiety, trauma, and various personality disorders.[18]

Over time, scientists learned that psychedelic substances act as amplifiers, intensifying the inner experiences and social realities of those who use them. Creating a positive outcome hinged on two elements: the individual's mind-set and the setting where the drug was administered. In retrospect, those CIA-funded MKUltra experiments that dosed unwitting subjects with LSD in a bid to find a mind-control serum probably would have caused a "challenging experience." Chances of a spiritual awakening might increase with better amenities.

● ● ●●●●●●●●●●●●●●●●●●●● ● ●

By 1970, scientists had produced almost two thousand articles about LSD. So I figured that somebody must have noticed a connection between psychedelics and headaches, right?

But exploring the possibility of a link between LSD and the treatment of persistent head pain proved somewhat elusive, which didn't completely surprise me given how few physicians cared to treat headache patients. Pain, generally, had never been something considered worthy of treatment. And patients who complained too often were easily categorized as hysterical.

However, some intriguing evidence can be found in the archives. Therapists employing psychedelic-assisted therapy sporadically reported a curious phenomenon: their patients' chronic headaches would vanish during treatment. In his book *Storming Heaven: LSD and the American Dream*, historian Jay Stevens notes instances where patients would exclaim, "Oh and the headache is gone too!" The therapists, initially surprised, would ask, "What headache?" only to be told, "Why, the headache I've had for ten or fifteen years."[19]

It's also likely that physicians presumed that patients undergoing LSD-assisted therapy would experience relief from migraine once their psychological issues had been resolved, given that in the late 1950s, physicians characterized almost all primary headaches as psychosomatic, or a "principal manifestation of temporary or sustained difficulties in life adjustment."

Consider the research report by Drs. Thomas Mortimer Ling and John Buckman, titled *Lysergic Acid (LSD 25) and Ritalin in the Treatment of*

*Neurosis.* This study details multiple patients, including a twenty-two-year-old woman whose migraine attacks dissipated after she underwent psychedelic-assisted therapy. "Inner-worry" created by childhood traumas, they argued, was exacerbating her tendency to have migraine. When her fear of abandonment disappeared after nine LSD sessions, so too did her migraine. The mechanism of action made complete sense to them since they believed that migraine was a psychosomatic disease produced by stress, tension, and trauma. Ling and Buckman attributed her healing to the reevaluation of her experiences, seeing her mother's actions as caring rather than abandoning.[20]

Such conclusions were logical at the time, given the prevalent influence of Harold G. Wolff's theory that a "migraine personality" was at the root of the ailment. The thinking was, if LSD could assist someone in adapting and improving their life, then it followed that the underlying explanation for migraine relief had to be psychological. Nevertheless, these observations between mental well-being and physical relief provide a fascinating glimpse into the potential role of psychedelics in treating a condition long misunderstood and neglected by the medical community.

●  ●  ●●●●●●●●●●●●●●●●●  ●  ●

My search to uncover evidence of a long-standing connection between psychedelics and head pain finally yielded results in the picturesque city of Florence, Italy. Here, in 1954, the first European headache clinic was born. Dr. Enrico Greppi, who believed the time had come for the medical community to take the extraordinary pain of migraines seriously, joined forces with his former medical student Dr. Federigo Sicuteri to found a center with an entirely different approach to care.[21]

Greppi and Sicuteri understood that migraine patients required medical attention, an opinion that contrasted sharply with the prevailing views across the Atlantic in Manhattan, where Wolff's theory of the "migraine personality" allowed far too many doctors to dismiss the disease as imaginary or self-inflicted. They saw their patients as victims of a disease, not individuals with flawed personalities.[22]

Sicuteri took issue with Wolff's vascular theory—equating the pain of migraines with the dilation of cranial vessels. He realized that two simultaneous occurrences did not necessarily explain a complex phenomenon. While it was true that ergotamine constricted blood vessels *and* stopped a migraine attack, correlation was not causation. And migraine, he pointed out, was more than head pain. It manifested in nausea, light sensitivity, sound sensitivity, and fatigue. The root cause had to be something more central, something deeper.

Wolff's research, ironically, provided at least one clue that challenged his own theory: people without migraines felt no ill effects when their cranial vessels were artificially dilated. This led Sicuteri to a groundbreaking hypothesis: perhaps a chemical was lowering the pain threshold in those with migraine.[23]

Sicuteri's attention was drawn to serotonin, a neurotransmitter discovered in 1935 by his compatriot, Italian pharmacologist and chemist Vittorio Erspamer. New scientific research on serotonin was revealing its role in a wide array of bodily functions, including digestion and mood. Could serotonin be the elusive agent responsible for the suffering endured by migraine patients?

Luckily, Sicuteri had the means to test his hypothesis. Sandoz had provided the clinic with an experimental drug known to block serotonin receptors: LSD-25.

● ● ●:●:●:●:●:●:●:●:●:●:●:● ● ●

Serotonin is now a household name thanks to the popularity of selective serotonin reuptake inhibitors (SSRIs) like Pfizer's Zoloft, a drug that had been marketed with the claim that a "chemical imbalance" caused depression. Yet few know that back in the 1950s LSD played a crucial role in unraveling serotonin's chemical structure and biological function. The profound impacts of even tiny doses of LSD on the human psyche led scientists to ponder the connection between bloodborne chemicals and behavior.

By 1955, researchers had identified a striking similarity between the chemical structure of serotonin (5-HT) and LSD. Both shared an *indole ring*, a distinct structure comprising a six-membered benzene ring fused to a five-membered pyrrole ring. This discovery positioned LSD as a powerful tool in understanding serotonin, and it became the most potent activator of the serotonin system known at the time.

Serotonin                                    LSD

Sicuteri's experiment with LSD had gone better than he could have imagined. The "selected patients" given oral drops of LSD returned to the clinic pain-free, "even in severe forms of migraine." The drug didn't just abort their migraine attacks—it prevented them. Nothing else in the entire pharmacopeia could do that. Although he reportedly used nonhallucinogenic doses, the side effects concerned him. He didn't see how LSD could be used to treat migraine.[24]

Luckily, Albert Hofmann had already anticipated that LSD's ability to block serotonin receptors might have therapeutic potential. His laboratory had been developing new derivatives of LSD that might affect serotonin without inducing hallucinations. These were the exact compounds Sicuteri was looking to test.

In 1963, Sicuteri's landmark study revealed that these lysergic derivatives, including LSD, could effectively prevent migraine and cluster headache. Among them, methysergide emerged as the standout and was subsequently patented and marketed under various names. It stood as a lone champion in preventing migraines for decades.[25]

The success of methysergide challenged the long-standing theories surrounding migraines, particularly those of Harold G. Wolff, who ascribed migraines to psychosomatic causes. Unfortunately, the stigmatized "migraine personality" idea persisted, despite this breakthrough.[26]

In 2002, Novatis, the company that then owned methysergide, voluntarily pulled the drug from the market. However, its legacy persisted, paving the way for new medications like sumatriptan (Imitrex in the United States and Imigran in the United Kingdom). Introduced in 1991, this medication was hailed as a "revolutionary" treatment. Little recognized was sumatriptan's molecular resemblance to serotonin—and by extension, to psychedelics like LSD and psilocybin.

The story of LSD's discovery and its connection to migraine treatments is a riveting chapter in the field of psychopharmacology. Hofmann's work with LSD opened new doors, illuminating not only our understanding of consciousness but also the potential for innovative treatments for some of the most difficult-to-treat disorders in medicine, including migraine and cluster headache.

## Chapter Seven

● ● ●●●●●●●●●●●●●●●●●●●● ● ●

# GERMINATING CURIOSITY

T SOMETIMES SEEMS LIKE PEOPLE BELIEVE ANYTHING THEY READ ON THE internet. So I found it somewhat reassuring to discover that Flash struggled to convince anyone to try his psychedelic treatment.

Flash would post about his use of mushrooms from time to time, but nobody seemed that interested. But his whiskey experiment germinated into conversation. In the fall of 1999, Flash posted a description of how he'd been able to use the mushrooms to abort his most recent fall cycle. When the pain started to hit, he dug out his supply of honey-preserved mushrooms and "boiled up a batch of 12 [Liberty Caps] for 10 minutes." He noted that he drank the solution slowly over the course of half an hour on an empty stomach. The tea "cleared" his head and lifted the pain that had been clouding his thoughts that cycle. He also reported almost no side effects. Not only did the tea terminate his cycle "there and then," but more importantly—however improbable it might have seemed to readers—he claimed, based on past experience, "That single dose is all the treatment I'll need for the next 12 months. Who said life had to be hell with CH? Wish my doctor would take an interest—perhaps then he could help some other poor bastard!"

The first people to respond were curious.

Max*: "What is Liberty Cap?"

Flash: "It is one of several wild mushrooms that contain the drug psilocybin."

Annie*: "Am I reading you right? You boiled up a batch of magic mushrooms, drank it as tea and this is your effective CH preventative, and it holds you over for a 12-month period???"

Not everyone was amused. One guy wondered why anybody would trust some random new guy who insisted on an alias. "Excuse me Mr. 'No E-mail.' Four years without CH. . . . What brings you here? My address is here if you prefer to remain invisible."

Flash responded, "CH almost destroyed my life." He detailed years spent as a university dropout, financial struggles, and relationships ruined. "Are you suggesting, that since I can treat my condition, I should keep the treatment to myself? . . . I am taking a big risk—AND I DONT HAVE TO!"

But weren't these "controlled substances"?

Yes, said June*, and in college her best friend had jumped to her death out of a sixth-floor window while on some sort of psychedelic trip. "Having known her, I don't think she would have done it without the 'shrooms.'"

A terrible loss, everyone agreed.

Annie piped in to say that a reaction this serious seemed moot given that Flash was recommending "a miniscule dose." And if he "prefers anonymity at this point, that's his right. Who knows? He could be our 'caped crusader'—kinda like Zorro!!"

Anyway, it seemed a little pedestrian to worry about the legal status of psychedelics given how much pain they faced. "We would be pain-free . . . and probably have a lot of fun while in jail. Wow!!! All the pretty colors."

Everyone jumped in with jokes now—a forum that overflowed with this much darkness and pain required a sense of humor.

At their next conference, they could serve an "organic buffet . . . with shrooms in the salad, and of course, we have the herbal tea."

"Ok, add bail money to the list [of things to bring]."

"Honestly officer," Annie joked. "It's for MEDICINAL purposes!"

People might laugh, but they also couldn't help but think, *What if the idea had merit?*

Bill Pahlow, founder and then president of the now defunct patient advocacy group Organization for the Understanding of Cluster Headache (OUCH), thought it might.

"Now I've poo-pooed a lot of 'cures' posted here. But I've got a feelin' about this one. He could be onto something (no not 'on something')."

Pahlow had been intrigued enough by Flash's initial post to dig a little deeper into the idea; thus far, his independent research into the scientific literature, starting with Albert Hofmann's synthesis of methysergide as a derivative of LSD, verified everything that Flash had said.

Flash was also right about the similarities between psilocybin and serotonin. Pahlow reported on the board, "I found an article today from a doctor . . . [who has] been testing the action of psilocybin on 5-HT (serotonin). . . . I'm going to wait to see what the doctors have to say."

But nobody needed to take Pahlow's word for any of this. His sleuthing included correspondence with a well-respected headache specialist who worked at one of the most prestigious headache centers in the world. The doctor responded positively to Pahlow's email inquiry regarding the therapeutic potential of psilocybin. "The claim of the gentleman from Scotland is very interesting, and maybe not so impossible. . . . there is evidence of psilocybin affecting 5-HT receptors and thus theoretically the process of headaches," adding that the Food and Drug Administration (FDA) had already approved methysergide (Sansert), an analog of LSD, for this exact indication.

Case closed. "I put more stock in Flash's shroom theory than anything else. I think he really may have stumbled onto the ultimate preventative," said Pahlow.

Pahlow's endorsement inspired a lively debate. At least a dozen people weighed in with opinions, some more informed than others, about the possibility that a psychedelic drug might work. Everything was on the table:

from the tangled history between psychedelics and headache medicine to the implications suggested by the biochemical similarities between LSD, psilocybin, ergotamine, methysergide, sumatriptan, and serotonin. They all shared an indole ring, but what did that mean? *Was cluster headache a disorder of excess serotonin*, Flash wondered? Pahlow thought this was a reasonable guess given that research had uncovered that "Clusterheads have high serum 5-HT levels and low platelet 5-HT levels, and elevated histamine and low melatonin. What does this mean, heck if I know."

The more they talked about the neurochemistry, the more excited people seemed to get. Two different people named Tom* recalled that they'd been pain-free when they'd experimented with psychedelics. Neither, however, seemed eager to test Flash's theory.

Theresa* had a completely different experience. "Mushrooms, for me, have actually induced migraines. They can be fun while you're out camping and you melt into the peace of nature, but the after-effects were never worth it."

Fred* was skeptical but intrigued. "I've never found those drugs to bring me any relief, not that I ever used it for medicinal purposes (well, any relief from an attack or a cycle)."

And Donovan* couldn't say because, although he enjoyed taking psychedelic drugs, he went out of his way never to take them when he had a cluster headache; he feared that psychedelics would magnify the pain. He'd once had a headache while on LSD and felt the drug made his "normal headache feel much like cluster . . . and worse." He couldn't imagine what a psychedelic would do to a cluster headache. "I shudder to think."

Flash empathized with those, like Marshall*, who supported psychedelic use but thought it too risky as a therapy for cluster headache; he had less patience for fearmongering. June's friend, he suggested, had probably taken PCP rather than LSD or psilocybin. "It's the drug that is responsible for making people think they can fly, lift up cars, generally behave like an angry cross between Superman and the Incredible Hulk." (I feel certain that Flash wouldn't have said this, had he known the connection between PCP and violence is a myth.[1])

For the most part, Flash treated people's reports about psychedelic use as data. By the end of November 1999, Flash counted three people for whom psychedelics had worked and two for whom they had not. Maybe his efforts constituted "the smallest (un)clinical trial in history," but he hoped they might discover a critical pattern. "Please keep the info coming in people," he wrote.

Nobody, however, had much else to say. Despite the frisson of excitement surrounding the topic, no member volunteered to try Flash's protocol on themselves. Still, Flash had managed to generate a few threads of mycelial interest.

● ● ●●●●●●●●●●●●●●●●●●●● ● ●

The board remained quiet on the topic until a guy named Gunner* showed up three months later, on February 15, 2000, with a memorable opening salvo: "Am I nuts?"

The previous week, Gunner's attacks made him so desperate that he drank a psychedelic tea made from magic mushrooms. "I DON'T do drugs," but he got the idea from a post on the forum from a guy who swore this would work. (He probably meant Flash.)

The tea brought considerable relief, but he was still getting a few mild attacks. A friend suggested he try again with a fresh batch, as the first dose was at least two years old and had likely lost its potency. But maybe he wasn't thinking straight. What did the forum think? Should he try drinking another cup of psychedelic tea?

The board's response was unanimous: Yes! Try it and report back ASAP.

Gunner dutifully obliged with updated results the next day. His second dose seemed to have stopped his cycle in its tracks.

Brianna* could hardly believe it. "What is this about a mushroom tea?" The previous few weeks had been hell. Her husband was in cycle, and he had nothing to use to abort an attack. "Jeff* couldn't take Imitrex because he'd previously had a heart attack, which was a contraindication for the drug. The O2 seems to be our only alternative and I am trying to get him to go to the Doc to get the Rx, but he is in pretty bad shape. Just wants to lay down and die and you know laying down just doesn't work so dying standing up is the trick."

The topic of suicide, as it does too often on the board, came up. "Jeff and I have talked extensively today about suicide, and he has assured me, in his words to me . . . 'If you can love me in spite of all of this horror I put you through, I can love you enough to never have you fear me taking my own life. Don't ever, ever think I will consider it. I love you and the kids too much to throw that all away, we will make it through this TOGETHER!'"

Still, it felt important to get his gun out of the house. Jeff called a friend to take it from them, but they had to wait for their son to come home since he'd already taken the initiative to hide it from his father. "Such a good boy!"

But the last straw was when their doctor refused to write a prescription for oxygen, the safest, most effective treatment he might take. "Jeff wouldn't even wait around to find out why, he just stormed out." Conditions had grown intolerable.

"So it's the shrooms!"

The results were dramatic. Jeff's head hurt the night he drank the weak tea Brianna brewed from the dried caps and stems of psychedelic mushrooms bought from a trusted source. At first, they worried it might not work and the pain was such that he'd been rocking back and forth, crying and moaning.

But then something changed. Brianna described it as a chill that came over him. First, "he began to complain about being cold, very cold, rocking with his head clenched in his hands from a sitting up position to his head on his knees and up again, moaning 'oh God, oh God,' then he came up and said, 'Oh MY GOD!'"

The headache was gone. Somewhere in between his upright and kneeling positions, the headache had disappeared. Jeff, she reported, rubbed his head in disbelief, smiling and wiping his tears away, in utter disbelief that the pain had finally passed.

The transformation wasn't merely physical; it was as if an oppressive fog had lifted from his mind. For weeks, Jeff had been speaking of a suicide he swore he'd never actually carry out. But now, something had shifted.

Collapsing into Brianna's embrace, he burst into laughter, a sound so infectious that she found herself laughing along. And that night, for the first time in what felt like an eternity, they both slept—really slept—free from the specter of agony and despair.

A jolt of pain woke Jeff the next morning. A second cup of tea did what weeks of prescriptions had failed to do: it stopped the pain in its tracks. The shadows still lingered, but their edges seemed softer now, less menacing. The experience seeded a hope for the future they hadn't felt in weeks. "We are on the right track in my opinion. I don't know for certain scientifically why it works but I do know BEYOND a doubt that it DOES work! I saw it with my own eyes and nothing, and I mean nothing has come close to working this well for Jeff in 20 years." Brianna's enthusiasm rippled through the forum, igniting a rare spark of optimism in a space more often filled with despair.

Mushroom tea? Could the solution be this simple? Clusterhead Derek Garlin* had located a neurologist from Missoula, Montana, who had done some research about how "other plants" might treat headache disorders, but "the frigging research bucks and federal laws" were stopping it. He sent the guy an email describing the conversation happening on CH.com and asking if he had information about plant- or fungi-based treatments (e.g., mushrooms) that might help cluster headache patients. Everybody on the forum, Garlin assured Russo, would deeply appreciate his help.

● ● ●●●●●●●●●●●●●●●●●●●● ● ●

Dr. Ethan Russo, board-certified neurologist, psychopharmacology researcher, and sometime ethnobotanist, sent Garlin an encouraging reply. After the usual caveats about how he "obviously" couldn't recommend a risky, illegal drug, Russo explained that he'd been studying for a decade how indigenous people use plant medicine and had noticed a pattern: every psychoactive organism that produced a psychedelic effect in a high dosage treated headache at a low dosage.

He ticked off the examples: cannabis, peyote (mescaline), ergot alkaloids (which give us LSD, methysergide, and others), and *Psilocybe* mushrooms.

Indigenous people in the Amazon used several plant medicines that did the same.

The efficacy of these drugs, Russo explained, could almost certainly be explained by neurochemistry—specifically, the affinity of psychedelics for certain serotonin receptors. A broad range of evidence supported his hypothesis: he'd heard that indigenous cultures in Mexico aborted migraine by putting small pieces of mushroom under their tongue, and there'd been reports about peyote as a treatment for migraine as early as the nineteenth century. Biomedical research identifying the ideal serotonin receptors for treating migraine and cluster headache only underscored the point. Flash had stumbled on an idea that was old and new at the same time, echoing ancient practice, even as it jutted against modern medical dogmas. So Russo, frustrated with barriers to continuing his studies, asked Garlin to share a call to action with as many patients as he could: "What is needed in this country is for groups like yours to rally politically so that work in this area can proceed to provide safe and effective treatments for cluster and other diseases."

Ethan Russo had spent years slogging around the Amazon to bring back countless promising species of psychoactive plants. He knew better than almost anyone how much knowledge could be lost if we didn't ask the right questions of the right people.

● ● ●●●●●●●●●●●●●●●●●● ● ●

We often think about scientists as people who "discover" new drugs—or at least "discover" new uses for drugs we already know about. But every drug has a backstory. These histories can be difficult to see—but those tiny little pills that the doctor prescribes have so many stories to tell about power, inequality, and deceit.

In the sixteenth and seventeenth centuries, colonial explorers opened an exchange between an Old and New World that would radically transform the global biome. The indigenous people in the New World were decidedly shortchanged in the deal. Christopher Columbus and his contemporaries might have brought domesticated animals like horses, cattle, pigs, and chickens to the Americas, but their expeditions unleashed a devastating wave of infectious diseases like smallpox, malaria, and measles that decimated indigenous populations.[2]

European explorers eyed the New World's exotic flora from their initial voyages, but by the eighteenth century, the lure of botanical "green gold" exceeded even the appeal of precious metals. Along with significant cash crops—sugar, potatoes, tomatoes, cacao—the Western world also discovered potent medicinal plants, including quinine, coca, sassafras, ginger, aloe, and tobacco.

Then, as now, bioprospecting often came in the form of *ethnobotany*, a term coined in 1896 to describe the study of an indigenous people's plant lore. Many commonly prescribed drugs in contemporary life come from plants or fungi, their discovery made possible because scientists noticed indigenous populations using them as medicine. Pharmaceuticals derived from plant medicines have rarely, if ever, produced value for the indigenous peoples who taught us their worth.

The same is true of the magic mushrooms used by Clusterbusters. Psychedelic mushrooms are native in regions across North America, Europe, and Russia, but as Andy Letcher describes in his excellent history of magic mushrooms, *Shroom: A Cultural History of the Magic Mushroom*, nearly all Western cultures considered these fungi toxic until the early to mid-twentieth century. Those who ate hallucinogenic mushrooms by accident, by and large, considered the aftereffects to be undesirable poisonings.[3]

Spanish colonists who observed Aztecs consuming a psychedelic mushroom as early as the sixteenth century considered the practice to be blasphemous. Locals called this fungus *teonanácatl*, a word, colonists noted with disgust, that translated to "God's flesh." The Spanish prohibited its use given the obvious conclusion that this mushroom assisted the idolatrous in witchcraft. Westerners' knowledge of these fungi faded so much that by the twentieth century, academics questioned whether *teonanácatl* had ever existed. This otherwise obscure academic debate only came to a conclusion when ethnobotanist Richard Evans Schultes's research identified *teonanácatl* as a mushroom called *Panaeolus sphinctrinus* still used by indigenous healers in Oaxaca.[4] But put a pin in that story, because the next mycelial thread passes through Peru before it stops off in Mexico.

● ● ●●●●●●●●●●●●●●●●●●●● ● ●

I called Dr. Russo to learn more about the indigenous people he studied. Who knew what other connections he'd point me toward?

Russo remembered receiving that email from Derek Garlin, the Clusterhead who had contacted him to ask if Flash's theory about psychedelics might have merit. It helps that he saves every email he receives from people who get relief from plant medicines.

Plant medicines, Russo told me, had always interested him, but it took him seven years of practicing neurology before he decided to study their therapeutic use. Prescribing "increasingly toxic drugs . . . with less and less benefit" was burning him out. His migraine patients seemed to bear the brunt of it.

There had to be an alternative. So he started by digging into ethnobotanists' research on headache. This is when he first noticed that psychedelic drugs, taken in a low dose, could treat headache disorders. His first article on the topic, published in 1992, offered a review of potential headache treatments used by indigenous people in the Ecuadorian Amazon.[5] His next step would be to learn from the people themselves.

In 1995, Russo spent several months living with the Machiguenga, an indigenous tribe residing in the middle of Parque Nacional del Manú, a reserve in the Amazon famous for its biological diversity. Peru keeps it that way by forbidding access to everyone but its indigenous denizens and a few researchers who must apply for permission to enter.

Russo left Peru with a deep appreciation for the Machiguenga, whom he called "geniuses." Following the "ancient ways of their culture" seemed to keep people in excellent health. So far as he could tell, the biggest risk to the community came from contact with Westerners who brought infectious diseases.[6]

As for plant medicine, the Parque Nacional del Manú might be famous for its biological diversity, but the real opportunity for an ethnobotanist like Russo wasn't in the flora or fauna but in the people. The Machiguenga knew how to use the plants in the jungle, and one of their practices that really caught his attention involved a plant called *Psychotria sp.* (*Rubiaceae*). He learned that hunters would drip juice of the leaves into their eyes. The liquid stung, but it sharpened their senses: sight, sound, and smell became more acute. Russo thought the plant contained dimethyltryptamine (DMT), the hallucinogen in ayahuasca. But using it as an eye drop didn't cause a psychedelic effect—the experiences included no hallucinations at all. Intriguingly, the Machiguenga used the same plant when they had a migraine. The process was simple: wrap the leaves in a banana leaf and squeeze, filtering the liquid through cotton. The resulting drops could go straight into the eye. It would sting, but the headache and all its symptoms—nausea, sensitivity to light—would disappear in about ten to fifteen minutes.

Did it really work? Russo has migraine, and a self-experiment gave him confidence that, yes, it's a great way to abort an attack. But he wanted to learn whether a DMT-containing plant medicine could offer a useful preventive medicine for migraine or cluster headache.

He collected five hundred different plants with the help of a research assistant while in the Peruvian Amazon. When they returned to Montana, they screened each one. Nearly all exhibited serotonin-receptor activity. The experiment made him realize that DMT is not available just in that little corner of the Amazon, either. Rather, he concluded, it's pretty widespread in nature. "If there's some grand design to all this, there's quite a trickster involved."

Was he onto something big? Something that might help his patients? He knew the right person to ask.

●  ●  ●●●●●●●●●●●●●●●●●●●●  ●  ●

In 1997, Ethan Russo sent a handwritten letter to Basel, Switzerland, via airmail. Did the recipient, Dr. Hofmann, think it possible that a subhallucinogenic dose of LSD could prevent migraine? Russo received a reply a few months later.

Dr. Hofmann's hand-typed letter, dated May 19, 1997, apologized for his delayed response.

"Your idea, that LSD in low doses may be effective in migraine prophylaxis, seems to me very reasonable." He too once wanted to study the "effects of daily use of low, no hallucinations producing doses of LSD, but only came to very preliminary studies." Hofmann—a company man—had stopped his formal investigations of LSD once Sandoz Pharmaceuticals abandoned its production in 1965. Nevertheless, he was "very interested in [Russo's] upcoming investigation."

Russo was ecstatic to receive Hofmann's "ringing endorsement of the idea." (He still had it, of course—a keepsake like that is something to preserve. See Appendix.)

Russo might not have managed to get his research on psychedelics and headaches off the ground, but he never gave up on plant medicine. He shifted his attention toward medical marijuana. Rick Doblin's Multidisciplinary Association for Psychedelic Studies supported Russo's early efforts to obtain National Institutes of Health funding for a clinical trial testing smoked marijuana as a treatment for migraine and, when that failed, a subsequent safety study of prolonged marijuana use.[7] Between 2003 and 2017, he worked as senior medical advisor, medical monitor, and study physician at GW Pharmaceuticals, where he played a pivotal role in developing cannabis-derived treatments for cancer-related pain and intractable epilepsy. Every position he has held since has been on the same trajectory: transforming the cannabis therapeutics industry.

People with cluster headache, Russo assured me, were on the right track. But getting the FDA and the biomedical establishment to pay attention would be difficult. Clusterbusters' method of self-experimentation with plants, he told me, should continue. "Ethnobotany doesn't have to originate in the jungle; it can originate in the concrete jungle, too."

## Chapter Eight

● ● ●●●●●●●●●●●●●●●●●● ● ●

# UNDERGROUND WORLDS

ARK HAYWORTH* ENJOYED HIS INDEPENDENCE.

In the 1980s, he found the peace he was seeking in Cabarete, a small town on the northeastern shore of the Dominican Republic. He owned a small shop, Pink Shark Windsurfing, and he loved nothing more than gliding across the blue sea on a board with a small sail and a strong wind, acres of whitewater foaming and booming, hissing, roaring, and crackling just behind him.

Paradise lost a bit of its shine when his pain spiraled out of control. His "migraines" had turned out to be cluster headache. He usually felt fine. Up to eighteen months could pass without an attack if he was lucky. But every cluster cycle disabled him. So he closed the shop and started bartending instead.

Hayworth, a vocal libertarian, liked that the Dominican Republic didn't tax him like his native Canada, but regular healthcare was hard to access. Finding appropriate care on the island seemed impossible, so he started working with a neurologist in Canada who was willing to treat him long distance, and his parents shipped him whatever the doctor prescribed. But that solution was getting expensive.

If he was honest, none of the drugs worked well against a pain he described as a "testicle being squeezed [through his eye socket] while a white-hot poker is being rammed through it simultaneously." So, at a certain point in every cycle, he'd start looking for something else to ease his pain.

Finding CH.com in March 1999 felt like opening a door to an entirely new world. Just yesterday, he had thought he had the worst pain on earth. Now he wondered if he had it all wrong: maybe he wasn't cursed after all. At least his cluster headache attacks came in cycles that eventually ended. The thought of living as a chronic like these people online was unimaginable. Maybe each of his episodic attacks made him suicidal, but at least he could always count on there being some amount of relief on the other side.

Hanging out with sick people on the internet wasn't his idea of a good time, but he needed help. A global community with experience using alternative treatments could be a good resource. So, he created an account using the name "PinkSharkMark" and drafted a post that explained, "I'll bet we could all write a book on the symptoms, [not to mention] the failures of the medical [and insurance] system."

"Pinky" spent the next six weeks asking questions: Had anyone else used prednisone, a medicine his neurologist in Canada had prescribed him. Would they recommend Demerol or morphine instead? "It's GOTTA be cheaper, and I know I can get them on the island here." Everyone was happy to offer advice, even if, like him, they had more questions than answers about their disease.

He left the forum the minute his cycle disappeared. Who could blame him? He much preferred working at the bar, and the water beckoned. No time for hours upon hours spent hunched over a computer, commiserating with people even more miserable than he was.

Pinky didn't reappear on the forum until May 2000, at which point he'd been back in cycle for several months. "I've had six visits from the beast in just under 96 hours. Extremely discouraging." His 1999 cluster headache cycle had lasted sixteen weeks and cost him a ton of money in medications and lost wages. He added with more than a bit of sarcasm, "[Had someone] heard of a new treatment? Extract of Amazonian toad's toenails? Poisonous shellfish toxins to be applied cutaneously? Dancing naked under a banyan tree while chanting Jewel lyrics backwards?"

Ironically, people had indeed been discussing a miracle treatment, one that PinkSharkMark happened to know how to grow at home. Even better? Pinky also knew how to reach the kind of people who could help other Clusterheads make their own medicine. He didn't know it yet, but he was about to become the mycelial thread connecting these two subcultures.

● ● ●●●●●●●●●●●●●●●●●●●●●● ● ●

The relief experienced by both Gunner and Jeff, Brianna's husband, sounded far too good to be true. What did a case or two prove, anyway? An anecdote was different from an actual experiment. People on the forum debated the possibilities: Maybe they had a strong placebo response? Most people dismissed this out of hand. Cluster headache was too severe to succumb to belief. (Randomized clinical trials later prove this wrong, but placebo plays a powerful role in the therapeutic power of most medications.[1])

It was also difficult to know whether their cycles might have ended naturally, regardless of whether they'd taken a dose of magic mushrooms. Clinical trials testing treatments for cluster headache often find it challenging to distinguish between the effects of the medicine and the natural, occasionally unpredictable cycle of the disease.

Flash argued that they couldn't know for sure until someone with chronic cluster headache tried a psychedelic. Chronic cluster headache, by definition, was intractable. Testing psychedelics on chronics could reduce (although not eliminate) the possibility of the cluster cycle resolving on its own, thereby rendering the psychedelic response unknown. Placebo also seemed much less likely to work for chronics—they knew all too well that very little could help them. But even weeks after Gunner's and Jeff's success stories had been posted, nobody on the forum with chronic cluster headache stepped up to volunteer for the experiment.

Flash got the data he wanted in August 2000, when a woman named Stace* posted a message extolling the lifesaving powers of psychedelic mushrooms. Just existing, she explained, had been bleak for a long time, but it became unbearable when the attacks stopped going into remission. Nothing the doctor prescribed worked, and the relentless pain had taken a toll on what she'd once considered a full, active life.

The previous week she had brewed some mushroom tea—"The BEST TEA I HAVE EVER HAD!"—and drank it just as she was getting an attack. It reduced the pain of "a potential 8 to 10 (kip) . . . in thirty minutes." But most importantly, she hadn't had any pain since. "It's been a week—the best week of my life! I am happy, my boyfriend is happy, my job isn't quite so bad anymore, and even my dog has noticed the difference. What can I say? I owe it all to you guys!!!! THANK YOU!"

Stace's post inspired a new wave of experiments. Mushroom tea might really be an effective treatment if it stopped a chronic from getting attacks. Suddenly, people like Rory*, who'd been sitting on the fence, began to wonder aloud whether psychedelics might be worth the risk. "It'd be cool to see if this type of treatment could end what has been, at least for me, a six year, non-stop, no breaks trip to hell."

There was one remaining problem: How exactly would someone find a "magic mushroom"? So far, everybody who tried Flash's treatment had obtained their drugs from a trusted friend. But most people in the group, even those who had done drugs in their youth, were at a loss. They hadn't tried to rustle up a psychedelic since college, and few knew how to contact a drug dealer in their middle age.

Most people saw supply as just one more practical problem they needed to overcome in their medical care. But the supply issue presented an epistemological problem for Flash. How could he interpret the data that people provided him about taking psychedelics for cluster headache if they knew nothing about the drug they took? Unlike government-regulated medications, LSD and mushrooms lacked clear, trustworthy labels describing their content and dosage. Even when people felt certain they had taken the correct drug, questions often arose about whether the potency might have faded over time.

As more people began experimenting, quality began emerging as a wild-card in treatment outcomes. A report rolled in that mushrooms didn't do a thing: Should the group interpret this as a failure of the treatment? Or had the subject never taken the drug in the first place? Maybe there was a third explanation: a drug interaction rendered the psychedelic drug ineffective.

Flash felt confident that he could help people source psychedelic mush-rooms in the United Kingdom, where Liberty Caps were easy to identify and harvest. But the United Kingdom was a small, domesticated island. A landscape free of large predators and a climate that supports identifi-able plants and fungi helped foragers feel comfortable trudging through the countryside in their Wellies. In contrast, the wilds of North America, with its rugged terrain and greater variety of toxic species, seemed far more daunting. Plus, Britain's legal approach to mushrooms was far less punitive than that of America's brutal carceral state.[2]

So, for all his confidence about the therapeutic potential of psychedelic drugs, Flash understood his limits. He was cautious, repeatedly refusing to provide advice about mushroom foraging beyond his comfort zone. Advis-ing someone to eat the wrong mushroom could have fatal consequences. He certainly couldn't have been reassured by the naïveté of some of the ques-tions he fielded, like the guy who asked whether he could use the mush-rooms growing under a dead log behind his house. "God has cunningly disguised the North American variety to be easily confused with deadly ones," Flash reminded the group.

When people asked where they could get the magic elixir that Flash had been promoting, he suggested a reputable drug dealer. Or if they were will-ing to risk foraging and the possibility of accidentally consuming a fatal fungus, he recommended they go out and procure "a hippy and a textbook."

Caution, he emphasized, was needed. The drugs themselves weren't dangerous, but sourcing them could be. Finally, and most importantly, he warned everyone against engaging in behavior likely to get the entire group

shut down: "DO NOT START TRADING THE GODDAMN THINGS OVER
THE NET OR WE'LL ALL END UP IN JAIL."

● ● ●●●●●●●●●●●●●●●●●●●● ● ●

Back home in the Dominican Republic, PinkSharkMark pored through the
posts on psychedelic therapy that had stacked up in his absence. It was a
topic that had long fascinated him, but he took extra time to read up on the
latest psychedelic research before disclosing his background to the group.
In the 1970s, he'd been a "former magic mushroom hobbyist." He therefore
felt uniquely qualified to help the community solve one of its most intractable problems: finding a safe, predictable, trustworthy way to obtain psychedelic substances. People could grow their own crops, and he could teach
them the correct technique.

Growing shrooms in the late 1970s hadn't been easy. Although Timothy
Leary extolled psilocybin as a source of profound insights, magic mushrooms never achieved mainstream status in the countercultural movement. During that period, black-market purchases often led to deception,
as buyers frequently ended up with ordinary mushrooms laced with LSD
or PCP—altered and preserved until they were barely recognizable. Those
seeking the experience had to either venture to Mexico or develop foraging
skills, which became more accessible only when ethnobotanists released
specialized field guides in the 1970s.[3]

Techniques for cultivating *Psilocybe* mushrooms at home began to cir-
culate in the mid-1970s. But the process was difficult. Growing mushrooms
necessitated the kind of time, money, effort, and patience that only a true
enthusiast might possess.

The most tedious part, Pinky knew, was locating appropriate spores.
Most growers had to search for *Psilocybe* mushrooms in the wild to collect their spores. The spores would be germinated on a sterilized medium
known as agar—a gel-like nutrient used in laboratory settings. The next
step involved the selection of mycelial threads with a sterile scalpel.[4]

This entire process demanded considerable effort. Anyone can order
agar plates online now—they cost about two bucks apiece. But in the 1970s,

a supply like that required a friend who worked in a laboratory. So most hobbyist growers improvised with homemade recipes. This made it even more important to pay fastidious attention to the maintenance of a sterile environment since the same warm, moist conditions needed to cultivate mushrooms encourage the growth of all sorts of molds and fungi, some of which cause unwanted or even dangerous health effects.

Pinky's internet search revealed that, in the years since he'd been growing mushrooms, much had changed. New techniques made home cultivation more straightforward and accessible. In almost every US state, spores could be obtained safely, legally, and cheaply via mail order and then easily, if illegally, grown in the privacy of one's home. Pinky hadn't tried this new cultivation technique yet, since he wasn't confident that mail-order spores would make it through the Dominican Republic's customs.

But Pinky felt confident he could teach people on the forum how to grow their own shrooms, especially since he'd been chatting with lots of experienced cultivators who were willing to help. Sick people were far from the only subculture gathering online: message boards had provided refuge for drug geeks and psychonauts for years.[5] It's not surprising, really, that drug users would be early adopters of internet technology. The people who invented the internet had strong ties to the counterculture: marijuana was the first thing ever sold online.[6]

The internet provided the kind of safe, unregulated space that nurtured drug subcultures, enabled a black market in drug sales, and offered spaces where drug geeks could create their own repositories for the kinds of drug information difficult to obtain elsewhere.[7] The key to producing a safe stock of psychedelic drugs would be as simple as providing those in CH.com with a hyperlink to the broader psychedelic underground—a network that had been streamlining the home cultivation of psychedelic mushrooms for years.

So once Pinky had caught up with the latest psychedelic postings, he had good news to share with his fellow Clusterheads: "The safest way to get your hands on REAL psilocybin mushrooms is to grow them yourself. It is absurdly simple, dirt cheap (less than the price of a single Imitrex injector), and requires less than four square feet of space. All you need is psilocybin mushroom spores, some half-pint glass canning jars, some powdered brown rice, and some vermiculite."

Psilocybin spores, he explained, could be legally purchased and shipped because they don't actually *contain* psilocybin. A few caveats: Georgia, California, and Idaho outlawed the sale of spores, and the products would be labeled "intended ONLY for microscopy and taxonomy purposes," with a wink and a nod.

It cost $10 to buy a single syringe that carried up to hundreds of thousands of spores suspended in sterile water. Spores would remain viable for up to a year so long as the syringe remained in a dark, refrigerated space. Pinky learned that some sellers had terrible reputations. So it might help to read online reviews to buy spores from a website that people trusted would send a quality syringe.

Instructions for cultivating spores into mushrooms were easy to find online. Hundreds of sites hosted directions for "PF Tek," a technique named after its inventor, "Psilocybe Fanaticus," who discovered mycelium grew much better when spores were "planted" (germinated) in a "soil" (substrate) that included vermiculite. Gardeners like mixing vermiculite into potting soil to hold the water and air that plants need to grow. PF Tek worked for the same reason: vermiculite provided mycelial threads the space required to develop their elaborate networks.

In short, cultivating mushrooms at home provided the perfect solution to their ongoing supply problems, while also allowing people to feel confident in the quality of mushrooms they consumed. "Growing your own eliminates any possible misidentification issues," Pinky explained. It also offered a relatively quick solution, since it didn't take long to grow a crop of mushrooms—"as little as a month . . . [and] only two weeks if you just eat the mycelium," which also contains psilocybin. He also promised it would be easy. "I do not exaggerate when I say that a ten-year-old child could do it."

Growing mushrooms, Pinky pointed out, was illegal but easy to hide. "We're talking about maybe six or eight small mason jars that can easily reside in a small box on the top shelf of a closet somewhere: no weird smells, no high voltage gro-lights, no noise." The setup looked like "a clump of white fuzzy stuff." If anyone asked, the jars looked like they contained "an exotic fungus (true) . . . used in holistic medicine (also true)." He also felt certain that police weren't looking for people who grew magic mushrooms at home, given they weren't "part of a drug-smuggling ring." Cops might "bust some guy at a concert or a rave for selling mushrooms" but weren't hunting down people like them.

It might be the perfect crime: easy, cheap, and moral unless their philosophy involved following a wrongheaded law instead of "growing some mushrooms for a beloved spouse who had been in unremitting agony for years."

• • •••••••••••••••••• • •

It was true that, yes, everything was easier now than it had been in the 1970s when Pinky had last grown mushrooms. But he would have to admit, it was hardly the cakewalk he'd promised others. To wit, very little of what Pinky said about mushroom cultivation applied to his own situation in the Dominican Republic.

Mail-order companies didn't operate there—nor did Pinky feel comfortable having anyone ship spores to his address. He figured he could only get them by traveling to Canada—a trip he couldn't complete for four months. Plus, having spores was just the first step—and he knew he'd have to ace cultivation given how difficult it was to obtain spores on the island.

Pinky was so concerned about his ability to grow mushrooms in the DR, given the molds in the air, that his first effort to do so included the following extra precautions: After showering, he tucked his hair into a clean shower cap and wore nothing but a face mask and bathing suit. He then rewashed his arms to his elbows and sprayed Lysol on his hands and forearms, as well as in the kitchen and the oven. He also attempted to sanitize a small work area using what he called "the oven trick," which involved preheating, then cooling, the six mason jars holding the growing medium in stages to kill errant molds. Finally, the needle attached to the spore-filled syringe required attention. He decided to pass the needle through a flame before inoculating each jar.

Pinky's borderline obsessive-compulsive attention to detail made sense, given the stakes. He was the one convincing everyone to grow their own mushrooms—but he hadn't done it himself for years. He had to succeed to show everyone how easy it really was.

"If I have a successful result under these Keystone Cop conditions [in the DR], it should be a piece of cake for those of you who are better at planning things out beforehand." Plus, Pinky had continued advocating for using psychedelics as a treatment without ever using them. He "knew" they worked—they'd worked for all who'd admitted to experimenting with shrooms since Stace* had reported success, but as he put it, "Until I try them myself, I won't know for sure."

There was an urgency too. The velvety creep of shadows was threatening what felt like an all-too-brief remission from his last cycle—a seven-month infernal descent that had nearly bankrupted him.

Luckily, the psychedelic underground, as always, stood ready to assist. Pinky's descriptions of psilocybin's salutary effect on cluster headache inspired posters on sites like the Shroomery and Drool Donkey to offer help. One reputable spore supplier offered to waive minimum-order requirements and shipping fees to anyone with cluster headache. A "knowledgeable grower . . . offered to ship pre-mixed and pre-sterilized jars of substrate (mushroom food) to Clusterheads at just a bit above his cost." Both sites welcomed Clusterheads to ask questions on their forum about cultivation.

Pinky warned, "MOST IMPORTANTLY, remember that these guys will gladly provide you LEGAL stuff . . . information, substrate jars, spores . . . but DO NOT ask them to put themselves at risk by sending you mushrooms. PLEASE PLEASE PLEASE don't sour a budding relationship with folks that are willing to help us all out by placing them in a position where they are forced to refuse your request, okay?"

● ●  ●●●●●●●●●●●●●●●●●●●  ● ●

Hope can be dangerous for someone who lives in mortal fear of their next cluster cycle. But living without hope grinds away at the resilience required to survive each attack. Go too far in either direction and the disease knocks you down. Best, I'm often told by old-timers, to live in the present and squeeze joy out of every moment without pain.

But even I could see hope growing every time Stace posted a report about her continued remission. Every pain-free day brought more cheers—how could it not? Stace delighted everyone with every detail of her new-found life. "Laughing as I enjoy a bottle of wine with someone I love. Laughing as I take high-altitude camping trips. Laughing as I think 'Geez, I can almost NOT remember what an attack feels like.' Laughing because of all the pain-free goodness in a tiny little mushroom. Laughing because it doesn't hurt to laugh anymore. BTW—seven weeks and counting, GUYS! I can hardly believe it!"

Neither could Stephen*, who hadn't had a pain-free day in years until a mushroom trip broke his cycle. Everyone cheered his good news.

Lonny* found it more difficult than either Stephen or Stace to break his chronic cycle, but everyone in the group helped him troubleshoot his dosage until he found a solution. Inquiries about the new mushroom treatment poured into the site.

Not to say that everyone was having success—plenty of people struggled to get relief even after Pinky attempted to resolve supply issues. But these failures were, by and large, understood as problems to solve rather than a sign that everyone should give up. Perhaps dosages required tweaking. Or maybe other headache medications were blocking the therapeutic effects of psilocybin. Flash wasn't particularly worried; he kept plugging away at the problem.

He figured that they needed two things. They needed a centralized web-site that could offer clear, basic instructions on the mushroom treatment, so they wouldn't have to keep repeating the same instructions to every newcomer on the board. And they needed a concerted data-collection effort so they could work out the most effective way to take psychedelic mushrooms while also documenting the treatment's effectiveness.

The seed for this data-driven approach was planted in December 2000, following a request for case studies from Erowid, a nonprofit organization that provides information about psychoactive substances on its website. Flash wondered if Erowid would also be willing to host a survey capable of collecting the research data they needed. In a serendipitous turn, Earth, one of the cofounders of Erowid, agreed to help. The data might come in handy one day. Jonas* volunteered to copy and paste all the "shroom stories" posted on the forum and save them in a file.

Now they just had to figure out why the treatment worked for some people but not others. It was a frustrating problem, especially since they kept finding hints that suggested that the pharmaceutical industry may very well have known that psychedelic compounds had the ability to treat cluster headache all along. For example, the chemical structures of classic psychedelics looked so much like the pharmaceutical drugs that Sandoz and Glaxo (now GSK) created for treating migraine and cluster headache. Pinky posted the similarities:

- Every single one had an indole structure.
- Sandoz derived methysergide from LSD.
- GlaxoWellcome's sumatriptan (Imitrex) looked a lot like sulphonated DMT. (DMT is the potent psychedelic substance found in ayahuasca.)

Albert Hofmann said that methysergide was an effort to "dehallucinogenize" a hallucinogen. Pinky wondered if GlaxoWellcome might have been trying to do the same with sumatriptan. Regardless of their intent, the result left much to be desired. Sumatriptan might be able to abort an attack, but it couldn't stop the next one from coming.

Did this mean the psychedelic effect was necessary? Pinky wasn't sure, but he wondered if corporations had thrown the baby out with the bathwater.

Maybe. Why would a corporation want a drug that people could take twice a year when they could create something that needed to be taken daily? But they might not have had any choice given that the government was dead set on criminalizing psychedelic drugs. "Reading this kinda' pisses me off," said a forum member named James*. "I don't see why more research into hallucinogenic therapy isn't done. . . . Well, I see why it isn't done, but it makes little sense." He lamented that they were right on the brink of a cure, but the government, so worried about the potential for abuse, couldn't care less. "In the 'War on Drugs,' both 'sides' in the battle are at a stalemate, and we Clusterheads are the ultimate losers."

I understood James's frustration. I'd be mad too. There was too much promise here to give up or give in. Despite the difficulties, the momentum of the movement carried the mission forward: the group would work together to figure out the best treatment protocol. They weren't ready to go back to the days without hope.

Chapter Nine

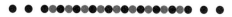

# THE FALL

F PSYCHEDELIC RESEARCH IN THE 1950S AND 1960S REALLY WAS AS
promising as people say it was, then why did it all end so abruptly?

The dominant narrative goes something like this: In the 1960s, the American public had tired of authority. The civil rights movement transitioned from nonviolent protests to race riots. The Vietnam War sparked widespread opposition and public protests. Political assassinations rocked the nation. Countercultural groups claimed LSD facilitated their revolutionary ideals, promising liberation from the establishment, a challenge to capitalism's logic, and a call for youth radicalization. Timothy Leary, the countercultural icon, cautioned the establishment to "be prepared for change" while telling followers to "tune in, turn on, and drop out." Marijuana and LSD seemed to be a common thread through all this social unrest.

After President Lyndon B. Johnson's decision to criminalize the recreational use of LSD in 1968, President Richard Nixon passed the 1970 Controlled Substances Act, then launched a War on Drugs, a series of policies directed toward punishing people who misused drugs that would have devastating effects on the entire world. The Drug Enforcement Administration's decision to categorize psychedelics, like LSD and psilocybin, as

Schedule I drugs, just created further collateral damage. Public health concerns had little to do with it; the policy changes were motivated by the government's desire to control its enemies: civil rights leaders and the antiwar left.

But neither LBJ's decision to criminalize nonmedical use of LSD nor Nixon's CSA fully explain why scientists stopped investigating the potential *therapeutic* effects of psychedelics. Clear-eyed historians have now demonstrated that Food and Drug Administration (FDA) reforms intended to protect consumers from dangerous pharmaceuticals did far more to stop this research than President Nixon's paranoia about losing political power. The utter collapse of potentially groundbreaking scientific research on the beneficial therapeutic effects of psychedelics is due in no small part to a new adherence to a technology widely regarded as quite useful: the randomized controlled trial (RCT).[1]

• • •••••••••••••••••••••• • •

In the early to mid-twentieth century, the development of effective pharmaceuticals created hope that people could live better, longer, happier lives. Diseases that used to mean certain death could now be treated with relative ease, thanks to the discovery of insulin, antibiotics, and steroids.

The pharmaceutical industry offered even relatively healthy people the possibility of "better living through chemistry."[2] Amphetamines marketed for obesity and "pre-obesity" flooded the market. Doctors prescribed Dexamyl, a combination of amphetamine and barbiturate, to treat the kind of everyday stress that middle-class businessmen and their wives experienced. By the mid-1950s, Miltown (meprobamate), a mild tranquilizer that promised to relieve anxiety while leaving consumers alert, became the most prescribed drug in America. Newspapers and magazines hyped the benefits of these new "wonder drugs." Finally, everyone could achieve tranquility and inner peace without the tedium of introspection.[3]

But by the mid-1950s, scientific reports began to raise questions about the safety of some of these "miracle cures." Long-term use of cortisone had severe side effects, bacteria seemingly became resistant to antibiotics over time, and drug overdoses were becoming a problem. Doctors gave out tranquilizers and amphetamines like candy. Prestigious medical journals began printing editorials asking whether it might be time to reconsider the safety and efficacy of how drugs were evaluated.[4]

Congress had already passed several laws to protect consumers from the pharmaceutical industry. The 1906 Pure Food and Drug Act, influenced in part by Upton Sinclair's muckraking novel *The Jungle*, marked a significant step in regulating consumer products. This act led to the establishment of a federal enforcement agency, which would eventually become the Food and Drug Administration, and required that all drugs be labeled if they contained ingredients considered dangerous: alcohol, morphine, cocaine, heroin, opium, eucaine, chloroform, cannabis indica, chloral hydrate, and acetanilide.[5]

The next major law was also inspired by a scandal. In 1937, more than one hundred people died after ingesting the widely used medicine Elixir Sulfanilamide. A federal investigation revealed the drug manufacturer was to blame—the company used a poisonous solvent to prepare a batch of the elixir. The 1938 Food, Drug, and Cosmetic Act required pharmaceutical companies to prove their products were safe before they could be marketed in the United States.[6]

Meanwhile, the pharmaceutical industry continued to flood the market with medications, which drove up healthcare costs. In 1940, Americans spent around $4 billion (4 percent of gross national product [GNP]) on health and medical care, about $29.60 per person annually. By 1960, those numbers had jumped to $26.9 billion (5.3 percent of GNP) and $146 per person per year.[7] American families worried about how they could afford all this medicine. Medications competed with groceries in their budgeting. Yet both seemed necessary.

Some of this increased cost was expected if the quality of treatments improved outcomes. Some new drugs, like insulin, truly saved lives. But the pharmaceutical industry had critics who argued that pharmaceutical marketing was excessive, misleading, and wasteful. People shouldn't need to pay such high prices for necessary drugs.

"Physicians," warned a 1956 editorial in the *New England Journal of Medicine*, "should be particularly careful in accepting drugs purely based on the manufacturer's evidence or based on testimonials provided to the manufacturer. They should demand clear, unbiased, well studied and adequately controlled evidence produced and interpreted by reliable observers."[8]

By the end of the 1950s, the industry faced scrutiny from the government over accusations of price fixing and misleading marketing practices. The pharmaceutical industry was about to face a reckoning that would fundamentally change medicine.

●  ●  ●●●●●●●●●●●●●●●●●●●●  ●  ●

In 1959, Sen. Estes Kefauver, a powerful Democrat from the mountains of Tennessee, turned his attention to the drug industry. This worried pharmaceutical executives a great deal. At first glance, Kefauver seemed benign, a soft-spoken man with a shy smile, thick glasses, and a disarmingly homespun personality, but he'd already gained a fierce reputation as a trustbuster.[9]

In his first term as a senator, Kefauver led groundbreaking committee hearings on organized crime, going head-to-head with the nation's most notorious mafia bosses. These confrontations were not only televised but also acclaimed, with the program winning an Emmy for its riveting portrayal of the fight against corruption. Americans, who tuned in en masse, gained so much respect for the man they were watching that, in 1951, Kefauver was chosen as one of the ten most admired men, alongside Pope Pius XII, Albert Einstein, and Douglas MacArthur. *Time* magazine put Kefauver on its cover three different times. So much admiration for a Southern Democrat who fought for desegregation and antilynching bills was unusual. He might as well have been Jimmy Stewart's iconic Mr. (Jefferson) Smith, the fictional character who goes to Washington in a relentless pursuit of justice.

No one could deny that the drug industry created important products, but price fixing and the questionable effectiveness of an increasing number of medications made people feel vulnerable and held captive by the industry. They wanted the government to protect them. Kefauver believed that it was the state's responsibility to ensure that innovative industries, such as pharmaceuticals, worked to the benefit of the average American, not just to line their pockets with outsized earnings.

From 1959 to 1960, Kefauver's hearings produced evidence that the American public spent more than $250 million on "useless drugs." Witness after witness detailed how poorly the FDA's attempts to rein in the misdeeds of an increasingly powerful pharmaceutical industry were going. Officials had little ability to keep dangerous drugs off the market, even in the absence of sufficient clinical testing. Worse, some insiders at the regulatory body felt their bosses had gotten a bit too cozy with industry. Medical officers sometimes received "orders from above" to approve a drug, no matter what the evidence indicated.

The drug industry, Senator Kefauver argued, must be held to higher standards than typical corporations because their consumers had little choice but to depend on the medicines the industry was creating and selling. They served "sick people . . . many of whom are people with small incomes. The consumers of the ethical drug industry are captives."[10]

Kefauver proposed an ambitious piece of legislation that limited pharmaceutical drug patents to a mere three years, regulated pharmaceutical advertisements, limited the number and type of "me-too" drugs on the market, and increased the safety of prescription drugs and competition in the field by insisting drug companies demonstrate their products were safe and effective prior to gaining the FDA's approval for sale.

The bill faced fierce opposition from the pharmaceutical industry and the medical profession—neither wanted to cede their power to determine whether a substance ought to be offered to the public. While the drug industry took advantage of Cold War politics to argue that Kefauver's efforts to limit its profiteering amounted to an insidious form of socialism, the American Medical Association (AMA) insisted that only physicians using experimental drugs in the real world had the expertise to determine their safety and efficacy.

Kefauver's bill was dead in the water until news about thalidomide sent shock waves across the nation. Thalidomide, a popular sleeping pill widely considered "harmless as a sugar cookie," caused thousands of European mothers to give birth to babies with severe defects, stunning an American public. Most fetuses exposed to thalidomide were not likely to survive. Those that did were often born with missing limbs, twisted hands, disfigured ears, and distorted facial features. Media reports shared macabre images of naked infants, splayed out for the public as freak shows. US families, according to news reports, had been spared this fate for one reason: Dr. Frances Oldham Kelsey, a skeptical physician who worked as a medical officer at the FDA, had refused to approve thalidomide for sale in the United States until the manufacturer produced more convincing data on its safety. Sadly, her hunch about the potential risks of the drug proved correct.

However, no matter how diligent Dr. Kelsey may have been, neither she nor the FDA had the power to keep thalidomide entirely out of American medicine cabinets. The FDA could only keep drug companies from *marketing* their products. The couldn't stop companies from distributing experimental drugs directly to physicians, who could then use them as they pleased (which, of course, was exactly how American physicians and psychotherapists received LSD and psilocybin from Sandoz Pharmaceuticals). This loophole offered unethical companies a surreptitious path to unsuspecting consumers. The FDA couldn't be sure, but it was possible that doctors had already given thalidomide to about twenty thousand Americans, including 624 pregnant women.

Public trust in the FDA plummeted. If thalidomide, widely believed to be safe, could disfigure newborns, what other poisons were lying in wait in Americans' medicine cabinets at home?

President John F. Kennedy, under pressure to act, demanded that Congress pass legislation that provided the FDA with more funding, staff, and power. Kennedy argued,

New drugs are being placed in the market every day, without any requirement of advanced proof that they will be effective in treating the conditions for which they are recommended. Over 20% of the new drugs available since 1956 were found to be incapable of bearing out one or more of what their sponsors claimed on what their effect would be. An extensive underground traffic exists in habit-forming barbiturates and stimulants. Drugs which could often be sold by a simple common name are too often sold by complex scientific names, which confuse the purchaser and raise the price.[11]

None of this, of course, could deal with the issue at hand, which, as one member of the White House press corps put it, constituted a "period of anguish" over the thalidomide scare that had women "asking for abortions" well before a time when the procedure was legal.[12] The public demanded that the government keep them safe.

Kennedy did his best to reassure the country. "The Food and Drug Administration have had nearly 200 people working on this; every doctor, every hospital, every nurse has been notified." But women would need to remain vigilant. "Every woman in this country, I think, must be aware that it's most important that they check their medicine cabinet, and that they do not take this drug, and that they turn it in."[13]

Women would have to look out for their own health.

● ● ●●●●●●●●●●●●●●●●●●●● ● ●

President Kennedy needed Congress to act fast, and Senator Kefauver had a piece of legislation he could co-opt. In 1962, Kennedy signed into law the Kefauver-Harris Drug Amendments to the Federal Food and Drug Control Act. The amendments bearing Senator Kefauver's name did not realize the cost-saving reforms that the bill originally intended. But this new consumer rights bill had several consequences—one of which was the unintended reduction in clinical research assessing the therapeutic potential of LSD.[14]

The FDA now had the power to mandate that the pharmaceutical industry prove the safety and efficacy of its medications before marketing them. Congress, however, left the details of implementing this important work to the experts. Finding an objective way to make these assessments was a priority. But there was a politics of determining what counted as "objective evidence."

The American Medical Association (AMA) argued that doctors ought to have the autonomy to decide what medication worked best for their patients. But the FDA worried that physicians might be too close to the pharmaceutical industry to make objective assessments, especially after Kefauver's hearings revealed how the pharmaceutical industry used marketing to persuade doctors to do their bidding.[15]

The FDA's new rules mandated that clinical researchers only study drugs that had an approved Investigational New Drug (IND) application on file. But there was a catch: only a drug manufacturer had the kind of information that the FDA required for completion of an IND application.[16] Every IND application requested the drug sponsor to specify the qualifications necessary to become an investigator and how the drug could be used in an experiment.[17]

LSD was hardly the most scandalous drug in 1963, but Sandoz had reason to worry, especially given the shenanigans happening at places like Harvard, where Timothy Leary had been conducting scandalous psilocybin research. In any case, its US patent was expiring in 1963.

Sandoz had always encouraged researchers to self-administer LSD "to gain an insight into the world of ideas and sensations of mental patients."[18] But critics had begun to question whether self-experimentation was the best way to produce objective data. And psychedelic researchers were making it hard to defend the practice. Their study results sometimes looked a bit too enthusiastic, like they'd been boosted by a "therapist-induced mystical experience similar to religious conversion."[19]

● ● ●●●●●●●●●●●●●●●●●●● ● ●

Self-experimentation has a rich history in science and medicine. Look no further than Albert Hofmann, the diligent worker who told his boss in advance that he planned to come to work on a Monday morning and take a drug that had *already* poisoned him. Making oneself a subject seemed like the ethical thing to do—it suggested that a scientist was willing to put the pursuit of knowledge before personal gain.[20]

In the 1950s, taking psychoactive drugs was just another day at the lab. Scientists considered self-experimentation a legitimate scientific research method. Some, like Albert Hofmann, sampled drugs to screen for toxicity and dosage. But scientists also hoped that these drugs might also give them a glimpse of their patients' inner lives.

What was it like to experience delusions? Psychoactive drugs offered an important way to bridge the chasm between the observer and the observed. How else could they access the subjective lives of the people they most wanted to understand? If LSD mimicked insanity, then perhaps researchers—most of whom were psychiatrists who treated the mentally ill—might experience the ineffable interiority of those who could not represent their own experiences.[21]

A package in the mail brings a vial filled with a potent drug that promises the experience of temporary psychosis. A compelling offer. What could go wrong?

The FDA's first investigation into serious ethical violations involving LSD research occurred in 1961. According to reports, therapists at Hollywood Hospital had been offering their clients psychedelic therapy using the free vials of LSD that Sandoz provided them for research purposes. None of them could claim to have any training in the field—the therapy was, after all, still experimental. Nevertheless, business was lucrative. Sessions cost as much as $500 apiece—nearly $5,000 in today's dollars. Some of the clients accused their therapists of abusive behavior, including sexual assault.[22]

Enter Timothy Leary, the controversial public intellectual cum folk hero whose antics have so often been blamed for the fall of psychedelic science. In the 1950s, Leary had been the director of psychological research at Kaiser Foundation Hospital in California, where he published nearly fifty papers in psychology journals and a widely lauded book titled *Interpersonal Diagnosis of Personality*. But a tumultuous period of his life, combined with his disillusionment with the field led him to a brief departure from academia. In late 1959, the Harvard psychology department invited him to join their faculty as an invited lecturer.

Leary's infamous Harvard Psilocybin Project, which he began almost as soon as he arrived, was seen as so weird, wild, and problematic that he came to represent everything topsy-turvy with experimental medical research specifically and the counterculture in general. In one dramatic instance, David McClelland, chair of Harvard's Department of Psychology and Social Relations, called Leary into his office in the fall of 1961, the weekend after a particularly rowdy psilocybin "experiment," during which the writer Allen Ginsberg had stripped naked and declared himself the messiah, just before attempting to broker a peace deal between Kennedy and Nikita Khrushchev over the telephone (neither could be reached).[23]

"What the hell is going on, Tim?" McClelland demanded. Two graduate students had apparently lodged a complaint that Leary wasn't conducting research so much as he was hosting wild drug parties. Their complaint included words like "Beatniks. Orgies. Naked poets. Junkies. Homosexuality . . . Queers. Beards. Criminal types." Leary attempted to assure his chair that the experiment had gone quite well. "I'll send you the reports from the session as soon as they are typed. . . . We're learning a lot."[24]

In the dorm room—one of his labs of choice—and in the classroom, Leary had been teaching graduate students that psychedelic tools rendered traditional methods of studying psychological processes obsolete. Experiments took place off campus, in living rooms decorated with candles, cushions, books, and drawings that Leary hoped would enhance the therapeutic effects of the psilocybin.

Leary's colleagues at Harvard insisted that the drug hadn't been the problem. He later wondered if the real problem with his Harvard Psilocybin Project had been a genuine intellectual disagreement about the role of self-experimentation in science. This seems unlikely given that many of Leary's colleagues had taken the drug themselves as part of the scientific method. A bit more self-reflection might have led him to the more obvious conclusion that taking psilocybin *with* subjects and then having sex with them was a bit far afield of normal science, especially if the press caught on.

Leary also violated a more serious norm in science by crossing the line between objectivity and evangelism. In spring 1963, Harvard dismissed Leary for his failure to fulfill his teaching contract (which, in truth, was about to expire and neither party wished to extend).

● ● ●●●●●●●●●●●●●●●●●● ● ●

Scapegoating a man as mischievous and destructive as Timothy Leary for the downfall of psychedelics is far easier than explaining that the real collapse of psychedelic research was the result of a bureaucratic accident—an unintended outcome of the FDA's effort to keep the public safe.

But rogue researchers and an emerging black market in LSD didn't make Sandoz eager to maintain the free distribution of a drug that was going off patent that year. You can see the company's reluctance in the tight restrictions on the number and type of researchers allowed to study LSD in the IND it submitted to the FDA in 1963.[25] Most American psychedelic researchers failed to meet the full criteria outlined there. (Timothy Leary would certainly have failed the test even if he had managed to remain at Harvard.) The chilling effect on psychedelic research was immediate: in 1963, the number of authorized research studies in the United States fell from a few hundred to seventeen.[26]

Over the next two years, Sandoz expanded its IND to allow a few more researchers the ability to study LSD and psilocybin. But the FDA's insistence that drug development use randomized clinical trials presented a new set of challenges.

By 1962, experts had largely agreed that a "randomized double-blind placebo-controlled trial" offered the ideal method to produce an unbiased, comprehensive evaluation of the safety and effectiveness of testing new drugs.[27] The method offered an appealing facade of objectivity. An investigator might exhibit bias, but data produced from an RCT could be analyzed using statistics. Math—rather than individual physicians—would decide if drugs were safe and effective.[28]

An RCT is an experiment with a few key components. Randomly assign one group of patients (aka "human subjects") to a control group and another group of subjects to the treatment group. The control group receives a placebo that looks identical to the treatment under study but won't affect any of the outcomes being measured.

This presented a problem for psychedelic science. The success of an RCT hinges on the believability of the placebo. According to the logic of an RCT, it's essential that both the subject and the investigator remain oblivious to which group has received the actual intervention and which has been given a placebo.

Of course, it's nearly impossible to find a believable placebo for a drug like LSD, which creates obvious effects on perception. So, it's worth pausing a moment to consider why, exactly, the placebo was—and continues to be—considered such an important factor in assessing whether a drug really works.

Researchers and medical professionals have long known that the mere belief that a treatment will be helpful can improve a person's symptoms on its own. The more a patient believes a treatment will work, the greater the placebo effect. Likewise, the placebo effect can be dampened by giving patients fewer reasons to believe that they will improve.

It might seem like a doctor would want to boost the placebo effect if it helped improve outcomes. But the placebo effect presented the medical profession with a problem. How could a doctor control the placebo effect? Unlike a drug, a placebo doesn't have a dose that can be easily tweaked or standardized. Doctors built their reputations as men of science.[29] If they relied on something as ephemeral as a placebo, they might as well have been shamans.

Clinical trials, therefore, must include a placebo group so that researchers can distinguish between *perceived* improvements, driven by the expectation of receiving treatment, and *real* biological effects of the treatment. The only drug that mattered was the drug that worked its magic inside the body.

But psychedelic psychiatrists believed that LSD-assisted therapy worked because it evoked a transformative shift in people's consciousness. It was difficult for them to understand how or why they'd want to dampen that experience.

● ● ●●●●●●●●●●●●●●●●●●●● ● ●

Yes, psychedelic substances are a particularly poor fit for the randomized clinical trial, but they are not the only therapy that struggles to meet the so-called gold standard for scientific evidence.

Imagine, for example, trying to evaluate a surgical technique using a randomized clinical trial. How would an investigator ensure that every patient's surgery proceeded in the exact same way? Surgeries always include a bit of variation. A patient might react in an unexpected way to an anesthetic. Surgeons have varying levels of skill. Procedures in some surgical fields advance so quickly that the process of assessment by RCT provides data on obsolete techniques. Further complicating matters is the use of a placebo, which in this context would necessitate a sham surgery, an ethically questionable approach.[30] The very essence of an operation defies the standardization required for rigorous scientific studies.

The limitations of clinical trials aren't exclusive to surgery and psychedelics; they extend to conventional medications as well. A clear illustration of this came to light during the HIV/AIDS crisis in the 1980s and 1990s.[31] This catastrophic epidemic highlighted the inherent drawbacks of the clinical trial system. Activists in the gay community, triply marginalized due to the deadly combination of homophobia, fear of contagion, and a lack of credentials as scientific experts, pressed the biomedical community for a more dynamic research approach that prioritized urgency, inclusivity, and innovation.

Nobody, they argued, should get a placebo given the deadliness of this disease. Study participants insisted on this fact by making RCTs impossible: they pooled together their pills and redistributed dosages to ensure that everyone got at least a little bit of the medicine. Others established "buyers clubs" to import and distribute unapproved drugs, allowing them to circumvent the stringent clinical trial and regulatory process.

AIDS patients made clear that the will to survive was stronger than an altruistic desire to produce "pure" science for the FDA. So they forced the FDA and other regulatory bodies to revisit their methods. Clinical trials, it turned out, *could* be streamlined. The FDA *could* increase patient involvement. And when push came to shove, the government *did* have funding to pay for overlooked diseases.

Alas, people with cluster headache still feel very much overlooked.

• • ••••••••••••••••••• • •

In the wake of all the controversy, Sandoz did not remain willing to expose itself to legal liability for long. In 1965, Congress passed the Drug Abuse Control Amendments to rein in an expanding black market in the manufacture and sale of amphetamines and barbiturates, but the legislation included language about "hallucinogens" that worried the pharmaceutical manufacturer.

Sandoz could see that the black market for LSD was just getting worse. If Timothy Leary bears some blame for the end of psychedelic science, here is the spot in the narrative where we can insert him.

The media weren't making the political climate any easier, either. Prior to the mid-1960s, LSD tended to receive positive press coverage— sometimes overwhelmingly so. Consider, for example, the extraordinary response to Cary Grant's declaration that weekly LSD sessions had transformed him into a happy person, saved his marriage, and offered him peace of mind. The story prompted years of optimistic stories about the therapeutic possibilities that LSD might offer.[32] Then the media suddenly decided that LSD presented a mortal threat to the country's youth.[33] Journalists no longer bothered differentiating between medical and black-market versions of the drug, the latter of which was likely to be laced with something potentially deadly. LSD, if headlines were to be trusted, made people suicidal, sex crazed, murderous, psychotic, or worse: revolutionary.

Sandoz no longer held a patent for LSD. Why continue to sponsor a drug that exposed the company to so much legal liability?

Fifty-eight psychedelic studies were forced to stop their research midstream after Sandoz pulled its sponsorship of LSD because they no longer met the FDA's bureaucratic requirement that every drug under investigation have an approved IND. But the US government maintained sufficient interest in maintaining research into LSD that it negotiated an agreement with Sandoz that enabled psychedelic research in the United States to continue. Sandoz would transfer its remaining stock of LSD to the National

Institutes of Mental Health (NIMH), which would now take over the role of distributor.[34]

The gambit worked for a short time. But scientists no longer wanted to study LSD. New psychiatric drugs, like Thorazine, seemed like they could snap people out of dark, delusional states. And a moral panic about the dangers of LSD made studying it far too stigmatizing.

The federal government's decision to list LSD and psilocybin as Schedule I drugs in 1970 had only been the cherry on top of a series of policies devastating psychedelic research. The last psychedelic study in the United States—at a site funded by the NIMH—closed its doors in 1976.

● ● ●●●●●●●●●●●●●●●●●●●● ● ●

Sen. Estes Kefauver had hoped his new law would make pharmaceuticals safe, effective, and affordable. He successfully managed to make medicines safer and more effective. But the law ended up making drugs *a lot* more expensive. FDA regulations, aimed at protecting consumers, gave the biggest, richest pharmaceutical companies an even bigger leg up. Smaller firms were disadvantaged, unable to bear the financial burden of the new experimental requirements set by the FDA for drug approval. A few years after the enactment of the amendments, policy analysts noted an ironic twist. The regulations meant to ensure safety and efficacy had inadvertently spurred a greater focus on profitability among drug companies. Randomized controlled trials, the gold standard for determining if a new drug was safe and effective, were so expensive that only the largest and best-resourced firms could afford drug development.[35]

All this presented a challenge for the individuals connected through CH.com, who had none of the resources of a drug manufacturer. They weren't even an organization themselves, merely a loosely connected group trying to navigate the complex world of drug development. They believed they had valid evidence for the efficacy of psilocybin, but how could they possibly convince the FDA of the legitimacy of their claims, especially given the stigma still attached to psychedelic experimentation?

Clusterheads needed to survive no matter what it took. A clinical trial would be welcome, but rules and regulations made this seem like a dim possibility. If the powers that be would not offer the help they needed, then they would reclaim this power for themselves, clinical trials be damned.

## Chapter Ten

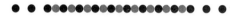

# THE PROTOCOL

*C*HICAGO, *SPRING 1978*

Bob Wold's first cluster headache interrupted a glorious spring day, the kind that fills Chicagoans' hearts with optimism that summer might soon return. He was playing catch with his oldest son in the backyard when a strange sensation tingled up his spine to his head. Something felt wrong. He turned on his heel and stumbled toward the house.

By the time he reached the sofa, the tingling had escalated into a relentless, searing roar, and now it felt as though someone was rattling a hot bayonet in his eye. His swollen eye began to tear, and snot poured out of his nose—not a few drips but a waterfall.

He paced. He considered slamming his head against the concrete outside. He might have screamed. Thirty minutes later it just stopped.

The next twenty-three years of his life should sound familiar by now. Dozens of therapies, including over sixty prescription medications and four in-patient hospitalizations, all failed. He could usually manage, but that resilience began to wear thin when, in 2001, the cycle of pain never stopped. The disease, his doctors explained, had become chronic. He began spending every night pacing the short length that stretched across his living and dining rooms in a fruitless attempt to shake off the pain.

Life became unbearable when the oxygen stopped working. His family pretended they couldn't hear his screams or the sound his head made as he bashed it against the bathroom tiles, but of course they could—and it frightened them. Mary tried to shield the kids, but when Bob was in pain, he was "in his own world."

Wold's doctor suggested he consider having his trigeminal nerve destroyed using Gamma Knife neurosurgery. Little evidence supported the procedure, but the doctor didn't have much else to offer. Wold kept seeing people with chronic cluster headache posting horror stories online about how the procedure made their attacks worse. It didn't seem like a great idea.

A second surgeon suggested a microvascular decompression operation that would involve the placement of Teflon around his nerve. This option seemed worse, given the four- to six-week recovery period and the accompanying risks that included cerebral spinal fluid leak, hearing loss, facial numbness, and, in rare cases, bleeding, infection, seizures, or paralysis. He couldn't find anybody online who felt better after this procedure either.

That's when the UPS box filled with mushrooms arrived at his door.

●  ●  ●●●●●●●●●●●●●●●●●●●●●  ●  ●

Wold knew about Flash. He knew about most headache-related things happening online. Patient forums had been a lifeline since 1995, when he first plugged his computer into a phone line and let 'er rip. I wouldn't be surprised if he spent more time hanging out online than he spent with Mary.

But the thought of taking a psychedelic scared him. He'd never done it before. Was he really going to start now that he was a grandfather? He had a lot of mouths to feed. But getting brain surgery seemed like a much more frightening proposition.

He tore open the package, tossed the mushrooms into boiling water, and gulped down the brew. Sure enough, his head cleared in about thirty minutes, which offered him his first twelve-hour break from pain in over a month.

Wold tried again the next day, despite advice from those on the forum who suggested that he wait a few days for the best results. The pain, once again, "drained" from his skull.

"I could tell it was definitely different than anything I'd ever experienced before with any other medication," he told me. His headache didn't just disappear; the drug seemed to clear his mind. "It was just an amazing feeling. I wasn't . . . hallucinating at all. My head just cleared."

The best part? He giggled the whole time. The tea didn't make him feel "trippy," but he did feel incredibly light. A bit like he'd had a couple of beers. His family loved seeing him so happy—it had been a while since they'd seen him smile.

His attacks returned the following day, but he could see potential. The mushrooms did what nothing else he'd taken had ever managed: break the worst cluster headache cycle of his life.

"I canceled all of my appointments for the scheduled surgeries and decided mushrooms were what I was going to do."

Unfortunately, the package contained only enough mushrooms for two doses—not enough to break his cycles. At times like this, he told me, "it was nice to have teenagers around the house." Wold's kids took about a month to find him some more. "To be honest, I found that a bit reassuring. Imagine how upset I'd be if they came home with them the next day!"

Wold felt more confident this time around. His attacks had returned, but they were less intense than before, and he'd done his best to stay off his prescribed drugs (all fifteen of them) to make sure that a drug interaction didn't undermine the effectiveness of the mushrooms, which was a subject hotly debated on the forum.

Wold was also considerably less frightened of what might happen once he drank the tea on his third go-around. Unlike with the previous, somewhat rushed attempts, Wold took the time to make sure the set and setting would amplify the pleasure of his experience. He would take his third dose during his town's Fourth of July celebrations.

There's a luxury in a summer evening spent outdoors. By the time the sun went down that Thursday, a gentle western breeze had cooled Madison Meadow Park to eighty degrees. How marvelous it must have felt to sink into his lawn chair after months upon months of agony. His family laid out blankets and snacks as his daughters quieted their young children. Wold put on his headphones tuned to Pink Floyd; the band, always his go-to, had been his online alias years before clusterheadaches.com existed. As the mushrooms began to take hold, he allowed his face to tilt gently toward the darkening sky.

People often say that psilocybin changes them, allowing them to see, experience, and understand the world differently. I sometimes wonder what he saw in those fireworks that night—a sensation, perhaps, of weightlessness, as psilocybin transformed "Comfortably Numb" into an ethereal, synesthetic rendering of individual streaks of light popping into shimmering allium-shaped molecules, a mycelial mat knitting the sky.

A capricious hope expanded into the space once consumed with pain.

After the parade was over and the visions faded, Wold waited to see what would happen. The headaches didn't return. He made it past his usual fall season headache-free, and Christmas passed without incident. Around New Year's, he noticed the telltale shadows appearing, so he re-treated himself on the six-month mark. That treatment "wiped out the shadows." The pain remitted for another six months, but then the shadows gathered. He would have another psychedelic July 4th in his town park.

Maybe his hope was justified. Maybe it was time to declare his independence from cluster headache.

Wold didn't realize it yet, but this experience would change everything going forward, not just his pain. His entire life would soon be taken over by a battle to pull cluster headache out of its obscure corner of medicine and into the spotlight.

● ● ●○●○●○●○●○●○●○●○●○ ● ●

Daren "DJ" Johnson, like Bob Wold, searched for connection in patient forums. He founded clusterheadaches.com (CH.com) in 1998 to create a dedicated space for people with cluster headache. He rarely engaged in any of the conversation about psychedelics: discussing a federally illegal drug on a website he created seemed like a bad idea, given that he served in the military on active duty. But he allowed the conversation to continue. Free speech mattered to him.

Maintaining that freedom couldn't have been easy. Over time, disagreements about psychedelic experimentation threatened to poison the entire community. Some suggested that those in favor of developing psychedelic treatments should build their own website. DJ wouldn't censor posts on the topic at CH.com, but a dedicated site seemed like a great way to reduce drama. And much to his delight, everyone on CH.com thought it was a terrific idea.

But the effort to build a new website was beset with problems. If Wold's memory serves, their webmaster quit after a Clusterhead who opposed the use of psychedelics threatened to file a lawsuit. DJ suggested that Wold, a friend from his days on migraine patient forums, might be interested in helping.

Wold had to think it over. He knew how to build plenty of things. A website was not one of them.

On the other hand, Wold felt that he owed his health to people who refused to allow challenges get the best of them. Where would he be without the help of people like Flash and Pinky? It made him angry that anyone would threaten someone else for trying to get information out to people. Plus, Wold felt confident that the law was on his side. The way he put it to me was, "You can get online and learn how to build a bomb."

He'd also seen other websites from the psychedelic underground successfully fend off legal problems. "It's a free speech issue."

So Wold got to work. He wanted a site where anyone could obtain background information about the use of psychedelics for cluster headache, including a uniform set of instructions about how to bust. Ideally, the site would be useful to patients, doctors, researchers, and legislators: a one-stop shop.

He made it sound simple, a boring administrative task that he'd be willing to manage: a compilation of the information people had already shared on CH.com. But the project he had in mind was far more ambitious: a website containing accurate, up-to-date information that anyone, anywhere could use to treat cluster headache with psychedelic mushrooms required that the group first develop recommendations for a therapeutic dose, along with safety regimens. Pharmaceutical companies take years to do the same kind of work.

Wold was also pushing hard to get the work the Clusterheads were doing informally onto the radar of more legitimate—in other words, well-funded—organizations. Treating people at scale required that they partner with the pharmaceutical industry. This would take money—a lot of money—and alliances across medicine, nonprofits, and industry. Decriminalization was off the table for now. It would be hard enough to get magic mushrooms accepted as a medicine.

● ● ●●●●●●●●●●●●●●●●●●●● ● ●

The first step would be to create a new group, separate from the main CH.com website, where people committed to developing psychedelic therapy for cluster headache could meet privately. No more time wasted with squabbles.

Luckily, the internet made it easy to create a space where people from around the world could meet away from prying eyes. Wold just needed to sign up for a group through Yahoo!, which had just begun offering the public free online forums where members could post files, share photos, and create polls.

Wold formed a new Yahoo! group called The Cluster Buster, and invited a few dozen people who he thought would be committed to the cause. On August 4, 2002, Wold sent them an email.

Hello fellow clusterheads and keepers of the flame!

Welcome and thank you for joining us here. This message board and email service has been started to join together people interested in advancing psilocybin and related therapies, for cluster headache. . . . Our purpose here is to take a proactive role in researching the treatment, spreading the word, and beginning the long road to acceptance of the treatment as a "legal" way for people to treat their headaches.

Those who received the email, he explained, had been chosen for their ability to contribute to this mission. He welcomed suggestions from new members, but he alone would control access to the forum to maintain the quality of their discussions.

I'm the only one that can invite people for automatic membership. That way, no one can just "drop in" and cause any trouble, and we can make sure that people here are interested in helping the cause. I won't mind people with differing views. . . . We need to be able to look at everything from every angle if we're going to get this right. But I'd rather not devote a large amount of our time to fighting over whether or not this is a worthy undertaking, with nonsupporters (or spammers . . . or trolls).[1]

Their first point of order would be to choose a mission. Everyone immediately agreed that they could not afford to wait for medicine. The severity of their disorder demanded urgent action. They would prioritize self-experimentation with psychedelic drugs, no matter its legality. Their initial project would be simple: develop their own data-based protocol—medication that anyone could grow at home.

Wold suggested they start with an FAQs section, something easy to produce, a task the group might complete within weeks if everyone took responsibility for "a section or two." "I've written FAQ's before and have experience in what works, but if there are a couple of you that are willing to take this on, I'd be happy to just be a proofreader and coordinator," Wold added.

A cluster squad sprang to action, sending rapid-fire messages offering help.

"I'm in on a FAQ. . . . Anyone want to be my partner?"

"I'll help!

"I'm not much of a computer whiz, but I would be willing to help compile and put into writing some of the necessary info for the FAQ and/or help brainstorm what should be in it."

The questions were easy—everyone agreed on what needed to be in there:

How do I obtain mushrooms?
How much psilocybin do I need to take to treat my CHs?
How often will I need to dose?
Will my meds interact with psilocybin?
Do I need to detox from my meds for mushroom therapy?
Will mushroom therapy help chronic cluster sufferers as well as
   episodics?

The more complicated problem would be developing answers. Questions like these would require in-depth responses, and for some they didn't currently have full answers. This straightforward task would turn out to be anything but. How could a group of nonscientists, working in tandem, and in secret, from homes around the world, create instructions that would produce a safe, effective, standardized treatment from spores that they cultivated in their closets?

First, there was the basic information, including a rationale for taking *Psilocybe* mushrooms and information about how to source spores, not to mention grow, harvest, and store mushrooms at home. Then they needed to grapple with the fact that psilocybin, the substance they were taking, came in the form of a homegrown mushroom rather than a pharmaceutical-grade drug.

A drug protocol would, by definition, need to explain to readers how to take this medication. But how could they provide a set of standardized instructions for taking a mushroom? They would also have to figure out drug interactions. CH.com board members had long suspected that many of the drugs regularly prescribed for cluster headache interfered with psychedelic therapy. But it was difficult to ask people to detox from the kinds of medications, like prednisone, that Clusterheads had long relied on to suppress attacks.

Questions remained: Did Clusterheads need to detox from all drugs prior to taking *Psilocybe* mushrooms? Was there a way to use mushrooms to help with this detox? Could side effects like nausea and anxiety be minimized? Was the psychedelic trip necessary, or was a subhallucinogenic dose an option? And most importantly, despite all the success stories they'd heard, why did some people still struggle to get relief, despite multiple attempts at using mushrooms? Could the dosing structure be tweaked to be made more effective?

The more questions they asked, the more they began to realize that for this FAQ to help anyone, anywhere self-treat with mushrooms, they would need to answer a whole lot of previously unsolved problems.

● ● ●●●●●●●●●●●●●●●●●●●● ● ●

The pharmaceutical industry grapples with a similar set of questions when developing drugs. Biomedical researchers answer them using a series of systematic experimental procedures. Preclinical testing, which occurs in animals and computer modeling, provides important information about dosing, side effects, and drug interactions and can answer complex questions about absorption and metabolism. Clinical trials in human subjects provide specific answers about dosing, including the optimal frequency of doses, and additional information about safety and efficacy.

Pharmaceutical companies, of course, are forced to do this much testing because of regulations like the 1962 Kefauver-Harris Act. But as we've learned, pharmaceutical research and development is notoriously slow and expensive. It takes an average of fourteen years and $1 billion for drug candidates to make it from the laboratory to the pharmacy. That only accounts for drugs that make it to market. The vast majority fail to make it through clinical trials.[2]

But the people gathering in Bob Wold's new forum had none of the resources available to scientists working in pharmaceutical companies. No animal studies or lab analyses. No brain scans or blood tests. And most importantly, they lacked the most basic ingredient for conducting these experiments: a standardized drug that could be taken in a consistent, measurable dosage.

Standards, in science, are everything. They serve a variety of functions, ranging from the pragmatic to the epistemological to the political. Standards convert "messy" varied outcomes into something predictable and reproducible, thereby ensuring reliability and validity.[3] But they also provide science (and therefore the researchers who conduct it) with power and authority, institutionalizing and legitimating the value of the work.[4]

But standards were also really useful, a fact that people in Clusterbusters realized, right away. The group began to discuss whether they *could* or *should* run their own version of a small experiment, controlling as much as they possibly could. Doing so would require that they standardize the intervention. What strain of mushroom would they choose? Would they source their spores from the same place to ensure they all took the same strain of psilocybin mushroom? Would they all take the same dose? Would their effort to standardize dried, ground-up mushrooms satisfy a doctor? Would they be testing whether the mushrooms stopped a cycle or prevented a cycle? How often would they take the shrooms—they'd have to agree on a protocol; no more free-wheelin' it. Were they really going to randomize people to take a placebo?

They certainly had their work cut out for them, beginning with a deceptively simple question: How does a person measure a dose of a mushroom? Experiments, after all, are exercises in precision. A researcher who eyeballs variables rather than measuring them painstakingly will find it difficult to draw a conclusion about the experiment's results.

The same was true for Clusterbusters. Self-experimentation required detailed knowledge of each dose; otherwise replication would be impossible. But there were also risks to mismeasuring individual doses. Too little of a dose might mean continued attacks. Too much could make for an uncomfortable psychedelic experience.

And measuring a dose wasn't always easy. Clusterbusters wanted to test psilocybin as a treatment for cluster headache. But they didn't have psilocybin; they had mushrooms that contained the drug they hoped could ease their pain. Multiple species of mushrooms contain psilocybin. Some species grow large mushrooms, while others grow small mushrooms. Some species are reputed to contain a great deal of psilocybin, while others are weak in comparison.

Variation in the potency of mushrooms is attributed to a remarkable range of factors. Even defining a "mushroom" is difficult. Does a dose of mushroom include only the fungus, or should it also include the mycelium, the "root"? Do some parts of the mushroom contain more psilocybin than others?

Mushrooms can be grown in *flushes*, or harvests, from the same set of mycelia. Does the first flush differ in potency from the third? Members wondered whether the timing of their harvest might affect the potency of their doses. Did it matter, for example, whether the mushrooms they harvested had opened their caps yet? "The shrooms we harvested . . . after the caps opened and they blew their spores . . . were less potent. If I harvested JUST before they opened, they were pretty heavy duty," noted one poster.

Mushrooms are messy.

Additionally, members began noticing that the storage and preparation of each dose could affect its potency. Eating more stems than caps or vice versa could produce radically different results. Or, as one Clusterbusters member accidentally discovered when he ate his mushrooms on a peanut butter sandwich, fat ingested with mushrooms could render the drug completely ineffective.

An individual's "frame of mind" could also transform how he or she experienced the potency of a psilocybin dose. Members were encouraged to pay attention to mind-set and physical setting. Positive thoughts, moods, and expectations and the right ambience (think of Bob Wold watching fireworks to the tune of Pink Floyd versus Flash's belief that Pink Floyd was far too dark and heavy to listen to during a trip) went a long way in ensuring a positive outcome.

But everyone's soundtrack, metaphorically speaking, is a little different. And exact standards are vital for doing good science.

● ● ●●●●●●●●●●●●●●●●●●● ● ●

The first draft of the FAQ was published on Clusterbusters' website by the end of 2003. This version involved the standardization of multiple sources of ambiguity: contamination concerns, dosing amount and vector, potential drug interactions, legal issues, psychological mind-set and physical setting, quantification of "trip levels," and pain scales. None were simple to sort out.

In clinical trials, researchers must limit their experiments to drugs that have gone through the IND process and been approved by the Food and Drug Administration.[5] Pharmaceutical-grade drugs have guaranteed potencies and chemical makeups. Psilocybin-containing mushrooms used by Clusterbusters had no such guarantee. PinkSharkMark's decision, early on, to source psychedelics from spores bought online and cultivated at home offered more autonomy and power over the quality of their supply, but it also helped them standardize their dose.

Cultivation allowed each Clusterbuster to have confidence in the knowledge of which mushroom species and strain they would consume. But cultivation alone couldn't erase variance between strains grown by each member, between individual harvests (or *flushes*), or even between different parts of each mushroom.

Pharmaceuticals are usually measured by weight or volume and are made by companies who are legally obligated to manufacture a consistent product so that consumers can feel confident that every dose they take will be the same as their last.

So Clusterbusters did their best to divide their mushrooms into standardized doses. A reliable scale helped remove the possibility of subjective error: "I just got myself a new scale last week," wrote one member. "The amount I have been describing previously as 1/4 gram was actually only 1/8 of a gram. . . . It was all pretty much guesswork for the lower doses."

A dosing error like that presented a problem for a person who wanted to maintain a consistent dose. But it also made creating a standardized dose in the community more difficult. Wold recommended that anytime a person took an "itsy bitsy tiny quantity like 1/8th of a gram, really anything under a gram, about the only reliable way to weigh it would be really to use a triple beam scale that's been calibrated with weights."

But even careful weighing couldn't eliminate all the unknowns because, ultimately, people have very different responses to psilocybin. It's even difficult to predict how the same individual will respond to the same dose on any given day. As one person put it, "three doses of the same amount produced three completely different highs. Sooo . . ."

So while objective measurement was recommended, Clusterbusters found that their bodies provided the most reliable instrument for assessing the potency of each dose. Embodied standards were the next best thing to perfect doses: let your body tell you the right dose.

Institutionalized drug development does something similar, using embodied standards to determine success in outcomes that are difficult to measure with objective technologies, including both pain and psychedelic experiences.[6] The primary difference here is that Clusterbusters had to use embodied standards to assess drug dosage, not just outcomes.

Clusterbusters suggested that those using psilocybin "start low," taking just a single half gram of psilocybin, and wait to see how they felt before increasing their dose. Individual assessments of psychoactive response could be measured using a "trip level" scale—a metric ranging from Level 1, indicating a mild high in which enhanced mood is experienced, to Level 5, indicating a complete immersion in hallucinations.

Clusterbusters' flexibility in dosage marks a significant departure from rigid dosing procedures required in institutionalized clinical trials. This flexibility might undermine their credibility when working with scientists, but it made pragmatic sense given the urgency of their need for treatment.

Flash told me that this embodied feedback was key to their success, given that it provided immediate, actionable insight: "When you use yourself as your own lab, you get far more insight into what's happening. The doctor can only go by what the patient tells them or what the blood test tells them. They don't really know what it feels like inside. You've got a really sensitive instrument in there, telling you how well something is working."

The trick then was to create a standard protocol that could be tweaked as needed for each person. As one Clusterhead said, "Adjustment in dosing seems to be inherent in our cluster headache salvation." So they came up with a dose that seemed to work for the most people—one gram of dried psilocybin—with multiple caveats and a suggestion to start with a much smaller dose. And they offered an easy-to-remember dosing schedule. The psilocybin should be taken three times, but other drugs could block the effects:

> The conservative rule of thumb is to wait five days.
> Wait five days after stopping Imitrex or verapamil, for example.
> Wait five days after dosing before returning to conventional meds such as Imitrex, etc.
> Wait five days between doses of tryptamines [psychedelics].

This wasn't a perfect system. They couldn't, for example, test whether the effects were caused by placebo. Nor did they have a perfect way to capture their data. Bob Wold always encouraged people to submit their results to the survey that still existed on Erowid's website, but hardly anyone ever followed through.

Was this clean, pure science? No. But it was helping people survive. The laboratory was never confined to sterile rooms of steel and glass; nor were the scientists always dressed in lab coats and protective goggles. In bedrooms and basements, in garages and makeshift tents, Clusterbusters found reprieve in a community willing to forge ahead where medical institutions had failed, in the process creating a novel participatory science woven from not only data but human connection.

Pain, they'd been taught, couldn't be measured objectively. But the members of Clusterbusters understood, deeply, that numbers alone could not define their agony or guide them toward effective treatment. So they cultivated psilocybin with the care of first-time parents, treating each spore as a fragile hope. For what is pain, if not a denial of hope? A constant, excruciating reminder of vulnerability. They operated without the luxury of waiting for a medical breakthrough, taking matters into their own hands.

Messy as it was, by 2003 Clusterbusters had accomplished a feat that most scientists would have found challenging, even if there hadn't been a prohibition on psychedelic research: a standardized protocol for treating cluster headache with a fungus they had cultivated in closets around the world.

Their efforts would prove groundbreaking. Psychedelic self-experimentation on the internet not only revolutionized what doctors knew about cluster headache but also created entirely new ways of doing science.

Part III

# Psychedelic Citizens

## Chapter Eleven

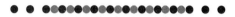

# HARVARD OR BUST

LAUNCHING A WEBSITE WITH A FULL SET OF INSTRUCTIONS ABOUT HOW to self-treat with magic mushrooms gave everyone something to celebrate. But Bob Wold could already see the limits of outlaw medicine.

Ainslie Course was neither the first nor the last person with cluster headache he would doctor. And the bigger and more successful the organization's reach, the more relentless the requests. He'd find an email begging for help in his inbox five or six times a week: "You're my last hope." How could he say no? Medicine had failed them. They needed something, anything, for relief.

Doctoring people at risk of suicide would stress out anyone. But knowing that each person he helped represented, at best, a drop in the bucket kept Wold up at night. A thought lodged itself in the corner of his brain: every single day, someone, somewhere, might die from this miserable disease because they had run out of hope. And yet, the treatment was both simple and cheap. It was like they were crawling through a desert and dying of thirst in full view of an actual oasis.

Publishing Clusterbusters' protocol online ought to have been enough, but Wold continually found that people needed more help than a static website could offer. Sometimes they found it hard to grow mushrooms. Sometimes they needed support weaning themselves off sumatriptan or prednisone. Sometimes they needed their dosing tweaked.

He should have predicted as much. DIY medicine was a bit like asking someone to choose their own chemotherapy based on a website FAQ. No matter how well the user interface on the "pick your own poison" oncology dashboard, it would feel a heck of a lot better to talk it through with an experienced doctor.

But even the most sympathetic doctors (and the Clusterbusters had met a few) either wouldn't or couldn't provide the individualized, flexible care that Wold had become so experienced in delivering.

The most frustrating challenges were always the conversations with desperate people who wanted his help but feared what might happen if they took an illicit drug. "A certain portion of the population," he told me, "still trusts the government and won't believe a drug is safe until the [Food and Drug Administration (FDA)] has approved it." Government messaging about "how bad drugs are"—and the whole "This is your brain on drugs" ad campaign with the fried egg visual—had been wildly effective.

"So, you're starting off with, I don't know 30, 40, 50 percent of the population thinking that it's not safe, even if it were decriminalized. . . . There are a lot of people that are waiting for the government's safe stamp to be put on [it]," Wold told me.[1]

This reliance on the government's official certification—in the face of so much evidence that it was wrong on this issue—could be very frustrating. It paralyzed people who wanted to be "good citizens"—it's hard enough to live in agony. But we live in a world where health and wellness are a moral good. Imagine choosing not to take a medicine that might restore health out of fear of being found out.

Wold had more sympathy for those who believed mushrooms could work but couldn't risk breaking the law because their immigration status or the color of their skin made everything much more complicated. Psychedelic mushrooms might save them from pain, but being caught with them would present a different set of threats. The oasis was real, Wold knew, but a large portion of those with cluster headache wouldn't go near it unless a sign read, "The FDA has declared this water safe to drink."

Wold often tried to assure people that their risk of getting caught was low. Normal drug tests don't measure psychedelic drugs, partly because the body quickly metabolizes them. "I spent a lot of time trying to talk people into the fact that they really weren't going to get into trouble." But he didn't like to push that hard on the issue. How could he know any individual's risk tolerance, let alone their actual risks? Most police officers in his community knew he took psychedelics for cluster headache. But he also used to coach most of them in the town's Little League. Wold was a grandfather, a baseball coach, and a gentle presence about town. Perhaps more importantly, he was a white guy, and he knew it. He just didn't have the moral authority to lecture anyone else.

"You start talking to them about that kind of stuff and suddenly, you get this really kind of weird feeling like, wow, I'm a drug pusher trying to talk somebody into taking these drugs. You feel like you're kind of dirty, honestly."

Others in the forum tired of being outlaws too. Emotions oscillated between fear of potential legal repercussions and moral outrage at the judgment they might encounter from the authorities. One moment, people would worry that growing mushrooms was a felony offense that could be charged as manufacturing with the intent to distribute. And then in the next moment, the sentiment would shift toward resolute confidence that police officers and juries would agree they had reasonable cause for breaking the law. After all, they'd collected reams of data demonstrating the therapeutic necessity of their actions.

Fear of arrest aside, wouldn't it be great if they could get this medicine from the neighborhood pharmacy? Sure, some people developed a love of growing shrooms. Some people love brewing craft beer too. But half the posts on the forum had to do with cultivation. Struggling with mold contamination, mistimed harvests, and dose miscalculations was exhausting.

A standardized pill, purchased in a pharmacy, would help people determine their precise dosage. No more guessing whether a batch of mushrooms hadn't worked due to lost potency or accidentally brewing a stronger tea than intended. The unregulated market of the underground made the therapy far more dangerous than it needed to be. The ability to obtain a regulated form of psilocybin would calm their nerves, which would offer them more control over their set and setting—factors that made all the difference to the effectiveness of psychedelics.

This would also alleviate the recurring problem faced when trying to help someone in a desperate situation. "Sorry, you've got to grow your own" felt like inadequate advice to a person deep in the throes of a cluster cycle, when simply contemplating surviving the next thirty minutes was sometimes too much to bear.

Deciding how to fix the situation, however, was somewhat more complicated. Lobbying politicians seemed premature without "official scientific evidence," especially given that President George W. Bush's attorney general, John Ashcroft, had promised to escalate the War on Drugs upon his confirmation by the Senate in January 2001.

GeorgieT*, a Buster on the forum whose experience in journalism made him a powerful ally and advisor in Wold's efforts, finally put his foot down. The next best step *had* to be aboveground science. "All the lobbying in the world won't help unless we can show the bureaucrats and legislators this is the real deal. We need physicians, neurologists especially, to make a credible case. We need official research clinical trials. . . . So first we have to convince the doctors something real is going on here with these magic mushrooms."[2]

Clusterbusters had to turn magic into the kind of science that governments would recognize.

●  ●  ●●●●●●●●●●●●●●●●●●●●  ●  ●

Marsha Weil agreed. Weil rarely posted messages on cluster forums, but logging onto CH.com in 1998 had changed her life. The patients she met there had been more helpful than any of the doctors she'd seen in her previous twenty years of having cluster headache. Like so many, she'd initially been given a diagnosis of migraine, despite having four to six severe headaches per night. When she finally received the correct diagnosis several years later, the doctor remarked that she "had a totally classic case, other than being a female."

She stopped seeking help from doctors in the late 1980s when a neurologist, having exhausted the conventional treatments he happened to know about, told her that they had "tried everything." She later learned that at least some of these treatments might have worked if he'd understood how to prescribe them. It was the online patient community that explained the proper way to use high-flow oxygen to abort an attack—she just needed to replace the useless nasal cannula prescribed by her doctor with a non-rebreather mask, a simple yet life-changing adjustment. The experience underscored the powerful wisdom within patient communities.

Flash's early posts about his experiences with psilocybin caught her attention. The science behind it seemed to make sense, and her excitement grew when she saw that others experimenting with psychedelics reported that these drugs helped them manage their attacks.

Weil hadn't yet had the opportunity to try the treatment herself since her cluster headache cycle had gone into a long remission, but she felt certain she would try it if it were needed. After all, the alternatives were flat-out awful. "My overall feeling: the drug companies have us held as hostages. The pain is so severe that you are willing to try anything and everything, which comes with major side effects."

Weil, an eminently rational person, had come to the same conclusion that so many others with cluster headache had: magic mushrooms seemed a better choice.

At some point—she couldn't remember when—somebody had indicated that a clinical trial would cost about $50,000 and suggested the group begin to fundraise. She liked the idea that a study might turn their knowledge into a valid treatment so people wouldn't need to "illegally source this stuff." But she didn't think a drug company would come along and fund the project. Cluster headache never attracted much attention from corporations.

This got her thinking.

Wold knew he needed a scientist to help him develop a pharmaceutical option to reach more patients in need. But how? Cold-calling university professors didn't seem like it would work: "Hi, I lead a semicriminal network of psychedelic drug users. We have a great idea. Would you like to work with us?"

Several people in the group suggested that Wold reach out to Rick Doblin, executive director and founder of the Multidisciplinary Association for Psychedelic Studies (MAPS), a small organization that seemed to fund the few scientists who managed to conduct research on psychedelics and cannabis in universities. Various people had written to Doblin over the years to ask whether MAPS might be interested in supporting a psychedelic cluster headache study. He'd always seemed game. MAPS, Doblin explained, could help design, obtain permission for, and conduct a pilot study for about $50,000.

Wold, however, had rather hoped to align with an organization less closely associated with illegal drug use than MAPS, which had always been willing to allow mysticism and tie-dyes to bleed into its collaborative endeavors with science. Aboveground research only mattered if the FDA acknowledged its legitimacy. Wold wondered if a government agency would view a project associated with MAPS as a serious endeavor. Or did MAPS's support of decriminalization discredit and stigmatize everything in its orbit—even well-done university research?

So he decided to start with headache specialists—the doctors tasked with treating their disease. Many of them also ran clinical trials for drug companies. Wold already knew the biggest names in the field. He'd been reading their scientific articles for years, and he'd been a patient in many of their offices. And now that medical conferences welcomed patient advocates, he knew how to find them. Surely these experts would jump at the chance to investigate the drug that was making their hardest-to-treat patients feel so much better.

But this was 2003. Very little academic research had been conducted on psychedelic substances in humans in the thirty-three years since the

Controlled Substances Act went into effect. Most people didn't think the study of psychedelics would ever return to universities. Every discussion Wold had in the headache world seemed to go the same way: interest, even intrigue, but no commitment.

Wold posted about these encounters to the group's message board: "I've written and talked to several of the leading cluster specialists in the US. . . . It appears that they are even afraid to discuss this in email." He wondered if maybe they worried their emails would end up in the newspaper. It did seem like the War on Drugs and the emerging opioid crisis were frightening doctors.[3] "God help someone that professed legalizing psilocybin. . . . It would be akin to [arguing for the legalization of] heroin."[4]

Two decades later, we now know that all this would change. But at the time, none of them could see the shift that was coming.

There was another problem, besides the legal and social stigma of psychedelics. Headache medicine already faced issues obtaining funding because headache *itself* was stigmatized. Even the federal government barely allocated money for research on the topic. The entire field depended on the largesse of big pharma. GlaxoWellcome, headache medicine's biggest funder in 2003, held the patent for sumatriptan, which—when injected— could abort a cluster headache attack in fifteen minutes or less. Would doctors ignore a potential treatment like psilocybin because it might cut into their funders' profits? Wold got the sense from his interactions at headache conferences that magic mushrooms were viewed as having the potential to undermine big pharma's profits.

Wold explained on the board, "I tried to get someone to bring up the subject [of psilocybin] at a [professional headache conference] last year. The problem there, I was told, is that most of these meetings are sponsored by pharmaceutical companies. Paid airfare . . . hotel rooms etc. Try bringing up something that isn't going to make anyone any money . . . for years . . . and could hurt sales. . . . You would never be invited to a conference again."[5]

Physicians, according to Wold, seemed to be interested in the idea of the study, but none could see a way past practical matters like funding, legality, and the complications of dealing with the DEA and the FDA. But he found support. "Believe it or not . . . many of them would love to be able to [prescribe psilocybin]. Many of them are well-aware of the evidence on the side of its efficacy." But a research study testing psychedelics would be too risky—a potential career killer.[6]

MAPS was the next logical step if he could somehow manage to find $50,000. But nobody in Clusterbusters seemed to have a clue about how they might go about fundraising for such a thing. Many struggled to keep a job, let alone pay for their own medications. It never occurred to him that a multimillionaire might be lurking on the board.

● ● ●●●●●●●●●●●●●●●●●●● ● ●

"My husband and I are willing to contribute $50,000 to $100,000 to MAPS to complete a pilot study."

Wold didn't respond right away to Marsha Weil's October 3, 2003, email. He would later tell her that he preferred to proceed carefully. But the truth was, he thought she must be joking.

Luckily, Marsha Weil was very, very serious.

The Weils had been lucky in life. David, Marsha's husband, had become Microsoft's twenty-fifth employee in 1980, just after the company moved from New Mexico to Seattle, and continued to work there for the next seventeen years before retiring. Most start-ups fail. Microsoft had transformed its first several thousand employees into millionaires by the early 1990s.

The Weils support a variety of philanthropic efforts through their family foundation, but Marsha envisioned a psychedelic study as something she might do on her own. "This was going to be sort of my thing," she told me. Her husband supported her, just as she had always supported everything he'd done. This would be a project that she had chosen and that she would lead.

Weil also considered the possibility that a study like this might help get the word out to more people who needed this medicine. "I knew that we would get publicity. . . . There were a lot of people that probably would not be on the internet but who would want to find out about this. I thought this is a great way to get the word out beyond just our small group," she told me.

Wold's dream of the underground and the aboveground working together was about to come true. And it certainly wasn't going to hurt to have an angel investor on board.

● ● ●:●:●:●:●:●:●:●:●:●:●:●:●:● ● ●

Few people can claim as much responsibility for the success of the psychedelic renaissance as Rick Doblin. Over the last four decades, his political advocacy has paved the way for researchers worldwide to conduct clinical research into psychedelics for a wide range of diseases and conditions. Since its founding in 1986, MAPS has grown into a multimillion-dollar research empire able, via its own public benefit corporation (now called Lykos Therapeutics), to conduct cutting-edge clinical trials on psychedelics.

Doblin has never been camera shy. In fact, if anything, his strategy has always been to be as public (or, in his words, "as transparent") as possible so that everyone has "the right information."[7] And the press can't get enough of him. Michael Pollan's 2018 best-selling book *How to Change Your Mind* gave Doblin and MAPS a huge boost by introducing the public to the idea that psychedelic substances might be used for something other than "turning on" and getting high.[8] Doblin scored a TED Talk the following year, which gave him a global platform to discuss "the future of psychedelic-assisted therapy."[9]

In 2021, *Nature Medicine*, one of the top medical journals in the world, published results from a MAPS-sponsored clinical trial, which provided strong evidence that MDMA, when administered in combination with talk therapy, could effectively treat severe posttraumatic stress disorder (PTSD). Of the ninety people enrolled in the study, 67 percent of those given MDMA alongside talk therapy no longer qualified for a diagnosis of PTSD two months after treatment. The same was true of only 32 percent of those given a placebo. MDMA, according to the study's authors, worked by enhancing talk therapy rather than via altering an individual's neurochemistry in the long term.[10] As Doblin told the *New York Times*, "It's not the drug—it's the therapy enhanced by the drug."[11] The press went wild, running profiles that described him as a revolutionary, making Doblin as iconic in the current psychedelic movement as Ben & Jerry are to craft ice cream.[12] Like them, he provides the movement with a relaxed, 1960s-throwback vibe.

It's a public persona that has remained unchanged over the decades. Thirty years ago, *New York* magazine described him as "an unabashed prose-lytizer, a psychedelic cheerleader in the tradition of Dr. Timothy Leary," a glowing guru who "burbles with psychedelic illumination and good humor."[13] That description perfectly fits the person I've encountered over the years, a man who maintains a relentless cheer and optimism, even when faced with the bleakest political forecasts—or when dealing with the most difficult personalities.

His laid-back, beatific manner hints that something is different with Doblin. Although he has a PhD in public policy from Harvard, he wears his scientific bona fides lightly. Unlike many others in the psychedelic space, Doblin makes so many jokes about drug use that he always seems to have one foot planted in the tie-dyed world of the counterculture, even as he works with his other foot firmly in the "straight" world of lab-coat-wearing scientists. As he's often said, it was his use of LSD—a lot of LSD—that got him interested in psychedelic therapy. "I was an LSD user, so my identifica-tion was as this counterculture drug-using criminal. So that's kind of who I thought of myself as, who I was. I just kind of accepted that."[14] That is, until he decided that the aboveground had advantages. Like providing him with the tools he'd need to fight the system from within.

Doblin had never been one to let authority stand in his way, having learned the hard way that governments don't always lead with moral righ-teousness. Like many Jewish kids of his generation, the Holocaust cast a long shadow. He'd been lucky—his family had emigrated to the United States before unspeakable bloodshed ripped through Europe. "I was born in 1953. . . . I was very much educated at a young age about the Holocaust and that just terrified me; the dehumanization, the scapegoating, the irra-tional taking over rational thought," he has said.[15]

Similarly, he couldn't understand why the United States needed to fight the Vietnam War. The Cuban Missile Crisis and the ever-present potential for nuclear war between the United States and the Soviet Union deepened his resolve: it was better to act according to his own moral compass than to witness the world dissolve into "cultural insanity" invoked by fear of the other.[16]

Nor was Doblin inclined to let conventional thinking dictate his moral compass. He dodged the draft at age eighteen—a decision that made him a felon. The other option, filing for an exemption as a conscientious objector didn't feel honest, he has said. He couldn't claim to be a pacifist because he believed war had been necessary to stop Hitler.

He thought the decision might one day land him in jail, but he figured it made sense to go to college in the meantime. He moved to Sarasota to attend the New College of Florida, which—back then, anyway—had a reputation for its unconventional, freewheeling approach to undergraduate education. That's where he began experimenting with LSD, a drug that flowed freely on campus despite its recent criminalization. It was a bumpy ride. He reveled in the vivid colors, intense sensations, and collective ecstasy of an all-night party. But these experiences left him feeling unsettled. Each trip peeled back layers of self, revealing imperfections and inner conflicts deep within his psyche. He had no idea what to do with these revelations until a guidance counselor at the school suggested he might benefit from reading the work of Stanislav Grof, a psychiatrist who'd conducted LSD research for years. Doblin would soon drop out of college so he could hitchhike to California, where Grof would be teaching a weeklong seminar about LSD therapy.[17]

Psychedelics, Doblin explained during his TED Talk, "gave me this feeling of our shared humanity, of our unity with all life. . . . And I felt that these experiences had the potential to help be an antidote to tribalism, to fundamentalism, to genocide and environmental destruction."[18] The law, he decided, wouldn't stop him from finding a way for LSD to heal the world. An inheritance from his grandparents and support from generous parents allowed him the time and resources to build himself a custom house, which he designed to maximize comfort during an acid trip.[19] He would

then become a full-time contractor specializing in the construction of custom homes. But the business ran into trouble when interest rates peaked at
18 percent in the late 1970s. He closed shop and reenrolled as an undergraduate at the New College of Florida. Maybe he could still become an underground psychedelic therapist.[20]

If LSD had transformed Doblin's world, with its ability to produce cos-
mic, mystical connections, he would soon discover that MDMA produced
something even more powerful: profound love and self-acceptance—an
essential medicine for the kind of psychotherapy that quickly healed even
the most serious traumas.

In the early 1980s Doblin began to wonder whether MDMA could do
even more. "Adam," in his experience, inspired open-minded, radical thinking, the antidote to dehumanization that he'd been searching for his whole
life. Doblin became such a believer that he started preaching the gospel of
MDMA to anyone who would listen; he even began mailing tablets to political and spiritual leaders, convinced they could use a drug that promoted
empathy to do good in the world. His outreach bore fruit when one recipient, a Benedictine monk named Brother David Steindl-Rast, was quoted
in a *Newsweek* article: "A monk spends his whole life cultivating the same
awakened attitude [that MDMA] gives you."[21]

Not every pie-in-the sky effort landed. Doblin's attempt to smuggle a
package of one thousand pills to members of the Soviet military who would
be negotiating with US President Ronald Reagan in 1985 only got as far as
Moscow. Too bad. It was worth a try.

But this advocacy did gain him entrance to somewhere big: the Esalen
Institute.

Laura Huxley learned about Rick Doblin after seeing a copy of his correspondence with Brother David. She sent him an invitation to Esalen
and yadda yadda yadda, the young Rick Doblin decided to take over the
underground's efforts to keep MDMA legal. It's fair to say that the DEA had
not anticipated Doblin when it announced its intention to place MDMA in
Schedule I of the Controlled Substances Act.

Doblin, on the other hand, had not only anticipated the DEA but had already prepared a strong defense. The best way to fight the system, he decided, would be to work within the system, not to mention play by the system's rules—a policy jujitsu of sorts. He convinced the psychedelic elders to take some essential actions while MDMA remained legal, like collecting data about its safety and efficacy from the therapists who had been using it. That and hiring David Nichols to synthesize two kilos of the stuff during a prohibition were strokes of genius. How could the DEA categorize MDMA as a drug with no therapeutic usefulness given how much evidence experts had already accumulated? MDMA-assisted psychotherapy, according to their data, could be administered safely and had clear medical benefits for those they treated.

By 1984, Rick had gone from proselytizing about MDMA by mail to an even more audacious gambit. In August of that year, he hand-delivered a package to the DEA's headquarters in Washington, DC, containing the petitions that he'd collected from experts and a request for an administrative hearing in front of a judge.

Doblin sees this act—the decision to engage with the system he had long avoided—as an important milestone both in his career and in the psychedelic movement. He often shows audiences a self-portrait captured just before he walked into the DEA office. It's a hazy, sepia-toned photo of his image reflected in a street-level window emblazoned with the sign of the ruinous federal agency. He hasn't yet stepped inside and discovered how its agents will react to a confrontation from a hippie draft dodger. And the window offers no hint of what is to come, a curtain obscuring whatever transparency into government power it might have offered.

Doblin wore a business-casual button-down shirt for his mission but decided to carry the petitions in a Huichol peyote bag—a subtle yet powerful symbol of the direct action he was now taking. "As I knocked on the DEA's door and stepped inside, I felt I was crossing a boundary," Doblin explained to a journalist writing for *Alternet*. "I was transitioning from a hidden underground existence to a visible, aboveground one."[22] He brought the social mycelium—dormant for so long—straight to the enemy, and prepared to emerge into the light.

Inaction was not an option, not in a world that always felt like it was teetering on annihilation. And the more he committed to making the world safer, the less he worried about the personal risk of his involvement. His moral compass pointed in one direction: the creation of a more peaceful and tolerant world. Psychedelics would be the bridge.[23]

Rick Doblin's brazen strategy caught the DEA off guard. Nobody had told them that doctors and therapists had been using MDMA in their clinics while it was legal. Their credentials presented the DEA with a serious challenge. Prohibition would be more difficult than they thought if MDMA wasn't just a drug used by kids getting their rocks off.

In the end, the courts sided with Doblin's nonprofit twice, ruling that "the overwhelming weight of medical opinion evidence received in this proceeding concurred that sufficient information existed to support a judgment by reputable physicians that MDMA was safe to use under medical supervision."[24]

But it was all for naught. If the DEA wanted to criminalize MDMA, it was going to do just that—courts be damned. In fact, the DEA didn't have to listen to the courts, whose role was simply advisory. The agency not only decided to ignore the court but also opted to change the definition of "medical benefit" to a set of criteria mirroring FDA approval, which would make it nearly impossible in the future to change how a Schedule I drug was categorized in the absence of clinical trials "proving" its safety and efficacy as a medication.

Doblin, ever the true believer, saw this frustrating turn of events as nothing more than a minor setback. So far as he was concerned, he had found a winning strategy for fighting the War on Drugs: work the system to fight the system. First, he founded MAPS to provide an organization from which he might advocate for the return of psychedelics. His next step would be learning how the system's machinery worked in order to throw sand more effectively in its gears.

Doblin completed the undergraduate degree he had started in 1971, choosing a senior thesis topic that would help him understand how to conduct rigorous research: a critical evaluation of Walter Pahnke's famous 1962 double-blind, placebo-controlled Good Friday Experiment demonstrating that psilocybin could induce mystical experiences when administered in the right setting. What's more, Doblin wrote a thesis good enough to be published in a peer-reviewed journal—the principal currency traded in academic circles. Doblin was beginning to learn how to speak a language that aboveground scientists and regulators understood and appreciated.[25]

Doblin hoped to continue his education in a clinical psychology department where he might pursue a PhD, but graduate programs, he said, were put off by his determination to conduct clinical research on MDMA. He couldn't help but notice that politics kept interfering with science. So he made a decision: if politics was the barrier to psychedelic science, then he'd better learn how to become a politician in the most mainstream, credible institution he could think of: Harvard University.

In the 1990s, Doblin enrolled in Harvard's Kennedy School of Government, where he wrote a doctoral thesis under the direction of Mark Kleiman (Kleiman, intriguingly, has been identified as a quiet but powerful supporter of the reemergence of psychedelics).[26]

The Kefauver-Harris Drug Amendments of 1962 had only been the beginning of increased government oversight into scientific affairs. Scandals continued to plague scientists. Some studies, like the Tuskegee Syphilis Study—in which the US Public Health Service spent decades observing what happened when syphilis went untreated in a group of African American men, who were neither informed of the disease they carried nor offered treatment for it—were breathtaking in their depravity. In response, policymakers enacted increasingly restrictive bureaucratic measures designed to ensure scientists behaved in a responsible, ethical, and legal manner.

Drug laws, combined with a culture of fear, made this bureaucracy even more complicated for those wishing to conduct clinical trials on Schedule I substances. And to make the task more difficult, federal funding generally only existed for drug research demonstrating the extent to which

Schedule I drugs caused harm. Doblin knew that MAPS would be one of the only private philanthropies funding the kind of work that the government wouldn't touch—the studies that examined the potential benefits of these substances.

Doblin used his time at Harvard to master the art of the aboveground by devising solutions to the most difficult of these policy problems. He chose a complicated topic for his dissertation: regulation of the medical use of psychedelics and marijuana. In it, he provided a policy road map explaining the most productive way to obtain permission from the FDA to study these compounds.[27]

A far cry from his impassioned calls to save the world through psychedelics, Doblin's dissertation is written in the dispassionate language of the "respectable" world. Two of its chapters are dedicated to the inner workings of an FDA program that, between 1989 and 1995, established the FDA's current policy of evaluating psychedelic and marijuana protocols. Another two chapters tackle difficult questions involving the methodological challenges of studying psychedelics. A final chapter offers a hypothetical policy designed to guide how prescriptions might be written and distributed safely in the case of legalized psychedelic psychotherapy.

As a university professor, I've read dozens of doctoral dissertations, sometimes as the primary advisor for a doctoral candidate in my own department but often as part of an awards committee assessing dissertations from candidates across the United States. Rick Doblin can sometimes come off like an extra from *Dazed and Confused*, succeeding despite how high he is, but he wrote a solid, well-researched dissertation, perfectly designed to assist his psychedelic quest.

Doblin's research process for the paper presented an excellent opportunity to conduct interviews with current and former government officials at the FDA—contacts that I'm sure would prove useful to the executive director of MAPS. Because, of course, Doblin couldn't just study science—not if he wanted to change the world. Ushering the psychedelic renaissance into existence would take more than just facts: it would take a politician, which is why Doblin often says that MAPS doesn't "really do science; we do political science."[28]

It's easy to see how pragmatic politics shaped, and continue to shape, Doblin's decisions—like the choice to pursue medicalization as a path to legalization or his more recent decision to partner with veterans who have PTSD. He's open about the political choices he makes—his goal has always been to use medicalization to legalize psychedelics more generally. He often tells journalists, "It's a fundamental human right to explore your consciousness."[29] As Doblin saw it, gaining FDA approval to use MDMA as a medicine was just the first step. He has always been playing the long game.

MAPS may have still been a small operation in 2003 when Bob Wold first contacted him, but it had already made some real progress. It even had a few clinical trials underway.

●  ●  ●●●●●●●●●●●●●●●●●●  ●  ●

Doblin still remembers the first email exchange he had with Bob Wold back in 2003, shortly after Wold started to take Weil's emailed offer seriously. "Wold was like we're doing psychedelic research, and we don't want to be criminals. Can you help us try to study this?"

Doblin had set up MAPS to do exactly what Wold was requesting—to organize clinical research on the health benefits of psychedelics. In addition to sharing this goal, Doblin also liked the fact that funding already existed. He hit reply.

"I'm glad to hear of the progress you have made in obtaining funding for research. MAPS would definitely be interested in being involved. MAPS could help you organize the research and could advise on how best to work with FDA."[30] MAPS offered consultants who could help connect an organization like Clusterbusters with academic researchers, assist with developing protocols for clinical trials, offer advice about handling the university's regulatory affairs, and provide expertise in handling the FDA and the DEA; it could also offer a much broader platform for communication about the study. They'd have a lot to discuss. "This is a complicated issue. Please call me to talk this over."[31]

That was Wednesday, November 12, 2003. They spent that Friday afternoon on the phone discussing, at length, how their two organizations might collaborate. Wold posted a detailed description of the conversation to the Clusterbusters message board just two days later.[32]

Doblin began by asking questions aimed at learning more about Bob Wold and the organization he represented.

Were they a legitimate nonprofit? "Not just yet, but in process."

Was cluster headache rare enough to qualify for "orphan drug status," which the US federal government offered to diseases affecting fewer than two hundred thousand people in the country? If it was, that could mean millions in federal funding. "Possibly. It's pretty unusual."

Doblin also had questions that seemed more specific to *his* interests. For example, as a man who'd always prioritized issues related to consciousness, he wanted to know if the psychedelic experience mattered in treatment. Wold explained people didn't need that big of a dose to treat themselves, but he speculated that the psychedelic effect of a larger dose might help with the trauma associated with cluster headache. It had certainly helped him.

Doblin also floated the idea of testing LSD, instead of, or in addition to, psilocybin in the clinical trial, which struck Wold as an odd choice, motivated more by Doblin's personal predilections than practicality. In principle, Wold agreed that LSD might be a better treatment than psilocybin based on reports from the few people in their survey who had tried it. But people were already frightened to try magic mushrooms. It would be even harder to convince people to take a drug as stigmatized as LSD. Plus, how would anyone source LSD? (Wold, I think, always envisioned academic research as a helpful resource for people to treat themselves.) Still, Wold said he'd consider the possibility.

Doblin later told me that he'd liked the idea of working with Clusterbusters from the get-go. The group told a good story about psychedelic medicine—a story that fit well with the "political science" he practiced at MAPS. Who, after all, could be more sympathetic than people suffering from a rare, debilitating disease? People still believed that psychedelics created the kind of neurotoxicity that could make someone suicidal, Doblin knew. But Clusterbusters used psychedelics to *avoid* suicide. "They were saying the opposite, that they're working for people who are suicidal because of the cluster headaches, that this is helping them cope," Doblin told me.

Better yet, Clusterbusters' desperate medical need presented a great counternarrative about criminality. If Bob Wold was a criminal, it was only because he was courageous enough to do the right thing despite the law. And Wold led an entire group just like himself: people who had come to the same conclusion that he had decades prior. According to Doblin, it was like they were saying, "We don't want to be criminals, but we're willing to do it because the medical community and the pharmaceutical industry have nothing for us. This is causing people to commit suicide and causing people to suffer incredibly. . . . We're criminals only because of medical necessity."

It's perhaps ironic that Doblin's embrace of criminality—however righteous—made Wold uncomfortable. Wold still worried about harming Clusterbusters by collaborating with MAPS. Did it make sense to work with an organization intent on keeping one foot in the underground if their primary goal was getting their own work aboveground?

"I'm still not convinced that MAPS is the place to do this but am interested in hearing more from them," he added in his post about the conversation. "I spoke to [Doblin] about my reservations with MAPS and the impressions that different organizations may give. Obviously, he didn't see any such problems with MAPS being involved and how that might be perceived by the 'establishment.'"[33]

The question, it turned out, was moot. Nobody in headache medicine felt equipped to take on a study with this much political and cultural baggage. Even Doblin, the most connected guy around, struggled to locate available psychedelic researchers with the necessary skills to conduct psychedelic research on cluster headache.

He did, however, have an idea that might work if Clusterbusters was willing to be patient. Over the past few years, Doblin had been cultivating a strong working relationship with John Halpern, a rising star in psychedelic medicine and a faculty member at Harvard Medical School's McLean Hospital. Doblin hadn't originally considered Halpern as a candidate for Clusterbusters' project since he was already quite busy working on a MAPS-sponsored clinical trial studying the therapeutic benefits of MDMA for those experiencing anxiety related to late-stage cancer. But he had his eyes on an emerging talent, a new physician who had recently accepted a position as a postdoctoral fellow at McLean Hospital, and who had an active interest in working with Halpern on psychedelic research.

Collaborating with Dr. R. Andrew Sewell, Doblin explained to Wold, presented a mix of opportunities and challenges. Sewell was much more junior than any of the physician-researchers they'd hoped to attract to their project. In fact, he was so junior, he was still completing his medical training. On the plus side, one could hardly ask for a physician with a better pedigree. Sewell was just finishing a distinguished dual residency in neurology *and* psychiatry at Massachusetts General, the original and largest of all the teaching hospitals affiliated with Harvard Medical School. Sewell's unusual decision to complete two residencies had lengthened his training by two years, but he would graduate soon. If Clusterbusters could wait until September 2004, they would land a veritable superstar on the rise. Halpern's mentorship would bridge the gap between potential and expertise.

But there was another problem. Although Doblin and Halpern had been instrumental in Sewell's decision to take a postdoctoral fellowship at Harvard's McLean Hospital—Sewell, apparently, had long harbored a desire to study psychedelics—neither had the funding to hire him. Instead, Sewell accepted a fellowship paid for by McLean's Alcohol and Drug Abuse Research Center. His new supervisors, the codirectors of the addiction center, agreed that Sewell could collaborate with Halpern in his spare time. Sewell didn't mind additional work. He had been prepared for this sort of thing—he knew that becoming a psychedelic researcher would be hard.

If they were looking for advantages, McLean stood out as an exceptional choice. Imagine having Clusterbusters' research conducted at Harvard Medical School's largest psychiatric hospital—an institution that ran the world's most extensive neuroscientific and psychiatric research program.[34] And its reputation was stellar: McLean has long been a refuge for celebrities, artists, and Boston's elite, including Ray Charles, James Taylor, and Sylvia Plath.

Doblin wished he could do better, but he was also out of ideas. He wrote to Wold, "I don't know of anyone else interested in undertaking such research, so am temporarily at a loss about how to proceed."[35]

Wold considered this new information carefully. He knew nothing about this new postdoctoral fellow, but he knew people took Harvard University seriously. Marsha Weil told Wold that she felt much the same: "If we could work with Harvard, with MAPS help, that would be great. To have a major university conducting our trials would be a major bonus for us."[36]

●  ●  ●●●●●●●●●●●●●●●●●●●●●  ●  ●

Sewell, for his part, seemed enthusiastic about the possibility of collaborating with Clusterbusters.

He emailed Bob Wold right away: "Your results are very intriguing! I'm sure I don't have to tell you that dihydroergotamine [DHE], one of the treatments we use for cluster headaches, is derived from ergot just as LSD can be. Prophylaxing against future headaches is something we have no other drug for, however, and I can't help but think that if we studied this, we might learn a lot about the pathogenesis of cluster headaches, as well as helping those who currently suffer from them."[37]

Wold liked Sewell right away. Only the best kind of nerds were this enthusiastic and knowledgeable about cluster headache. Maybe this guy was worth the wait. "We have no delusions of this becoming a pill to take with a prescription any time in the next couple of years. We understand the obstacles and the time involved. We just want to get the ball rolling, so to speak, and make sure it keeps rolling," Wold replied.

Sewell understood. He replied, "[I do] not share Dr. Doblin's optimism regarding the speed that we can get approval for clinical trials, however—I'm steeling myself for a long and enervating bureaucratic slog before we can get this off the ground. But psychedelic research is not for dilettantes."

Sewell kept saying the right things.

It would only take a few more emails and phone calls before Doblin made the relationship between Clusterbusters, MAPS, and Harvard official. A letter signed late February 2004 confirmed their agreement to "work together to conduct FDA-approved research into the use of psilocybin and LSD in the treatment and prevention of cluster headaches."[38] A subsequent memo of understanding laid out the financials. The Weils would donate $25,000 to MAPS in April or May 2004 "for the protocol design and approval process and for the study itself" and "up to . . . a $25,000 matching grant," which would be used for fund-raising purposes. "If the project is not approved by either the McLean [Institutional Review Board] or the FDA, MAPS will, subject to the donors' instructions, return all funds remaining unspent to the donors or retain them for other efforts approved by the donor."[39]

● ● ●●●●●●●●●●●●●●●●●●● ● ●

Feb 29, 2004.
Cyberspace.

Congratulations to all members of Clusterbusters. I [Bob Wold] received the hard copy of the confirmation letter from MAPS today. We are officially underway for Clinical Trials. . . . You are all allowed to smile and receive a pat on the back.

Cheers rolled in from the far corners of the internet. It seemed an almost unbelievable achievement. "Congratulations Bob . . . amazing," wrote GeorgieT. "And Harvard, too. Don't know how you pulled it off."

"How?" Wold replied. "I don't know for sure." He just did what he could, as fast as he could. "Taking the night off."

Wold deserved a break that night, but he'd be back at work tomorrow. Everyone else on the forum would need to get back to work too. The sales pitch to Harvard included more than just funding. Wold had promised data. Lots of it. Evidence that psychedelic therapy worked better as an abortive than sumatriptan. Evidence that it worked better as a preventative, "easily outscoring IV DHE, IV histamine, or anything else available." And evidence that "single-maintenance doses taken [in] three- to twelve-month intervals stop the cycles from returning in any way."[40]

Getting that data in order by the time Andrew Sewell started working at Harvard in October would take *a lot* of work. But they needed to celebrate every step in the right direction if they had any hope of enduring the long road ahead.

## Chapter Twelve

● ● ●●●●●●●●●●●●●●●● ● ●

# THE HEALER

Doctors must also be healers.

Treating people with substance use disorders, John Halpern explained to me, required nothing less. "Suffice it to say, back in medical school I got blasted for encouraging people who were opiate dependent to come to my clinic in the evening."

"What are these junkies doing in our clinic, Halpern?"

Wait, what? Halpern couldn't believe the attending physician was angry that he'd been successfully encouraging people to get the medical help they needed. Nor did he appreciate hearing patients derided as junkies. But even brash young med students know that a combative attitude won't get them anywhere. "I saw them in the emergency room and referred them to the clinic," he'd told his attending. People who use intravenous drugs often get infections from dirty needles. Their wounds would get gnarly if he didn't convince them to get treatment. "I communicated with them well."

"Fuck these patients," Halpern remembered the physician saying. "We don't have the resources to treat them. These people create problems."

Halpern didn't understand. He might have been new to medicine, but he'd seen enough to know that intravenous drug users only checked themselves into the emergency room under the most desperate of circumstances. Everyone deserved care. He had a moral imperative to tell patients how to get safe, nonjudgmental treatment. But he was "told that if [people who were opiate dependent] continued to come in, this guy was going to flunk [him.]"

Halpern slogged through the rest of his rotation, feeling terrible about the whole thing. There must be a better, more humane medical system that treated everyone, even so-called junkies, with care and compassion.

Halpern knew exactly whom to ask. His father, Dr. Abraham Halpern, a leading professor of psychiatry, was known for both his intellectual contributions as a forensic psychiatrist and his work as a lifelong champion of human rights. Halpern adored his father, "a very sweet, compassionate, brilliant person . . . far, far smarter than anyone else I know."

Halpern could remember his dad playing chess blindfolded against multiple players. "He could play three games simultaneously. He would turn his chair. Table one, table two, table three. He couldn't handle table four. And so, if you had a fourth game, he'd still win the three, but he couldn't . remember the moves on the fourth one." He beamed with pride when listing his father's accomplishments. Highlights included a flight to Selma, Alabama, in 1965, where he provided medical support to protesters marching with Dr. Martin Luther King Jr.; a decades-long record of protesting the death penalty; and a long alliance with the Falun Gong.

For Halpern, being able to visit his parents more often was a perk of attending medical school in New York. Respite from the hustle of the city was just a short train ride away. Mamaroneck, his hometown in Westchester County, lay twenty miles north of the city, but its verdant parks and sandy coastline made it feel like a different world.

On one of his trips home, Halpern's father invited his son to join him in conversation with an old friend who happened to be staying with the family that weekend, an Indian Canadian psychiatrist named Dr. Chunilal Roy—a perfect opportunity for a young med student to ask for advice, really.

Halpern could hardly have anticipated their response to his most recent experience in medical school. "They wound up talking about psychedelics in the sixties and [how] they actually showed a lot of promise for treating addiction."

At first, Halpern couldn't believe what he was hearing.

Psychedelics worked wonderfully, Dr. Roy explained, but the government shut down the research once the drugs left the laboratories for the street. Dr. Roy knew about their healing power firsthand from research he conducted in the 1960s into the prevalence of alcohol addiction among First Nations peoples in Saskatchewan.

Roy's results had been alarming: nearly everybody surveyed fit into his operational definition of an alcoholic. Intriguingly, the only exceptions he found were those who belonged to the Native American Church, which Roy attributed to their ceremonial use of peyote.[1]

Dr. Roy's story ignited Halpern's curiosity. Halpern returned to medical school, determined to read everything he could find on psychedelic medicine.

Halpern's research revealed signs that a crack might be forming in the prohibition against psychedelic research. Three years earlier, in 1990, the federal government had permitted Dr. Rick Strassman, a Buddhist and a clinical professor of psychiatry at the University of New Mexico, to inject dimethyltryptamine (DMT), a powerful hallucinogenic substance, into healthy human subjects to help understand the relationship between psychedelics and mystical experiences.

Reading this, Halpern knew he'd stumbled upon a unicorn. Strassman's research was the first—and for a long time the only—clinical trial testing psychedelic substances in human subjects that the federal government had approved since the 1970s.[2] He sent Strassman a letter of introduction to ask if he was accepting research interns. "I wound up doing a research subinternship with him in 1994, for six or eight weeks, while finishing up my fourth year at medical school . . . administering DMT to people," Halpern told me.

Halpern graduated medical school in 1994 as one of the only medical doctors in the United States with experience administering psychedelics to human subjects in a clinical trial. In 1996, he published an article reviewing existing research on the use of psychedelics as a treatment for addiction and pointing toward their promise.[3] By 1997, he was conducting his own research on the use of peyote as a sacrament in the Native American Church, under the mentorship of Harvard Medical School professor Dr. Harrison G. Pope Jr., one of the most prestigious drug researchers in the country. Halpern's star was on the rise.

●　●　●●●●●●●●●●●●●●●●●●●●　●　●

As I discussed in Chapter 7, scientists like Dr. Roy have been learning about the medicinal use of psychoactive plants and fungi from indigenous people for centuries. In fact, psychedelic historian Erika Dyck has described how in 1956, at Weyburn Hospital in Saskatchewan, Humphry Osmond and Abram Hoffer's participation in a Native American Church peyote ceremony helped inspire their pioneering research on LSD-assisted therapy for alcohol addiction.[4] Given all this, I began to wonder if my entire premise regarding Clusterbusters might be wrong: Did they deserve credit for their "discovery" of psychedelic medicine for headache disorders, given how much of what we know about these drugs came from indigenous populations?

Most people interested in psychedelics have heard the story about how, in 1957, an investment banking executive and amateur mycologist named R. Gordon Wasson brought knowledge about "magic mushrooms" to Westerners when *Life* magazine, one of the most popular publications at the time, published his beautifully photographed travelogue describing his experience taking the fungi with the Mazatec people in Oaxaca, Mexico, during one of their ritual ceremonies.[5] But as historians have pointed out, even this narrative excludes the contributions of Wasson's wife, Dr. Valentina Wasson, who was not only his collaborator on this project but also a physician and a scientist with an extensive background in mycology. *This Week* magazine published Dr. Wasson's account of the journey to Oaxaca, alongside an interview describing her belief that the mushroom would become an important medication that she thought might be especially useful as a treatment for "terminal diseases associated with severe pain."[6]

The Wassons had a mutual interest in the relationship between mushrooms and culture that inspired their travels around the world. In 1952,

Gordon Wasson received an irresistible tip. A Harvard professor had confirmed that the ancient Aztecs' *teonanácatl* referred to the *Panaeolus sphinctrinus* mushroom still used by indigenous healers in Oaxaca. Wasson immediately started making plans to get to Mexico.

In 1953, the Wassons brought their daughter to Oaxaca for their first of ten expeditions to Huautla de Jimenez, the town where the divine mushroom had originally been spotted. Traveling the narrow roads to the northern mountain village from New York required physical stamina, tenacity, and at least one pack mule to carry their belongings once the route became impassable by car. It must have also been expensive.

Upon arrival the family learned that generations of persecution had made the locals reluctant to talk about their mushroom rituals. Still, they managed to observe a local mushroom ceremony during their first visit to Huautla by duping their guide, Aurelio Carreras, with a sob story about their son's declining health and emotional well-being.[7]

Much to their delight, Carreras turned out to be a *curandero*, a traditional healer who held sacred ceremonies for the locals. Carreras would allow the Wassons to observe one of these *veladas* so long as they understood Westerners were not permitted to consume these mushrooms themselves.

The Wassons had better luck on their third trip to Huautla in 1955. This time, Gordon Wasson gained the trust of a local official, using the same pretext that worked with Carreras—he was worried about the health of his son. The official introduced him to a local *curandera* named María Sabina, whose skills of divination he so admired that she often acted as his advisor. Sabina, in turn, trusted the official and agreed to allow Wasson and his friend, a professional photographer, to attend that evening's *velada*.

Like her ancestors, María Sabina couldn't say with precision what year she was born, but her mother, María Concepción, told her it was in the morning of the day they celebrated the Virgin Magdalene in Huautla, the Mazatec village in Oaxaca close to where they lived. (Alvaro Estrado, her biographer, a Mazatec Indian from Huautla who recorded this information via interviews he conducted with her, would later discover in records that she was born on March 17, 1894).[8]

Sabina's father had suffered from an illness for years before dying young. Their family brought him to a variety of healers, which, in an isolated place like Huautla, meant he would be treated by *chjote chinje*, that is "people of knowledge," "wise men," or, in Spanish, *curanderos*.

*Curanderos* used the divine power of local mushrooms—which they sometimes call "child saints"—to travel to the spiritual world and ask for help healing the ailing. The spirits could then choose to provide the wise one with chants and songs, herbs and salves, or other modes of healing to cure those seeking help. But little could be done when the spirits refused their help, as was the case with Sabina's father.

It was a familiar scenario in Mazatec healthcare. The wisdom of divine mushrooms wasn't heritable, but like Sabina's father, most people had a familial relationship—however distant—with their *curanderos*. Similarly, most people sought mushroom vigils for help with health problems. However, illness for the Mazatec might be caused by several problems. Sometimes they just had a backache. But other times, poor health might be connected to either the psyche or the spiritual world.

Sabina and her younger sister, María Ana, began eating the local mushrooms when still children. Sabina knew she could eat the mushrooms because her grandparents spoke of them with great respect, and she had witnessed a wise man using them to heal her uncle. The mushrooms, she said, made him sing in a language that "spoke of stars, animals, and other things unknown to me," and "he danced while he said that he 'saw' animals, objects, and people."[9]

Two weeks after she had seen her uncle healed by the wise man, she found the same mushrooms under a tree and thought, "If I eat you, you, and you . . . I know that you will make me sing beautifully."[10]

She also liked how the mushrooms made her feel content and sated her hunger. One day while eating mushrooms, her dead father appeared and asked her to kneel and pray. She would eventually learn that "the mushrooms were like God. That they gave wisdom, that they cured illnesses, and that our people, since a long time ago, had eaten them. That they had power, that they were the blood of Christ."[11]

"In truth," she told her biographer, "I was born with my destiny. To be a Wise Woman. To be a daughter of the saint children."[12] She would fulfill this destiny all too soon when her only sister, María Ana, fell ill. Sabina, who couldn't bear to lose her sister, decided to heal her using the saint children. As was customary, she gave her sister a few pairs of mushrooms to eat during the ceremony. But Sabina ate many more, about thirty pairs, because she knew she would need "immense power."[13]

The mushrooms worked: she prayed while the saint children told her exactly what to say, how to sing, and how to use her hands to assist her sister. Her sister hemorrhaged while Sabina chanted and sang. But the visions continued. The "little ones" offered her a large white book filled with the wisdom of her people. She couldn't read, but she understood its knowledge just the same. The saint children's book provided her with the language to speak to God and, when possible, to heal the sick with her chants and songs.

Sabina knew she had become one of the wise ones when María Ana recovered. But unlike other curers and sorcerers, whom she considered "frauds," Sabina always maintained allegiance to Catholicism and believed that healing ought to be provided for free. Those seeking treatment were, however, expected to pay for the *hongos*, or fungus, and most brought gifts for the saints on the healers' altars.

Gordon Wasson believed Sabina was the real deal. Sabina, he wrote, had "a spirituality in her expression" and a "presence" that struck him as ancient in quality. Everything about the ceremony—even the chocolate the children drank that night—oozed with the authenticity he expected to find in a primitive ceremonial rite.

Dressed in her finest *huipil*, Sabina allocated pairs of mushrooms to all those taking them, reserving twice as many for herself and her daughter.[14] Wasson gnawed on his mushrooms, noting they "tasted bad—acrid with a rancid odor." In an hour or so, he would begin to see visions, first angular and vivid and then more intense and resplendent. In the meantime, Sabina chanted, invoking the mushroom in the name of Christ and the saints. She may not have been able to read, but every line purified Wasson with its poetry. Wasson said the experience left him "awestruck." "For the first time, the word ecstasy took on real meaning."[15]

A few days later Wasson's wife, physician Valentina Pavlovna Wasson, and their adult daughter joined him in Huautla to assist in his investigations. But heavy rains marooned them in town for two weeks—the roads were too muddy for travel, and their plane had no place to land. When Gordon Wasson offered his family the chance to take the mushrooms he'd found, they decided that hallucinations seemed like an improvement on their current situation: huddled in sleeping bags on the dirt floor of a small, damp, chilly, and windowless hut.

Plus, Dr. Wasson came up with a scientific justification for trying the mushrooms: Would they work without the presence of a shaman? They did. "It was as if my very soul had been scooped out and moved to a point in heavenly space, leaving my empty physical husk behind in the mud hut," she wrote.[16]

Neither of the Wassons' articles mentioned that Sabina only agreed to allow their participation in exchange for secrecy, including the promise never to publish the photos they had taken. Nor did they mention the false pretext used to convince Sabina to invite them to the ceremony in the first place: they never did have any concerns about their son's well-being. And while Wasson did use a pseudonym in place of María Sabina's real name and kept the name Huautla out of the popular press, the Wassons revealed her real name and the location of the mushrooms in their 1957 book *Mushrooms, Russia and History.*[17]

Given our history of stealing knowledge from indigenous people without thought or remuneration, perhaps we shouldn't be surprised by the devastation that followed. But sure enough, their disclosure of Sabina's identity and the location of her town would have tragic consequences for the *curandera* and the healing practice her people had engaged in for as long as we have recorded history.

Within months, travelers began seeking "magic mushrooms." By the 1960s, the formerly quiet mountain town was overwhelmed by hippies who couldn't have been more different from the Mazatec in behavior, dress, and values. Legend has it that celebrities like Bob Dylan, John Lennon, and

Mick Jagger joined the hordes of long-haired, poorly behaved visitors seeking adventure and spiritual renewal in Huautla.

María Sabina may have provided many of these travelers with *veladas*, but that didn't mean that she liked them. By the end of the decade, a veritable tsunami of countercultural pilgrims had transformed Huautla into a tourist destination, where travelers could easily purchase Sabina's saint children in open markets. It was like the naked hordes from Woodstock arriving in New Guinea, bathing in sacred streams, and having sex on the hillsides. Residents grew so frustrated that the municipality requested assistance from the Mexican government. In response, the army created military checkpoints to keep foreigners out of Huautla and the surrounding region between 1968 and 1976.[18]

Our collective memory considers the 1960s counterculture a revolutionary moment aligned with the values of the civil rights movement. However, the true narrative is more complex. Yes, hippies threatened the status quo regarding certain values: sex, drugs, music, marriage, religion, and military service. Embracing new spiritual practices, like meditation and yoga, promoted a sense that the counterculture really did want to transform the world. But as the swarms of tourists in Huautla demonstrate, romanticizing "exotic" spiritual and cultural practices is not the same as respecting, including, and offering reciprocal benefits to the people at the very heart of these cultures. People went to Huautla to experience a *velada* on their terms, as consumers rather than as welcome guests, and took more than they offered, ignoring how their own behavior contributed to the problems in the town.

María Sabina's newfound fame made her a countercultural icon. Her image was painted on murals across Mexico and emblazoned on T-shirts. In turn, this fame brought tourist dollars into the town, showering Huautla with revenue. But the townspeople were not altogether happy with the changes they saw in their community. Only the wealthiest businessmen seemed to benefit from the cash brought in from tourists, and the community blamed Sabina for ruining their Mazatec customs.

Their retribution was harsh: they burned her wooden house and store to the ground, leaving her family to eat wild tubers to survive. Worst of all, Sabina felt that the foreigners weakened her powers of divinity. "Before

Wasson, I felt that the saint children elevated me. I don't feel like that any-more. The force has diminished. If . . . the foreigners [hadn't come], the saint children would have kept their power."[19]

María Sabina remained poor until the day she died.

In a foreword to Sabina's biography, Gordon Wasson wrote that he had "winced" when reading her words and wondered if Sabina, in her wisdom, had been right. He even asked, rhetorically, whether he was "responsible for the end of a religious practice in Mesoamerica that goes back far, for a millennium."[20] But he felt certain he had made the correct decision. If he kept his experience to himself, the world would know "vaguely" about the sacred mushroom but not its vital importance. Spreading this knowledge, he added, ensured Sabina gained the "prestige" she deserved.

Never mind that his actions exposed the Mazatec people's land, language, customs, and culture to appropriation and extraction.[21] For Wasson, the pur-suit of expanding knowledge was paramount, a quest that he pursued with a zeal that often overshadowed the profound contributions and rights of the indigenous cultures at the heart of his discoveries. Gordon Wasson also neglected to mention that he had a commercial motivation to share his expe-rience and knowledge with the public. It turns out that the Wassons' essays were little more than a publicity campaign for their newly published book.

Whether one agrees with the Wassons' actions or not, their decisions likely played a sizeable role in our burgeoning knowledge of the healing powers of mushrooms decades later.

Upon return from their visit with Sabina, Gordon Wasson invited the prestigious mycologist Professor Roger Heim, from the National Museum of Natural History in Paris, to assist in the identification and description of the mushroom species growing near Huautla. Heim joined Wasson on his next trip to Mexico to collect samples for his French laboratory, but he also eagerly participated in one of Sabina's *veladas*. Once Heim had propagated enough mushrooms, he sent samples to Albert Hofmann, the Swiss chemist who had discovered LSD fifteen years earlier in his lab at Sandoz.

It was from mushrooms collected from Sabina's village that Hofmann isolated psilocybin and psilocin. In 1958 and 1959, when Sandoz filed three patents under Hofmann's name for psilocybin and psilocin, Wasson was not credited. However, he presumably benefited financially from these patents, as evidenced by Sandoz appointing him as a director in one of its American subsidiaries.

The rush to patent, let alone profit from, a healing cure that has existed for millennia hasn't slowed down since then. Plenty of others are lining up to snag a piece of the psilocybin pie: The US Patent and Trademark Office has granted seventy-eight patents related to psilocybin since Roger Heim and Albert Hofmann's 1958 patent. But they only represent about a fifth of the applications that have been submitted for consideration. One can only imagine how many more will follow.

It's difficult to overstate the extent to which Gordon Wasson profited from this extraction, given that he receives most of the credit for the "discovery" of *Psilocybe caerulescens*, even though he'd learned about its existence from ethnobotanists, and they, of course, knew that the indigenous people of the region had been using it for centuries. In fact, he is now known as the "father of ethnomycology." Two *Psilocybe* mushroom species are named after the Wassons: *Psilocybe wassonii heim* and *Psilocybe wassonorum guzmán*. Wasson was named an honorary research fellow of the Harvard Botanical Museum and elected a fellow of the Linnean Society of London. He also received Yale University's Addison Emery Verrill medal for outstanding contributions to natural history.

There are, you might not be surprised to learn, no mushroom species named after María Sabina.

● ● ●●●●●●●●●●●●●●●●●●● ● ●

Gordon Wasson behaved poorly. But was I judging him too harshly, given a comfortable sixty years of hindsight? Was the inequity in his exchanges with María Sabina par for the course for researchers in the mid-twentieth century? Did the rediscovery of psychedelics need to be so one-sided, extractive, and exploitative?

It turned out that I needn't look far to locate a different model of scientific engagement with indigenous people in the Americas.

Richard Evans Schultes (1915–2001) was the Harvard biology professor whose original research had provided the Wassons with the location of the divine mushroom that they had been seeking for decades. However, descriptions of Schultes, known as "the father of ethnobotany," paint him as having a genuine humility and respect for the collective wisdom that indigenous communities held about the medicinal uses of local plants and fungi.

Take, for example, the relationship he nurtured with indigenous communities in the Colombian Amazon. After completing his dissertation research at Harvard in 1941, Schultes traveled to Colombia to study curare, a plant-based neurotoxin that certain indigenous tribes used in their poison arrows. Whereas some scientists might feel compelled to bring a weapon for defense when traveling into a jungle filled with jaguars and peopled with tribes that used poison arrows, Schultes expressed a more open-minded sentiment—albeit in somewhat cringey colonial language. He needn't fear, as there were no "hostile Indians." Everyone, he felt certain, would reciprocate his own "gentlemanliness."[22]

Schultes, therefore, brought little with him other than "a pith helmet, an aluminum canoe, a minimum of food and medical supplies, plant-pressing materials, and one change of clothes,"[23] preferring to rely on local hospitality. Shamans, he found, provided him with extraordinarily rich information. Building trust, he believed, entailed his participating in a tribe's activities, including ritual ceremonies.

His adventures in the jungle would produce a huge amount of knowledge. Indigenous people, he found, used over seventy plants and fifteen ingredients to make poison arrows. Collaborators would go on to discover that curare and its derivatives had practical medical applications as a muscle relaxant, as an anesthetic, and for the treatment of tetanus.

It's easy to see why biographers would later describe Schultes as a real-life Indiana Jones. He taught his popular class, Plants and Human Affairs, in a Harvard classroom so decked out with cultural artifacts collected during his travels that it could have been mistaken for an anthropological museum. Students wondering whether botany might hold their interest would discover they best not let their attention stray the first time Schultes chose to whiz a dart from his eight-foot blowgun over their heads.

But unlike the fictional Indiana Jones, whose modus operandi often seemed to be theft of cultural artifacts for consumption (Indy has always been transparent that he will work for whoever will pay him to retrieve items of value), Schultes worked to preserve the lands and protect the people he studied.

The "healing forest," as Schultes called it, contained plants and fungi that could be extracted for all kinds of uses.[24]

But he insisted that the best way to understand these resources would be to "take advantage of the store of knowledge in the possession of the . . . native practitioners of the world's so-called primitive societies." Sure, biochemists could do the work on their own, but this would take decades, if not longer. Instead, he implored colleagues to "take advantage of what aboriginal peoples have learned over the centuries . . . [as] a kind of 'short cut' for deciding which of the 500,000 or so plant species in the world most urgently demand examination."[25]

A cynic might read Schultes's advocacy for forest conservation as a kind of greenwashing so he and others like him could continue exploiting indigenous knowledge. I'm sure there are plenty of reasons to critique the man—he was a white, male Harvard professor in the mid-1900s who used artifacts from the Global South to shoot darts at students—but his overall conduct indicates a willingness to collaborate and reciprocate with the communities he encountered. Schultes's extraordinary exploration of the northwestern Amazon brought him into contact with awe-inspiring landscapes, remnants of ancient Andean civilizations, and isolated indigenous tribes who had never seen a white person. He'd been warned along the way of the viciousness of tribes, only to find that even the most feared offered their plant knowledge with generosity.

Schultes returned to America convinced that these lands and the people who called them home must be protected at all costs. His advocacy, combined with the authority of his research, was in large part the driving force behind the 1989 creation of the Serranía de Chiribiquete National Park, the largest protected tropical rainforest in the world. Three uncontacted tribes call this park their home.[26]

All this knowledge, gained—or stolen, depending on your viewpoint—from indigenous communities, led directly back to the profit-making halls of some of the largest pharmaceutical companies in the world. But unlike the indigenous peoples, who had generations of knowledge about the power and possibilities of these substances, the scientists had no idea what the hell to do with them at first.[27] Some of those researchers thought reciprocation mattered. Others didn't.

In the world of scientific knowledge, Harvard University sits prominently on the top of the mound of influence. Its red shield promises nothing less than *veritas*, or truth. If the credibility of scientific claims depends on institutional backing, then the "Harvard" signifier provides research with formidable strength in the marketplace of ideas.

*Was it difficult to become a psychedelic researcher at a Harvard Medical School–affiliated hospital,* I wondered? When I asked, Halpern assured me that his interest in psychedelic research posed no barriers to his career. "I told my residency director [at Harvard] up front that I wanted to study psychedelics for addiction. He's like 'You're here to do your psychiatry residence.' I said, 'Of course, but I just want you to know.'"

In the last year of his medical residency, Halpern accepted a scholarship as a research fellow to work with Jack Mendelsohn, one of the codirectors of McLean's Alcohol and Drug Abuse Research Center. That's how Halpern met his "key mentor" at Harvard, Dr. Harrison G. Pope.

Halpern described Pope, whom he refers to as "Skip," as a "Wile E. Coyote super genius" who could claim credit to a laundry list of discoveries in psychiatry. "First person to publish on steroids being abusable. . . . First person to write about serotonin syndrome. . . . First person to write about body dysmorphic disorder—people who think they're small when they're big. That was all discovered by him. First person to discover that Depakote [can treat bipolar disorder] . . . that's Skip."

Pope also had a publication record of studying some of the same psychoactive drugs that interested Halpern. One of Pope's earliest publications, a literature review about iboga, a plant with hallucinogenic properties found in Gabon, was originally written as a term paper for the course Plants and

Human Affairs, taught by Richard Evans Schultes. Pope, Halpern continued, also wrote a book called *Voices from the Drug Culture*, which offered an unusually neutral portrayal of illicit drug use.[28] According to Halpern, Pope had even published a first-person account of injecting DMT. (I couldn't find this, and Pope said it wasn't true. And while Pope is a highly respected figure in psychiatry, he hadn't discovered serotonin syndrome. Most everyone I interviewed had a faulty memory, but I would eventually discover that Halpern's tendency to exaggerate made him a particularly unreliable narrator.)

In any case, Halpern identified Pope as the "perfect person" at McLean Hospital to seek out for advice. Halpern, who has a knack for doing impressions, reenacted the fateful encounter, adopting Pope's "Boston Brahmin voice."

"You know, Halpern," he began, really laying on a thick accent, "I'm not really interested in your ideas of studying a cohort of hallucinogen users. I mean, you're never going to find a population of pure, hallucinogen users anyway."

Halpern replied, "What about Native Americans? Peyote users use peyote, and they've never used other drugs at all. So, there's the cohort."

Pope dismissed the idea. "Nah, when's the last time you heard anybody with a problem from peyote? Sorry."

But the next day, Pope called Halpern at the break of dawn. "'Halpern, when's the last time [the National Institutes of Health] had a study of just a couple hundred Native Americans in it?' I said, 'I don't know, Skip, when? How many? When was the last time?' He goes, 'I'll tell you, never. Come see me immediately.'"

Although the federal government seemed hell-bent on stopping university researchers from experimenting with psychedelics on human subjects, rules about collecting data from people who already used these substances were considerably more relaxed. The government funded this kind of research all the time, so they could better understand drug abuse. There were ethical considerations, of course, like ensuring the confidentiality of participants and avoiding any influence on their drug use behaviors. However, the ethical and legal implications of observing how people use drugs are much easier to navigate than the complex and stringent regulations involved in administering drugs to human subjects in a clinical trial.

If they played their cards right, Halpern could design a study of the Native American Church that would lay the groundwork for future research revealing the benefits of psychedelic use.

Negotiating access to the Native American Church, a community with reasons to be wary about nonnative researchers, took a while. Halpern spent a few years traveling to the Navajo (Diné) Nation to explain his intentions and earn their trust.[29]

Conventional wisdom held that the National Institute on Drug Abuse (NIDA) did not fund research investigating the positive effects of illicit drug use. (The phrase *drug abuse* in their name reveals some of this bias.) Pope and Halpern's research proposal to NIDA framed their study in the most pessimistic way they could muster, using neutral language as a title for their grant: "Cognitive Effects of Substance Use in Native Americans."

The proposal sailed through NIDA's review process, securing Halpern a "training" grant to study the Native American Church under Dr. Harrison Pope's mentorship. Their research, which found no evidence of psychological or cognitive deficits in Native Americans who used peyote in a religious setting, became a crucial piece of evidence in the struggle to maintain religious freedom to use peyote.[30]

Halpern's years spent with the Native American Church shaped how he approached the study of psychedelics and, at least to some extent, his life. The system of law might place constraints on the kinds of research he could do, but his study of the Native American Church provided a potent model for designing psychedelic research within the system's constraints.

The approach proved especially handy when it came to solving one of Rick Doblin's biggest challenges: demonstrating the safety of MDMA. A panic that Ecstasy caused lasting "brain damage" had gained a foothold at NIDA, and the mass media were running with it. But the research driving this fear didn't comport with the underground's experience using the drug. (One of the most influential of these studies was retracted from the journal *Science*.) Demonstrating the safety of MDMA, however, would be a challenge. Risk of neurotoxicity made it even harder to get approval for the clinical research they would need to test its safety on humans. But the other option—obtaining data from people who danced all night at raves—introduced all sorts of "con-founding" variables. The effects of staying up all night and taking lots of other drugs might look like a cognitive deficit.

A doctoral student from the University of Utah contacted Doblin with a solution. He, like many other young Mormons, refrained from using drugs that their religion explicitly forbade. But he felt free to take lots of MDMA, since it wasn't mentioned in the rules. No "polypharmacy" to muck up the research. Doblin introduced the student to Halpern.[31] Studying young Mormons like this student, Halpern explained in his grant application to NIDA, offered "a unique population of nearly 'pure' ecstasy users" that would allow him to assess the long-term effects of MDMA use. NIDA provided him with a $1.8 million grant to fund the study. That money would secure at least 60 percent of his salary between 2004 and 2009.[32]

Halpern, therefore, understood that solid, "naturalistic" data sources made it possible to do psychedelic research. Moreover, he knew early on that the internet contained a veritable treasure trove of the kinds of data that drug researchers like him had long sought.[33] So when he and Clusterbusters found each other, perhaps Halpern had lucked into a far more convenient way to conduct the research he'd already been doing so well. The internet simply offered a new way to locate, observe, and collect data from the communities that ethnobotanists had always studied—something more akin to *cyberbotany*, the study of knowledge created in online communities.

Did Halpern view Clusterbusters as Gordon Wasson, the bioprospector, might have—that is, not as a community of care or a group of people with problems that needed solving, but as a source of knowledge he could willfully extract? Or did he view Clusterbusters as Professor Schultes implored his fellow ethnobotanists to: as allies with whom we shared an interdependent relationship. If we wanted to continue learning from those who knew the most about "the healing forest," then shouldn't we also extend our respect and protection?

Unfortunately, as the story unfolded, Bob Wold and Clusterbusters would soon learn the same lesson as María Sabina did all those years ago. Sometimes science can break your heart.

## Chapter Thirteen

• • ••••••••••••••••••• • •

# WHOSE KNOWLEDGE?

B OB AND MARY WOLD ARRIVED IN BOSTON ON THURSDAY, OCTOBER 21, 2004, just over six years after Flash's landmark post on CH.com. It was near midnight when they made it to their suburban hotel, but Bob never needed much sleep. Mary settled in for the night, knowing that Bob would be better off outside pacing the parking lot, where the crisp air and a steady stream of nicotine could steady his nerves while he ran through their weekend's plan for the thousandth time.

Their mission—to bring psychedelics back to Harvard—seemed preposterous, but then again, so did the entire conceit of their organization. And yet they had already accomplished so much. Rick Doblin had already arranged a formal agreement between Clusterbusters and the Department of Psychiatry at Harvard Medical School's McLean Hospital. But as Wold was beginning to learn, they would need more than just an agreement to get this study off the ground. As estimates of the study's cost climbed, the reality of funding this project became ever more daunting.

Clusterbusters would need to enroll the full support of the university's administration—especially its Development Office—if it had any hope of success.

Wold had started finalizing plans for this trip a few weeks earlier. Tomorrow morning, he would eat breakfast with a group of Busters whom he had assembled to assist with his presentation at Harvard. Marsha Weil had traveled from Seattle to be there. Three others would be joining them: Mitch Derrick, a Texas musician and a key contributor to the board; Dan Bemowski, a Buster with years of experience working in nonprofits; and Stuart Miller, a lawyer and lobbyist based in the Washington, DC, area. Wold hoped they would look like the kind of people that Harvard administrators would respect. It would be all too easy for a skeptic to dismiss them as "addicts."

The "Boston Six," as they called themselves, would meet Doblin and Halpern at McLean Hospital for lunch before their conference with the higher-ups at the hospital. They would have two hours to make their case— if they were lucky. Halpern warned that their time with his supervisor, Dr. Harrison "Skip" Pope, might be cut short as he had other obligations.

Capturing his attention required strategy.

Doblin and Halpern decided Dr. Andrew Sewell ought to begin with a medical presentation about cluster headache. Wold understood their reasoning: Halpern might have been the more senior scholar of the two, but Sewell, a psychiatrist *and* a neurologist, would be leading the project. He was more than qualified to speak about headache disorders.

But Wold insisted that the agenda include a patient who could provide the lived experience of the disease to those gathered in the room. Wold had never given a PowerPoint presentation before—and the thought of presenting to a room filled with Harvard doctors terrified him—but he'd come to Boston for a reason. It would have to be him.

Wold took a drag from his cigarette, his ritual sacrament. Mary could pray for the both of them. He made up for his lack of faith by doubling down on preparation.

●  ●  ●●●●●●●●●●●●●●●●●●●  ●  ●

The next day, Wold considered each of the ten course credits he had earned from his local community college as he entered Harvard's McLean

Hospital. He was a mix of pride—*not bad for the son of a carpenter*, he thought to himself—and nerves. Whatever happened over the next two hours would not just reflect his own competence (or lack thereof). This represented important work for an entire patient community.

Stepping into the building felt like crossing into another world. He'd later describe the conference room as "a foreign land . . . a room full of history with portraits of old white men with white hair on every wall. The smell of aged wood paneling and that unmistakable air of academia" heightened the sense that he'd entered a new realm.[1] At least he had a cheering section in the Boston Six, including, as Wold often liked to quip, "the spirit of Timothy Leary . . . sitting in the corner."

The meeting went better than anybody could have anticipated. Halpern had ensured the room was filled with all the right stakeholders and political rainmakers: Pope, the senior faculty member who would need to sign off as supervisor, Jay Livingston from McLean's Development Office, and a representative from public affairs. Sewell opened with an overview of cluster headache as a disease. But the patients' descriptions of their struggles stole the show.

As Halpern remembers it, his colleagues found Wold's straightforward manner as compelling as he had. "His naivete . . . was a major advantage. He was very plainspoken, Illinois type, what you see is what you get. . . . He's got this way about him. He'll really listen carefully and respond accurately. He's got a technique of getting to the heart of the matter. . . . it's his own history. He knows that damn well. Might not have academic credentials like a professor but when it comes to what he's debilitated with, he's an expert on that."

If Wold knew one thing for certain, it was that while patient descriptions of pain may be harrowing, they are easily minimized. It would not be so easy, however, to turn away if they witnessed the visceral terror of an attack.

In retrospect, Wold wondered if he should have warned them about the graphic slice of verité documentary filmmaking they were about to see. But, instead, he let it unfold on the screen.

A man—let's call him Ben—is in a hotel room, becoming frantic as he adjusts the flow of his oxygen tank while pressing a non-rebreather mask to his face as the pain escalates. A moment later, a man, perhaps a friend, enters the room and begins to support Ben's upper body with one arm while using his free hand to press a cold washcloth over Ben's affected eye. Painful contortions push them both off the bed, around the room, and onto the floor in a morbid dance, set to the harrowing sound of Ben's moans.

Watching the video, Wold knew, would be distressing. People gasped. A few cried. Most everyone averted their eyes. Doblin called it "horrific."

According to those in attendance, Pope stayed after the presentation far longer than anybody anticipated, participating in a long, animated question and answer period addressing potential study designs. Had they determined the size of their initial trial? Which psychedelic substance did they plan on studying? Would they use a placebo in this early clinical trial, and if so, how would they find a convincing placebo for a psychedelic? How many times would each subject be required to take a psychedelic? Would volunteers need to undergo therapy before and/or after taking a psychedelic? Where would the experiment take place? What were the risks of taking these drugs? How did they plan to minimize potential harm to human subjects?

Brilliant questions on a topic that Rick Doblin loved discussing. Nobody yet needed to know that they'd been putting off the hard decisions about study design for months.

In the end, the meeting lasted twice as long as expected, ending only when the cleaning staff made it clear that the room was no longer available. A few days later, Halpern sent an email reporting, "Skip Pope is so moved that he will give Andrew and me any time we need with him, and he is fully on board. YES."[2] (Pope doesn't recall being "moved" but will concede that he "favored" the plan for this research.)

Halpern's report also included good news from Jay Livingston, whose office led fund-raising for the hospital. (I wasn't able to contact Livingston to confirm if this was true, but, according to Halpern's email, he had identified a major donor whose son had cluster headache, who might be willing to offer "seed money" for research.)

"Essentially," Halpern told the group, "we have the hospital in full support of what we are planning to start. Everything is falling into place so well, I am pinching myself wondering what we might have forgotten or when that other shoe is going to drop. Well, we will face definite uphill struggles on this, for sure, but we all are collectively bringing the fuel we'll need to get there."[3]

Doblin and Halpern treated the Boston Six to a charming weekend. Rick and his wife welcomed everyone to their home twice—first for a Friday evening Shabbat meal and then on Sunday morning for brunch. In between, Halpern invited everyone to Salem, Massachusetts, for a tour of the town, ablaze in New England's brilliant foliage, followed by a party at his sister's home. A perfect set and setting to create a partnership and develop plans to bring their clinical trial to Harvard.

The Boston Six returned home buoyed by their discovery of compassionate, empathetic, dedicated researchers who recognized that patients had insights worth championing. Bob Wold and Marsha Weil marveled at how easily everything had clicked into place in the end. Doblin, Halpern, and Sewell were the perfect people for their project—so perfect, it seemed "meant to be." Working with Doblin and Halpern felt like a new way to hack medicine.

The underground had found its perfect match aboveground. If only aboveground research weren't so slow.

●　●　●●●●●●●●●●●●●●●●●●●●　●　●

Wold delivered on his promise to bring plenty of evidence. By the time Sewell had arrived at McLean Hospital, Wold had compiled and submitted data from at least a hundred people who had experimented with the use of psychedelic substances in the treatment of cluster headache. By Wold's count, the outcomes were overwhelmingly positive. The only people who seemed to have any trouble at all with the treatment had chronic cluster headache. But even they usually managed to obtain at least a few pain-free weeks. And there was a bonus too. Those who also had migraine reported that the psychedelics worked on both forms of headache. It would be wonderful if their treatment had an application that helped even more people.

Rick Doblin, John Halpern, and Andrew Sewell said they were delighted. Publishing evidence like this would "help inform the various relevant agencies and individuals about our proposed study," according to Halpern.[4] Sewell agreed. "By way of comparison, a typical case series contains six to ten patients, so to have over a hundred is quite compelling." Doblin underscored how "essential" it was "to have case reports from your organization of people who were helped by their use of LSD," as well as "of course similar reports for psilocybin as well."[5]

In September 2004, Halpern assigned Sewell the task of reviewing Clusterbusters' "fantastically helpful" shroom stories, with an eye toward publishing a case-series study about the efficacy of this treatment in a peer-reviewed journal. He offered an ambitious timeline. Research on the case study would take about a month, at which point Sewell would invest his time in the far more important work of designing the clinical trial testing psychedelics as a treatment for cluster headache. Getting a clinical trial approved—which, after all, was their primary goal—and obtaining all the permissions they would need to begin could take up to two years.

Sewell got started right away. But he was almost immediately confronted with the enormity of the task. Clusterbusters' data had been collected in a piecemeal manner and in various formats. He had some great survey data, but it had some quirks, and there seemed to be a lot of missing data. He also had a pile of "shroom stories," which were qualitative narratives, usually written in the first person, reporting individuals' self-experiments and outcomes. Most everything had been submitted anonymously, so it was difficult—albeit not impossible—to match individual patients' stories with their survey results.

The first step was transforming the data into a single document. Sewell opened an excel sheet, labeling one "Cluster headache—LSD" and the other, "Cluster—psilocybin." Data for each person, who had now been assigned a single case number, could be neatly listed in a single row, and their entire history could be summarized in columns created for that purpose.

Case number: 75. Name: Eleanor. Age: 50. Sex: Female. Age of onset: 34. Maximum number of attacks per day: Six.

Sewell then combed through each report—regardless of whether it came from a shroom story or a survey—to locate the relevant data. This way, Sewell could make sure that everyone's data was in one place.

It didn't take long to realize how much vital information they were missing. Sewell sent an email to Wold describing all the missing bits and pieces. Some people, he wrote, offered very complete records of their attacks and the treatment. But others failed to include basic demographics like age and sex and details about the number of attacks they experienced. He could also see that medical histories were not complete. "Nonetheless, it looks as if the stuff does work, and the testimonials are impressive enough that I'm excited to begin a formal trial!"[6]

● ● ●●●●●●●●●●●●●●●●●●●● ● ●

Wold understood exactly why Sewell was having trouble.

When Wold took on the work of organizing Clusterbusters in 2002, he also inherited a half-finished data-collection project, which included a digital file stuffed with shroom stories and a link to a survey on Erowid. Other than including a link to the survey in their FAQs, he'd mostly forgotten about this side of the work—that is, until he made that big promise about all the evidence they had.

That's when he realized, with a growing pit in his stomach, that they'd never developed a system to collect new testimonials about the treatment.

Results reported in their forum—or worse, in CH.com's massive public forum—would be difficult to wrangle into something that looked like systematic data collection. And what were the chances that anyone had filled out that survey on Erowid if nobody was promoting the link?

Wold felt optimistic that his team would come through, but nearly everything in Sewell's possession had been pulled together in the previous nine months. The process had been messy.

He posted his first SOS in late November 2003. "We will be needing as much anecdotal evidence as we can muster. . . . Write a shroom story. Fill out the survey. Contact anybody you know who tried these drugs but isn't online anymore. Convince them to do it even if they are afraid of being caught. We need data."[7]

The response was dishearteningly tepid. Over the next three months, only thirteen people, himself included, heeded his call to complete the survey. Something must be wrong, but what? Clusterbusters were usually keen. Could it be a concern for anonymity? Because that seemed like a problem they could solve.

Wold suspected there might be an issue with the survey that Flash and Earth had designed. Most people, he noticed, skipped the section that asked how well the psychedelic treatment worked. This, of course, would present a problem if they wanted to document its effectiveness. But Wold also understood why someone might struggle to answer that set of questions, given the nature of self-experimentation. The survey made it seem like an experiment was a single, easily quantified intervention with a "before" and "after." But self-experimentation involved a lot of tweaking.[8]

The answer seemed to be a bit of both. People replied that they didn't understand *when* to submit their data. At what point in the self-experiment was it appropriate to submit a survey reporting an outcome? How should they submit a report if they were successful "busting" one cycle but not a second cycle? Should they submit a separate report every time they busted? If so, how should they identify themselves on an anonymous survey so that the surveys could be linked to each other?

Wold assigned everyone a case number and urged them to submit their experiences as often as possible, no matter the outcome. He encouraged anyone who forgot their case number to ask for a reminder—he could always look up their code in the master document he kept on file. Harnessing more data would only speed up the scientific process. He emphasized,

"This data is probably THE most important set of information we can gather at this point as far as getting government approval. Time is becoming an issue at this point."[9]

In the meantime, a volunteer offered to comb through both forums to find any testimonials they might have missed, which could then be added to the "shroom stories" that Jonas had begun collecting back in 2001. Piecing together these stories was no small feat. Each narrative had to be given the proper case number, then traced over time. It was detective work of sorts, tracking each person's step in their treatment—a painstaking process, requiring patience and a keen eye for detail, especially considering that search functions in 2004 were more hindrance than help.

● ● ●●●●●●●●●●●●●●●●●●●● ● ●

Wold's diligence, combined with the collective effort of patients around the world, produced a giant pile of disorganized reports. Half the data wasn't labeled with case numbers, so Wold spent most of that summer matching people's survey data with their shroom stories.

Even still, Sewell's analysis made it easy to see how much data they were missing. Halpern suggested a few options. The first possibilities would require that they obtain approval from their Institutional Review Board (IRB), which he described as a "straightforward" and quick process: "Speak with each individual on the phone" or "do all of this online." However, he also suggested that if Wold could "somehow find this additional information and let us know it . . . that might permit us to avoid the IRB"—a shortcut to the ethical oversight mechanism in hospitals.[10]

Maybe they should just obtain everyone's medical records, replied Sewell. He'd been considering this as an option, he said, ever since the head of their IRB mentioned that the medical community might be suspicious about data collected from the internet.[11] If they collected medical records, a peer-reviewed journal would be more likely to publish their research.

Halpern agreed. "I met 'Case 150' at the [Multidisciplinary Association for Psychedelic Studies (MAPS)] event in NYC. . . . Remarkable to hear how much he had been suffering as well as how much he has benefited from these treatments." Sewell ought to verify all the information from "this very exciting work . . . [that Wold has] been doing and . . . shared with all of us."[12]

(The idea that they ought to verify any of this information from the very doctors whose patients had decided to stray so far from conventional medicine struck me as ironic. Doing so, however, might have seemed unavoidable in a system that gives physicians so much authority to speak about others' suffering.)

Obtaining all medical records presented a new challenge: most people submitted their reports anonymously. Plus, even if they had provided emails, it would be unethical to contact research subjects who hadn't already provided consent to be contacted by a researcher for follow-up.

Wold, once again, seemed like a useful way to navigate around the rules that regulate science in institutional settings. After all, he had a key that connected case numbers to real identities. Maybe, Sewell asked, Wold could contact each of these people and ask if they'd give him a call or send him an email.[13] Of course, Wold agreed.

What about making use of Clusterbusters' collaborative relationship with Erowid, asked Sewell? If Earth agreed, people with cluster headache could be directed to Erowid and asked if they would consent to an interview with researchers.

Sewell liked the idea enough to email a request to Earth.

"Fantastic news!" Earth replied, adding that it seemed like an amazing opportunity, and added that he'd be happy to provide additional support given his "genuine enthusiasm" for the project. But he also expressed some "residual annoyance" that Clusterbusters had paid John Halpern for the work he'd done for free.[14]

Erowid has long been a vital resource in the psychedelic ecosystem, providing a safe place where knowledge could be cultivated beyond the reach of government authority. By 2023, the nonprofit, according to its cofounders, had published 41,919 "experience reports," which it had curated from 117,359 submissions.[15] That kind of knowledge served everyone, from psychonauts to policymakers.

● ● ●●●●●●●●●●●●●●●●●●●●●●● ● ●

Official collection of medical records stopped after they had a full set of information on fifty-three people who used either psilocybin or LSD to self-treat cluster headache. This would be a hell of a case study.

The results were remarkable. LSD and psilocybin, according to reports, could end a cluster headache, prevent a new cluster headache cycle (or at least extend the length of a remission), and abort an attack. A drug capable of preventing a cluster headache cycle *and* preventing a new cycle from recurring? Unheard of. Except, of course, on the internet, where patients had been doing this for several years.

Doblin, perhaps unsurprisingly, thought the case study results demonstrating the efficacy of LSD were, by far, the most extraordinary finding. The case study data on LSD was admittedly much thinner than the evidence for psilocybin: only eight people in the case study reported use of LSD versus forty-eight who used psilocybin. But seven of the eight people in the case study series who used LSD reported the drug ended their cycle early. In comparison, only twenty-five of forty-eight people who used psilocybin could report the same. Flash, of course, appeared as a success in both the LSD and psilocybin columns.

Naturally, there were limitations to the data. The lack of a placebo group and uncertainties about the precise composition of each dose introduced potential inaccuracies. Self-reporting bias could lead participants to either exaggerate or downplay the effectiveness of the intervention. Nobody thought that the FDA would consider self-reports from people taking magic mushrooms at home as seriously as a randomized controlled trial (RCT). But Clusterbusters' surveys and self-reports provided an important place to start, particularly considering the government restrictions that made launching an RCT testing psychedelic substances so difficult.

"I am delighted," Sewell wrote in a report to the MAPS membership in the spring 2005 *MAPS Bulletin*, "at the progress we have been making towards restarting LSD research at Harvard." The study "carries no scientific weight but can be used as a justification for mounting a more formal controlled trial to test if the phenomenon reported actually does exist."[16]

Despite the vaguely insulting dismissal of its lack of "scientific weight," the months' and years' worth of underground work that Wold and his fellow Clusterheads had pulled together was finally seeing the light of day. Clusterbusters wasn't just a self-contained, underground message board anymore. People out there, *up there*, were finally listening.

But I often wondered if too much gratitude behaved like the dense forest canopy that, for so long, obscured the indispensable mycelial network below, by blinding Clusterbusters to their own significant contribution to the field of research: an invaluable cyberbotanical wisdom that taught the rest of us how indole-structured substances like psilocybin and LSD could be used as a treatment for headache disorders.

● ● ●●●●●●●●●●●●●●●●●●●● ● ●

At the end of April 2005, Wold received a first draft of the case study, naming him as a coauthor alongside Sewell, Halpern, and Pope.

Wold's reply, sent a week later, offered thoughtful comments about the doses that people had taken and specific edits to the text—for example, corrections to the official diagnostic criteria for cluster headache. Sewell sent his next draft on May 10 to all three of his collaborators with a note that he'd incorporated "everyone's comments." The next step in the process involved a thorough internal review process within the hospital. Sewell's draft would be circulated to Halpern for comments and then on to their other colleagues for review.

In the meantime, Wold wondered what, if anything, had been happening with their research protocol. It had been nine months since Sewell arrived at Harvard—nine months dedicated to a case study. Academia worked more slowly than he had ever imagined.

(I could have warned him how long these things take, especially when the lead author has a full-time job working on other research projects.)

Sewell tried to reassure him. "We have set an informal deadline of Albert Hofmann's 100th birthday to get it submitted to the IRB."[17]

Plans had been made to celebrate Albert Hofmann's January 11 birthday with an international symposium held from January 13 to 15, 2006, in

Basel, Switzerland. Eminent figures from the psychedelic world, including the centenarian Albert Hofmann himself, were expected to attend. Doblin had even arranged for a panel that would showcase some of the few university-based psychedelic researchers in the world. The symposium could provide a global platform to announce the return of LSD to Harvard.

That gave them six months.

"Privately," Sewell's email to Wold continued, "I can't see why it should take that long, but I also have to note that I thought we would have this case series submitted back in February [2005], and here it is six months later, so my estimates of the length of time it takes to do these things are not to be trusted."[18]

Sewell's premonition proved to be all too true.

●　●　●:●:●:●:●:●:●:●:●:●:●:●:●:●　●　●

That September, Sewell sent an invitation to a dedicated listserv where people could debate and, hopefully, come to a consensus about the clinical trial design.

Clusterbusters didn't have the funding for a study yet, so the proposed trial would have to be small: ten to twelve people at most. Since experiments are essentially statistical exercises, the research question would need to be focused.

That meant making difficult decisions. Take, for example, the debate about which drug to study. Clusterbusters, of course, insisted the trial include psilocybin. The whole point had been to legitimate the use of magic mushrooms—a fungus they could grow in their homes. Doblin, who had a somewhat different political objective, wanted to ensure that the clinical trial included LSD—which, he was quick to point out, he believed was a more effective treatment. Sewell could see a logic in designing a study that included both drugs, since it "seems to be a lot more effective. . . . If Harvard turns down LSD research, it will be because Harvard turns it down, not me." But it wasn't always clear if a small experiment had the statistical power to include two experimental drugs and a placebo.

And that was just one issue. How should they choose a dosage? Would this dose be given just once or repeated multiple times over the course of several days? Would some people receive a placebo? If so, would they invite participants to return and take an active dose (aka a crossover design)?

By the end of the year, it seemed like they might be reaching a consensus: They would invite twelve people who were experiencing a cluster headache cycle to participate in the clinical trial. Half would receive LSD. Half would receive psilocybin. Nobody would receive a placebo. They hoped the intervention would shorten the cycle.

And then, nothing, until August 2006, when a message from Andrew Sewell seemed to emphasize the importance of a placebo control.

The stakes involved felt painfully high: sometimes it seemed like this might be their only chance to run a clinical trial ever. They weren't some big pharma company with endless funds to run a huge trial with tons of participants and countless expensive safety provisions. The pressure made it even harder to balance issues that mattered to patients while considering pragmatic concerns about the bureaucratic, financial, and political obstacles.

This was complicated and risky, and they had to get it right.

●  ●  ●●●●●●●●●●●●●●●●●●●●  ●  ●

Andrew Sewell had managed, however, to have the case study ready for submission by the end of 2005. The final product—just eight hundred words long—seemed to come as a bit of a surprise to Wold, despite an email from Sewell in late August about the internal review.

His August email had led with good news: "Nobody had any criticisms of the science."

But there'd been some bad news as well: "The links with Clusterbusters drew some vitriol."

Reviewer One decided to visit Clusterbusters' website and "was aghast to find collaborators named 'Flash,' 'Pinky' and 'Erowid' . . . and psychedelic pictures of mushrooms." Any medical journal editor would do the same and "have a good laugh." Reviewer Two "suggest[ed] that we had been duped by a bunch of acid-heads intent on pressing their own agenda."

At least, Sewell added, Reviewer Three had enjoyed the paper. He thought they should submit it as it was.

Sewell recommended that the next draft downplay or even "sever as many ties with Clusterbusters as possible."

He asked Wold, "How would you feel about moving your name from the list of authors down to acknowledgements?"

In the email, Sewell worried he might be overstepping with this request, given how often these disputes led academics into lifelong feuds. But he thought Wold "probably" wouldn't mind. "Publication" likely mattered far more than getting credit for the work, given that Wold wasn't "in an academic career." Success, he added, sometimes means "listening to the authorities."[19]

Wold made a characteristic offhanded joke and said he understood.

But maybe he didn't quite understand.

The final submission included a brief acknowledgment of Bob Wold and Earth. Funding for the study was attributed to MAPS, which was technically correct, since that organization handled the financial transactions. And, in an odd twist, the research methods not only neglected to mention that the case studies had come from a research collective working together to develop a drug protocol but introduced a new origin story explaining that the authors had been inspired to conduct the study after being contacted by a man "who reported a complete remission of his cluster periods when he repeatedly used LSD on a recreational basis between 22 and 24 years old."[20]

Everything else had been Sewell, Halpern, and Pope's research, according to this revisionist history, including the location "through cluster headache support groups and an Internet-based survey—[of] several hundred people with cluster headache who reported use of psilocybin containing mushrooms or LSD specifically to treat their disorder."[21]

This, of course, was a fiction, as was Sewell's choice to use Flash's story "out of respect for the fact that he was first [and] because his case also illustrates both LSD and psilocybin use."[22]

No wonder Wold was surprised. Here's how the research methods were described in the last draft he'd read: "Cases for this series were derived from three sources [including] . . . an Internet group, Clusterbusters . . . which has been systematically collecting [these] cases . . . [and] online surveys . . . hosted . . . at the Erowid website."[23]

Whose study was this?

•  •  •••••••••••••••••••  •  •

Over a period of seven years, hundreds of people engaged in a collective self-experiment to find a way to treat cluster headache. The article transformed these experiences into a summary of fifty-three case studies that could be published on two printed pages. Choices had to be made.

But how much reduction is tolerable? What, precisely, was lost when the text no longer mentioned Clusterbusters? Who, if anyone, was harmed by removing Bob Wold's contribution as an author to the acknowledgments section?

There are no easy answers to the question "What is an author?" But there are guidelines, and scientific integrity depends on transparency. Giving credit where it's due helps make sure that the benefits and the responsibilities of authorship are equitably distributed. And one of those responsibilities includes the identification of potential conflicts of interest. The authors' decision to remove information about the contribution that Clusterbusters made to the production of data used in this paper had been an explicit attempt to make the paper appear more objective.[24]

Andrew Sewell included Clusterbusters' contributions in their subsequent collaborations. John Halpern did not.[25]

Science might present itself as an objective, politics-free practice. But research, like any other kind of work, is a messy business filled with all the things that make us human: ambitions and curiosity, mistakes and frustrations, creativity and anxiety, politics and passions. The best science takes an honest account of how well the research methods it uses can minimize these biases, so that readers understand how to interpret findings.

But the biggest thing this paper misses? Wisdom.

By presenting a simple count of how many people found relief using psilocybin or LSD, the paper implies that the social context of their experiments had no relevance to the effectiveness of the therapy. But how can we know if this is true? This had been a *collective* self-experiment, conducted with the support and encouragement of an online forum. How much of the magic was in the drug, and how much was in the setting? Excluding Clusterbusters doesn't just deprive them of the credit they deserve for their work. It also made the results of the study less objective and more difficult to interpret.

Contemporary psychedelic research is fueled by an alchemic process of transforming a community's hard-earned knowledge into the commodities that academics care about: peer-reviewed publications, research grants, and the kind of fawning profiles in popular magazines that even those considered "stars" of academia rarely enjoy. Clusterbusters is far from the only group that's had questions and concerns about who ought to be recognized as an expert or the owner of intellectual property. Over the years, I've come to realize that it's not unusual for published research on psychedelic substances to erase the traces of citizen science and the innovations of outlaws. It's an almost inevitable problem, given that stringent regulations have, for so long, obstructed the ability of scientists to conduct clinical research on psychedelic substances.

● ● ●●●●●●●●●●●●●●●●●●● ● ●

When Wold expressed concern that Clusterbusters would be erased from the research, Sewell placed the blame on a seven-month review process that involved "intense debate" over "every word" of the article. "I've never seen such a lot of hoopla."[26]

Nor should he worry about Clusterbusters being written out of history.

"Odds are you'll be writing a book on it someday. And I tell you what. If I end up living in a cardboard box because this cluster headache tomfoolery ends my career, promise me you'll bring me bags of stale bagels so I don't starve, eh? I don't think there are going to be any trips or awards in this, not in the near future. Maybe in a few decades if it works out. But we'd better anticipate a lot of spit in the meantime."[27]

Chapter Fourteen

● ● ●●●●●●●●●●●●●●●●●●● ● ●

# HOW TO BECOME A
# PSYCHEDELIC RESEARCHER

C*HICAGO, DECEMBER 31, 2005*
Everything was taking too damn long. None of the rules at the university made sense. Who were they protecting? When would someone start to care about patients?

Bob Wold sank into a favorite chair, swallowed a mouthful of the bitter mushroom tea, closed his eyes, and allowed himself to follow Stevie Nicks's chocolate velvet voice where she wanted to go.

He normally wouldn't eat anything more exotic than a cheeseburger, but he'd tolerate anything that banished the looming shadows on this cold, cloudy New Year's Eve. Mary had arranged for Wold to be alone that night so he could immerse himself in the moment, allowing his thoughts to wander unbridled.

The whims of the lottery spared Wold from Vietnam, a fate his brother hadn't escaped. He'd soon get married and have kids. Wold never took part in anything remotely "countercultural," unless you count his silent cheers for the protesters who took over the streets. It could have been him over there. It shouldn't have been anyone. But he never engaged in the scene—except for the music, which became a sanctuary. Pink Floyd became an instant favorite. Lately though, "Whipping Post," a song by the Allman Brothers, had etched itself into his "tripping playlist." The song, with its searing agony and relentless bass, offered a wicked truth and fed a hidden fury.

Bringing that steady midwestern game face to every interaction took a toll.

And then he remembered their paper. Fingers crossed, it would soon be published. Progress might be slow, but he should have known it would take time to get the hang of the Ivy League's peculiar rhythm.

Everything seemed to be working well now. Clusterbusters was so delighted with Andrew Sewell that they had arranged to fund his full salary for a calendar year beginning in September 2006. Doing so would allow Sewell to work full-time on their research, which ought to help speed things up.

Wold had also noticed an uptick of scientific interest in psychedelics. He'd heard rumors of a Johns Hopkins University study aimed at replicating Walter Pahnke's Good Friday Experiment in a more controlled setting. In just a couple weeks, the Swiss city of Basel would be teeming with eager faces, gathered from around the world to celebrate Albert Hofmann's one-hundredth birthday.

Halpern would be there to talk about his study investigating MDMA-assisted therapy, and Sewell had prepared a handout about their research on cluster headache. Doblin wanted to make sure they emphasized that the clinical trial would test LSD. Who could pass up such a tantalizing setting, given the serendipitous timing of Hofmann's birthday? The symposium was meant to be a celebration—not just of Hofmann's life but of the potential rebirth of psychedelic research he had inadvertently fathered.[1]

Wold filled with gratitude when he considered how much his A-Team was doing to help people who needed so much. Would he have felt so much gratitude had he known what would unfold just two weeks later?

Almost two thousand people had flown to Basel from all over the world to attend Albert Hofmann's birthday symposium. Hofmann, as vivacious and engaging as ever, rewarded them with charming tales of how LSD had granted him "an inner joy, an open-mindedness, a gratefulness, open eyes, and an internal sensitivity for the miracles of creation."[2]

Doblin's panel didn't go quite as well. In fact, the scene, caught on video and distributed on YouTube, would become the biggest psychedelic controversy associated with Harvard Medical School since Leary's ignominious departure.

The crisis began when Mark McCloud, a well-known member of the psychedelic community, hijacked the panel just as Halpern announced, "Sometime in 2006, we should be starting this [MDMA] study at Harvard."

"Are you a DEA agent?"[3]

"No." Halpern flashed a bemused smile. "No, but I'd like to just keep on talking. Let me just give my lecture. There's a question-and-answer period at the end."

McCloud pressed on. "Are you a DEA agent?"

"No," Halpern repeated, and then, with a dismissive shake of the head, again said, "No."

Doblin called out, "If John was a DEA agent, we would have had this study approved a long time ago."

People started to laugh. Halpern a DEA agent? He looked every bit the Ivy League academic as he peered down at the crowd through a tiny pair of frameless glasses perched on his nose. He still wore his hair—what was left of it, anyway—a bit long and unkempt. But the herringbone tweed sports coat and tie distinguished him from those in the audience who looked like they had just stepped out of a time machine from a Grateful Dead show.

A woman from the audience asked, "How come you turned in Leonard Pickard?"

For a moment, Halpern looked serious. "I did not do that."

She continued, "Your testimony helped."

He raised his eyebrows, defending himself with a careful nondenial. "I never testified!"

McCloud interjected with sardonic contempt, "You haven't testified for the DEA since December 4th—*my birthday by the way*—the year 2000?" He shook a pile of papers in his hand. "This is public record, *Agent* Halpern."[4]

"If I'm not doing this work, then there's no going back to Harvard," Halpern rebutted. The effectiveness of this argument, however, hinged on how much one thought this goal justified collaborating with an alleged agent of the state.

The vibe was getting awkward as a collective murmur filled the auditorium. Could Halpern be a snitch? Were audience members themselves in jeopardy?

Doblin, who had now made his way to the front of the room, tried to redirect the audience's attention to the panel. "He's not a DEA agent . . . as soon as this is over, then we could sit down and talk about it. . . . All these people have come here for something different."

McCloud stood down, at least for the moment. But he resumed making allegations when the panel ended. John Halpern, he claimed, as a crowd gathered around him, had been a cooperating witness in the 2003 case of *United States of America v. William Leonard Pickard and Clyde Apperson*, which the Drug Enforcement Administration called the largest LSD manufacturing bust in history. Pickard, whom many in the psychedelic community considered a saint given how much he risked producing the substance they all cared so much about, was now serving two consecutive life sentences in prison. No chance of parole. (Pickard maintained his innocence.)

After the panel, warnings not to be seen in Halpern's company circulated around the symposium—even wealthy philanthropists warned one another about the possibility that he might be wired.[5] If one trusted collaborator was colluding with law enforcement, then who else might be a narc?

Even in the psychedelic world, where people tended to be open about their use of illegal drugs, snitching violated a norm so central to belonging that it hardly needed to be mentioned. Even the hint that someone might be an informant could make them a pariah.

• • •••••••••••••••••••••• • •

The trouble began back on November 6, 2000, when William "Leonard" Pickard, then age fifty-five, fled from a routine traffic stop in Kansas. Helicopters, DEA agents, and bloodhounds took eighteen hours to find him.[6]

At first glance, Pickard seemed like an unlikely criminal mastermind. He projected the preternatural calm of a Buddhist monk—a quality he might have developed while living in a Zen monastery. He worked with drugs, yes, but as the deputy director of the Drug Policy Analysis Program at the University of California, Los Angeles. The director, Mark Kleiman, had just moved there from Harvard's Kennedy School of Government, where he'd advised Pickard in his master's studies in public policy.[7] Short of a PhD, Leonard Pickard had earned most every signifier of respect in the academic world.

But Pickard, who maintains a reputation as a brilliant, underground chemist within the psychedelic community, was no stranger to the law. Records of his arrests began in 1964, when he was just eighteen, and included two convictions involving the manufacture or attempted manufacture of psychedelic drugs. He received his first prison sentence in 1977 after authorities discovered and shut down his small MDMA laboratory. His most recent stint in prison had ended in 1992—four years served after the DEA found him leaving a warehouse containing an acid lab and enough LSD to dose two hundred thousand people.[8]

According to multiple media reports, Halpern and Pickard met in the mid-1990s in New Mexico when Halpern volunteered as a medical resident for Dr. Rick Strassman. Pickard had traveled to Albuquerque to "do drug research."[9]

Halpern, according to reports, was not in good shape when the two met.[10] Pickard found him crouching in a dark corner of a mutual acquaintance's home, lost in a terrifying ayahuasca trip. Pickard, reportedly, reassured the young man that he'd done "more LSD than anyone on the planet" and could guide him to a more peaceful place.[11] The two men were the best of friends by the time Halpern sobered up.

At some point in their relationship, Pickard allegedly paid Halpern a huge chunk of cash in exchange for arranging a meeting with a wealthy childhood friend who could launder his drug money. Five years after Halpern's fateful meeting with Pickard, the feds found a drug lab in a former missile silo in Kansas, which had been renovated into an extravagant, kitschy, underground palace.

Everyone seemed to agree that Halpern had nothing to do with Pickard's arrest. The "real snitch" had been Gordon Todd Skinner, the man who owned and lived in the silo. Prior to meeting Pickard, Skinner had spent much of his adult life floundering from one misdeed to the next: a failed effort at large-scale drug trafficking that led to a dramatic arrest and an indictment, a history of cooperating with the DEA to avoid convictions, and a pattern of financial mismanagement that reflects not just misfortune but a deeper disregard for ethical boundaries and responsibilities. By all accounts, he had plenty of reasons to fear the law—including a possible manslaughter charge—when, in late 1999, the DEA came knocking at his door.[12]

Skinner secured immunity by providing evidence leading to Pickard's imprisonment. However, Skinner's freedom was short-lived. He received a four-year federal prison sentence after his arrest at the 2003 Burning Man festival for distributing MDMA. In 2009, he faced even graver consequences—a life sentence plus ninety years—after a Tulsa jury convicted him of kidnapping, assault, and conspiracy in a harrowing case involving the torture of a man for an entire week.[13]

It's a wild, salacious story that reads like the plot of a Hollywood blockbuster.

● ● ●●●●●●●●●●●●●●●●●●●● ● ●

"A lot actually did know [what happened]," Halpern told the crowd who had gathered around him after the panel in Basel. Halpern had also emphasized, in our conversations, that he'd always told those he worked with about his relationship with Pickard, and his subsequent problems with the DEA: "I told NIDA, I told Harvard, I told McLean." Rick Doblin knew this story too.

Maybe nobody noticed when Halpern's alleged relationship with Pickard had been covered by the *San Francisco Gate* in 2001.[14] But they sure did pay attention when the *Entheogen Review*, an underground magazine dedicated to psychedelic substances, published an exposé about "Halperngate" in March 2006. The article, written by Jon Hanna, investigated McCloud's accusations and offered an assessment of the case from the perspective of "the larger underground community." Hanna provided Halpern and Doblin a draft of his article with an invitation for comment. Doblin's full response was published along with the article. Halpern declined to comment in writing.[15]

Doblin talks about operating MAPS with transparency, and although he's often criticized for falling short of this ideal, he does tend to offer quite a bit more information than most leaders of major organizations.[16] His response to Hanna struck me as earnest, particularly when it came to articulating his reasons for working with Halpern.

According to Hanna, Halpern received a "proffer agreement," in exchange for providing the government with all the verbal, electronic, and written information they have about the case, including emails and voicemails. Doblin's reply began by clarifying that he did not take snitching lightly, and that he believed in "accepting whatever punishment may unfortunately come one's way for being involved [with] . . . illegal drugs," but he also believed in "forgiveness and redemption."[17]

There was also a larger politics at stake that needed to be kept in mind. Halpern offered the only viable path Doblin had to get to Harvard—the kind of symbolic victory that would signal "the beginning of the post-Leary era," which he argued that everyone in the community should agree was an important goal. Whatever risks Halpern might have posed to the community had not materialized, but how could they quantify the risk of *not* working with him? Doblin led MAPS with the bold vision of bringing psychedelic research back to university laboratories. Leonard Pickard agreed. Doblin had spoken to him by phone in prison to make sure he supported MAPS's decision to collaborate with Halpern.

Hanna, however, argued that Pickard's opinion didn't matter. Consider, for example, that Halpern had been accused of wearing a wire to record his conversations with some of the most beloved people in the psychedelic community, including underground chemist Sasha Shulgin. Nobody knew if it was true, but, he argued, in a "community of outlaws . . . trust is the most precious commodity."[18]

Hanna pressed Doblin: Couldn't someone else at Harvard do this research?

"I know of no other Harvard doctors interested in conducting psychedelic research," Doblin responded.[19]

Hanna's exposé offered two important pieces of news. First, John Halpern would not be welcome at Burning Man that summer due to a lack of trust, which meant he would miss MAPS's twentieth-anniversary celebration. Second, Harvard Medical School's McLean Hospital would no longer accept funding from MAPS. According to Doblin, Dr. Jack Gorman, the hospital's new president, felt uneasy about maintaining a relationship with MAPS, "in part" because he wanted to distance the hospital from MAPS's pro-legalization position, and "in part" because he worried that all research funded by MAPS would be dismissed as biased, no matter how rock solid the science.

Doblin had made sure that Peter Lewis, the philanthropist funding Halpern's MDMA research, would be able to donate directly to the hospital.[20] Nothing was said about the fate of their cluster headache research.

(In an ironic twist, Gorman resigned from his position at McLean a few months later after admitting to having had sex with a former patient.)[21]

Drugs are a messy business, even in the hallowed halls of Harvard.

●  ●  ●●●●●●●●●●●●●●●●●●●  ●  ●

Wold didn't learn about the scandal until April when a friend sent a link to an online video recording of McCloud screaming at Halpern. A quick internet search linked to Jon Hanna's article, which filled him in on the remaining details. Somewhere between Halpern's complicated relationship with the law and MAPS's estrangement from McLean Hospital, he started to wonder why Doblin hadn't contacted him about this ages ago. Apparently Halpern *hadn't* been upfront with all his collaborators.

Clusterbusters had risked everything—time, energy, money, and credibility, not to mention admitting to what some might call criminal activity—to elevate their underground research to the prestigious halls of Harvard. Wold never considered that the Harvard professor they worked with might be tangled up in legal issues far graver than eating a forbidden mushroom.

The news spread to Clusterbusters' forum by May, leading several members to post concerns that their group's collaboration with a "known DEA informant" might leave patients vulnerable. Hadn't they just given him hundreds of documents filled with evidence that they'd been using illegal drugs?

Wold did his best to tamp down these anxieties. Halpern and Sewell, he said, were consummate professionals who would treat their data as confidential. Wold trusted they'd safeguard their data as they would any other confidential medical research. But a scandal like this risked further eroding trust within a community that already felt betrayed by the medical establishment. Wold emailed Doblin about the concerns the scandal had raised in his community. "I wish I had been told about the McLean decision before my members read it in the MAPS newsletter."[22]

Doblin handled Wold's concerns with an ease that suggested this hadn't been the first difficult email he'd received on the topic.

"I apologize for not informing you ahead of time. The final stages of negotiating with McLean were very intense and difficult. . . . MAPS withdrew only as a last resort when only that would have worked."[23] But none of this, Doblin insisted, would affect MAPS's ability to support Halpern, Sewell, or Clusterbusters. MAPS, Doblin assured Wold, remained committed to fulfilling its pledge to fund Sewell's salary at Harvard for the upcoming fiscal year, which would free up his time to research the efficacy of psychedelic substances as a treatment for cluster headache.

Funding issues, Doblin reassured Wold, could be sorted out on the back end once Clusterbusters finalized its nonprofit status. MAPS would simply route the money raised for this project (most of which the Weils had donated) back through Clusterbusters. Doblin wrote that he still planned to raise an additional "$20,000 to $25,000" of funding for Clusterbusters "by selling art and books signed by Albert Hofmann."

Wold hoped that the Weils would find this reassuring, given they had designated half of their $50,000 donation as a matching grant. As far as he was concerned, MAPS was obligated to raise that money.

Wold knew he didn't have many options aside from trusting Doblin. So he took a deep breath and decided to believe that all was well in their little corner of the psychedelic world. And for a while, everything did proceed as expected.

●  ●  ●:●:●:●:●:●:●:●:●:●:●:●:●:●  ●  ●

In the meantime, Andrew Sewell wasn't in the least bit anxious about their collaboration. He was raring to be let loose. There was no denying Sewell's capacious enthusiasm and commitment to conducting the kind of research that mattered to cluster headache patients. That, combined with a profound respect for their knowledge, made him a force to be reckoned with.

Sewell was bursting with ideas for research. What about the twenty-two people in their cluster headache survey who said they used an herbal remedy called "kudzu" to manage individual attacks? Kudzu had multiple bioactive properties. He'd like to follow up on that.

Others in the cluster headache forums swore they could abort attacks by drinking gallons of water. Sewell proposed that the physiological basis for the treatment might lie in vasal stimulation. He would love to pursue that angle.

What about the Clusterheads who treated themselves using lysergic acid amide (LSA, or ergine), a psychedelic derived from inexpensive, accessible, and legally purchased morning glory seeds? A small study investigating the use of LSA would make a lot of sense. Not only were morning glory seeds easy to obtain, but those using seeds could legally mail a sample from their stock to Sewell so he could assess the potency of their doses.

Best of all, the July 2006 issue of *Neurology*, the flagship journal of the American Academy of Neurology, published their case study: "Response of Cluster Headache to Psilocybin and LSD." Finally, credible documentation that psychedelics could (anecdotally) treat their disease.[24]

The findings, according to Sewell, Halpern, and Pope, were noteworthy for several reasons. First, no medication on the market could terminate a cluster cycle so effectively. Second, a few doses seemed to produce long-lasting relief, which meant there was no need to take a daily medicine. And third, if some people really did get better with a microdose, then the treatment might not require an alteration of consciousness.

The findings offered a provocative new way to treat a notorious disease, the paper argued, before concluding with the classic "further research is warranted."

Wold sent an email to Sewell asking whether this was the first study on psychedelics and pain since the Timothy Leary days.

Very nearly. Only a few had been published. None within the last twenty years.

Sharing the news with Clusterbusters had been a highlight of that year. The forum lit up with praise and optimism: "It is a BIG stepping stone, and will do so much for those who feel so hopeless."

"I hope that SOMEONE is listening."

But the partnership that had gotten them this far was about to go into freefall.

● ● ●●●●●●●●●●●●●●●●●●●● ● ●

It is hard to trace the beginning of the spectacular collapse of the relationship between mentor and mentee. But a tense email that Halpern sent to Sewell on January 17, 2006, suggests their collaboration had already been fiery for a while before the conflagration truly began.

Halpern started his email with a blunt acknowledgment: "What is happening right now between us has been percolating for some time."[25]

Sewell, according to Halpern, had allegedly committed multiple ethical breaches, including failure to renew the cluster headache survey with the IRB and to obtain a certificate of confidentiality—a document that protects research subjects from subpoena—despite Halpern's clear instructions to do so. Halpern also expressed concern that Sewell had initiated a study on LSA and another on kudzu without asking a supervisor to review his application to the IRB. "I am trying to protect you," he cautioned.

The email continued, any research involving "hallucinogens" at McLean Hospital needed Halpern's approval as the director of the newly formed Integrative Biological Psychiatry Lab. Sewell needed to understand that it didn't matter who paid his salary—that wasn't how supervision worked at the hospital. Halpern also pointed out that "the money from MAPS for any eventual cluster study will be coming to my lab."

Would Sewell agree to obtain Halpern's approval prior to studying anything related to hallucinogens? Halpern insisted he must. Their work was too important to risk exposing it to this "nuttiness."

Sewell's reply dripped with disdain. "Anything psychedelic-related, John, I'm happy to run by you—that's your domain. But most of what I do has nothing to do with psychedelics."

In June, Sewell sent an email to Doblin and Wold that floated a proposal to move his research on cluster headache, including his funding from Clusterbusters, to the neurology department, where he'd eventually start a headache clinic. The chair of the department, according to Sewell, liked the idea. "The only stipulation," Sewell reportedly told the chair of neurology, was that he had "to lend his support and signature to a clinical trial of psilocybin for cluster headache to be submitted to the IRB."[26]

Doblin seemed fine with the arrangement, so long as "the experiment included LSD as well as psilocybin." But Halpern didn't like the arrangement at all. "The fellowship money is for research here [in his lab] on CH+LSD/Psilocybin . . . Correct, Bob and Rick?"[27]

Nobody replied.

Bob Wold just wanted the damn research to get done.[28]

●  ●  ●●●●●●●●●●●●●●●●●●●  ●  ●

The dream team imploded in early September, when Halpern discovered that Sewell had published an essay that summer in both the *MAPS Bulletin* and the *Entheogen Review* titled "So You Want to Be a Psychedelic Researcher?"[29] The short editorial, now considered a classic in psychedelic studies, provided guidance for those who aspired to join such a stigmatized profession. Undergraduates, Sewell suggested in the editorial, could look for relevant courses, which they might find in anthropology, or join a local chapter of a campus group, like Students for Sensible Drug Policy. In the meantime, he recommended they read accessible scientific literature, attend conventions, and support organizations like MAPS or Erowid by donating or volunteering.

Becoming an aboveground psychedelic researcher required a graduate degree. Sewell wrote that he had decided to become a physician so he might one day be permitted to "give these drugs to people," and that he liked the idea that the public allowed doctors to tell them about what was "good or bad" for them too. More practically, a doctor could always earn money by seeing patients. But pursuing a PhD in neuroscience, clinical psychology, or cognitive science would also provide the credibility necessary for success. As he put it, "The more rigorous and stringent your research and its interpretation, the harder it will be for people to argue with it, reject it, or not take it seriously."

Yet Sewell's words had an unmistakable undercurrent of defiance. He advised undergraduates to "lie low and infiltrate the system," explaining that sometimes it was necessary to conform to others' expectations to build credibility before branching out into more independent pursuits. This had been his strategy, he revealed in a conspiratorial aside: "I didn't breathe a word of my interests until I was already on the faculty of Harvard Medical School."

Not that Sewell was a snob. On the contrary, he acknowledged that "amateur scientists" were making some of the most "cutting-edge discoveries in psychedelic science due to the legal hurdles that hindered academic research in this field," adding recommendations of conferences where people working aboveground and underground often mingled.

As if to underscore the tangled relationship between these worlds, Sewell concluded by providing contact details for seventeen collaborators who had agreed to offer resources to those interested in the field. The fact that Sewell's list of contacts included Marc "Lord Nose" Franklin, a well-known photographer in the psychedelic underground, alongside Nicholas Cozzi, a professor in the Department of Pharmacology at the University of Wisconsin, gives a sense of how expertise in psychedelic research spanned institutions recognized as places of legitimate "establishment" research and less formal spaces.[30]

●  ●  ●:●:●:●:●:●:●:●:●:●:●:●:●:●  ●  ●

Upon discovering these essays, Halpern sent an email to Wold describing Sewell's decision to publish content of this sort in two of the most contentious psychedelic organizations—MAPS and *Entheogen Review*—as the "depth of stupidity."[31] McLean had *just* cut ties with MAPS. While it was true that Halpern continued to work with Rick Doblin—a necessity given that MAPS remained the sole organization funding MDMA clinical trials—their collaboration had to stay on the down-low. A *MAPS Bulletin* article featuring a Harvard Medical School affiliation could only invite trouble from their buttoned-up employers.

Halpern was especially bothered by Sewell's suggestion that he'd been deceitful toward his employer to secure his position. Halpern always disclosed his intentions to his employers at Harvard. Likewise, McLean's administration knew that Sewell arrived at Harvard intending to work in Halpern's psychedelic laboratory. Why pretend otherwise?

Wold wrestled with this new information. Halpern was right to be concerned. Maybe this was the business owner in him, but Wold couldn't stop worrying about Sewell's suggestion that people lie to employers about their true aspirations. A little common sense went a long way. Imagine advising a carpenter that taking a job would be a good way to seduce the boss's daughter? Why feed the beast in a field already rife with (often unfair) assumptions of questionable morality? (Sewell would later recant, and tell Wold that he'd been honest with Harvard.)

Once again, Wold found himself wondering how much it harmed Clusterbusters' research to work with people so closely aligned with the underground. Learning about Halperngate and McLean's decision to sever
relations with MAPS had been a one-two punch. Now he had to grapple
with Sewell. He understood the appeal of telling authority figures to fuck
off. And he appreciated that Sewell treated him as an equal despite his not
having the same academic qualifications. But Clusterbusters wanted to
work with a Harvard hospital for a reason. The underground needed people
like Halpern and Sewell if it had any hope of changing the system. So he'd
prefer that their aboveground partners avoid becoming personae non grata
in the accepted halls of academia.

But did this cross a line? Sewell had become a real asset. Not only was
he a driving force behind the research that they were doing at McLean, but
he possessed an extraordinary talent for engaging with the patient community on their terms. He listened to their stories, struggles, and aspirations, and he took their suggestions seriously. Clusterheads rarely found
this much empathy in medicine. Maybe some of that determination made
him headstrong, but young people could sometimes be stubborn. Everyone
needed redemption and forgiveness, right? Sewell might be a bit green, but
he had real determination. Wold hoped Halpern might see his way past this
incident.

No such luck. The rift that had formed between the two researchers
would only grow.

It didn't help matters that Sewell refused to admit wrongdoing. "I persist
in feeling that you're making a mountain out of a molehill here," he wrote
to Halpern. "For one thing, I don't believe I've done anything wrong that
I need to take lumps for, and I stand by everything I wrote." Sewell even
refused to concede that the essay broke their agreement that he run anything mentioning a hallucinogen by Halpern before publication. "It doesn't
even mention LSD or psilocybin research."[32]

Sewell had no interest in genuflecting to Halpern—whom he deemed a
disagreeable, narcissistic snitch seemingly so disliked in the psychedelic

community that he'd been disinvited from Burning Man that year. Sewell had gone to the festival and enjoyed himself, only to return to have Halpern give him shit for returning with a shaved head. (Sewell thought the hospital would prefer the shaved head to the mohawk he'd grown fond of in the desert.)

●  ●  ●●●●●●●●●●●●●●●●●●  ●  ●

Halpern's emails to Wold were now dominated by complaints about Sewell, including the allegation that Sewell, with Doblin's encouragement, had been planning "a wholly independent research group from me at McLean." Halpern told Wold, "I reminded Rick that there is a simple solution here: Andrew can work for me or he can get himself fired."[33]

None of this, however, seemed to be stopping Sewell from moving forward. In mid-October, Wold received an update from Sewell about the study on LSA and cluster headache that he'd been wanting to do. Halpern had been clear: McLean's IRB mustn't approve any of Sewell's research studies on psychedelics unless they had his signature. Sewell submitted a protocol anyway, which—he was happy to report—had just received IRB approval. "[Dr. Halpern's] proclamation that I should immediately cease all work on cluster headache or psychedelic research carries no weight," he wrote with confidence. "I don't have the patience for those sorts of shenanigans . . . [and] I'm reassured that his threats appear to be fairly empty ones."[34]

But Sewell's attempt to move his psychedelic research over to the neurology department backfired. The situation came to a head in late October when Halpern felt that Sewell had been "slandering" him in emails sent to a "Visionary Plant" listserv—a secretive discussion group limited to an inner circle of psychedelic VIPs. Halpern was no longer welcome in that circle, but he still had a few allies in the group.

Halpern, according to Sewell's emails to the listserv, bossed him around—but he was just a guy who worked in the same hospital. Sure, they had collaborated on a research study, but "since then we have [been] going our separate ways."[35] Sewell told the listserv that he found the behavior so confusing that he asked McLean Hospital's head of research if Halpern was somehow his boss. "He confirmed that although it has been understood by everyone that I am working with him on hallucinogen research, he is nowhere formally named as my supervisor."[36]

Yes. That was how it worked.

●  ●  ●●●●●●●●●●●●●●●●●●  ●  ●

Andrew Sewell, according to John Halpern, had worn out his welcome at McLean Hospital. Everyone he had talked to said Sewell was "unsupervisable."

Bob Wold couldn't quite believe that things had gotten so bad so quickly. Sewell had *just* told the Yahoo! group that he'd been making progress on a new study about LSD and morning glory seeds.

"Every seed-eater at CB is ecstatic," Wold emailed Halpern.[37] "I just hope [people] don't come away in the end feeling used and abused, [with] their pain, suffering and contributions, lost in a maze of bureaucratic mayhem. . . . I'm sure you, and hopefully Andrew, realize that it's not good to give people hope, accomplishment and progress, and then have it yanked out from below their feet."[38]

But Halpern and Sewell had locked horns in a battle that would yield only harm. Sewell would never agree to work under Halpern's supervision. Halpern insisted that all psychedelic research at McLean occur under his watch. And Wold had just about had enough.

News of death filled Wold's emails. He knew of at least six people with cluster headache who had died in the last ten months—two in just the last month: a suicide by gunshot and an accidental fentanyl overdose.

Each one weighed on Wold, but Eddie's* overdose troubled him especially. Eddie had experimented with mushroom therapy a few years prior but struggled with the dosage. He'd been in remission, but his cluster attacks had resumed a few months before. Wold forwarded his last, devastating message to Doblin, Halpern, and Sewell to give them a sense of the crises he was managing:

I am ready to try anything. A .45 sounds nice right about now. I live in [a place where psychedelic mushrooms don't grow naturally] and so just happening across some in the park is out of the question. I am asking out of sheer desperation. I feel as if I could pluck my eye out if it would end this. I desperately need an escape, only for a little while. I feel that I wish death would take me or god would spare me. I am desperate . . . Please help . . . ? God please help.[39]

Eddie's death had been ruled overdose by fentanyl. Wold believes that's how a lot of cluster headache–related deaths are categorized. Medical examiners just get it wrong. A bunch of insecure academics feuding over territory doesn't help anyone.

Would his friend have needed fentanyl if he'd had access to psilocybin or LSD? Could an approved clinical trial have given him the hope he needed to live another day?

"I don't know for sure . . . [but we] need to get these trials started. I don't know how many more friends I can lose."

All he could do was beg.

It would not be enough. Andrew Sewell was asked to resign at the end of November.[40]

● ● ●●●●●●●●●●●●●●●●●● ● ●

Bob Wold now faced a new set of problems. His inbox presented the most immediate issue: every day brought a new set of allegations and accusations from one member of the team-formerly-known-as-dream against the other. Wold likes to joke that he "never thought he'd have to be a psychologist to Harvard psychiatrists." And with the lead of the project gone, Clusterbusters would need to find someone to do their research. But nothing worried Wold quite as much as their financial situation, and MAPS still maintained control of their entire research budget.

How did Doblin want to redirect the $80,000 worth of funding that MAPS and Clusterbusters had set aside to fund a yearlong fellowship for Andrew Sewell?

MAPS, Doblin explained, only remained committed to a funding obligation so long as the possibility of the project existed. And MAPS, officially, had no capacity to assist their efforts at McLean. Doblin liked the idea of funding Sewell's fellowship, so he'd decided to make that happen. But that was no longer a possibility. Nevertheless, he would continue to offer support. Once a psilocybin/LSD study was approved, MAPS would donate $26,000 raised from the sales of items signed by Albert Hofmann.[41]

But apparently Hofmann had also had enough of Halpern. A week after Sewell's departure, Doblin received word that after learning about "recent incidents with and around John Halpern," Hofmann "strong[ly] wish[ed] all proceeds from the sales of the prints he signed . . . be restricted to LSD research and studies in Switzerland."[42] An edict like this from the "father of LSD" might as well have served as a formal excommunication from the psychedelic world.

"The main lesson here," Doblin explained, "is that the fights between Halpern and Sewell are hurting everyone, regardless of who is responsible for the fights taking place."[43]

Hofmann's decision meant that MAPS no longer had an additional $25,000 in its budget to allocate to cluster headache research. But Doblin assured Wold that he would fulfill his pledge, so long as Clusterbusters produced a project *worthy* of MAPS's money. Wold should know, however, that raising this money would be a challenge since MAPS's largest donor of unrestricted funds had also specified that none of his funds be directed to John Halpern.

Doblin's decision infuriated Marsha Weil, Clusterbusters' primary (and, in some ways, only) funder. The latter half of her $50,000 contribution to MAPS had been designated as a matching grant. As far as she was concerned, MAPS was now indebted to them for $25,000—money that MAPS had already raised but was now refusing to use toward Clusterbusters' priorities.

Doblin did his best to smooth things over, but Weil had heard enough. She would remain on Clusterbusters' Board of Directors and help Wold oversee research at Harvard. But she'd been thoroughly discouraged by the way this philanthropic effort had unfolded.

Weil didn't particularly care whether Halpern had snitched. But she worried about his reputation in the wake of "Halperngate." If, as she believed, people in the psychedelic community disliked the researcher they were depending upon, he would struggle to be invited to psychedelic science conferences. How would Halpern raise funds if he was banned from attending meetings where the people who cared about this research networked? Would the psychedelic world sneer at Clusterbusters too? They needed all the allies they could get.

In the meantime, neither Wold nor Weil understood how Harvard had managed to spend over $14,000 to produce a protocol for a clinical trial that, to date, did not exist (it had paid for the salary of a consultant provided by MAPS). Halpern tried to reassure Wold that he would personally ensure Clusterbusters' research was completed to satisfaction. But nothing either Doblin or Halpern said ever won back Weil's trust. She had no intention of throwing good money after bad.

Cash was shorter than ever, important alliances had been irreparably damaged, and the number of people who could accomplish the task at hand was becoming smaller by the day—because psychedelic researchers, it turns out, were getting awfully hard to come by.

●  ●  ●●●●●●●●●●●●●●●●●●●  ●  ●

Despite the fallout from Sewell's article on becoming a psychedelic researcher, his question about how to do such controversial research in universities is both important and difficult to answer. Ironically, given their feud, John Halpern might've been one of the few scientists with the expertise to answer this question in 2006. Not many others could boast that they had a funded clinical trial testing a psychedelic underway.

Halpern had always been careful to emphasize the importance of good science. But he also understood that science occurs within a political context that associated psychedelics with a freewheeling, rule-bending, socially disruptive, tree-hugging, orgiastic, draft-dodging counterculture.

Countering these stereotypes required that he present himself as a respectable, law-abiding citizen. Halpern made a point to emphasize that science meant more than conducting well-designed experiments. It also included paperwork, public affairs, and approval from senior faculty. As he told one journalist who asked about the legacy of Timothy Leary, "We have seen how not to do it, haven't we?"[44]

Halpern had good reason to worry. Running a tight ship was an absolute necessity in his line of work. For instance, McLean's decision to distance itself from MAPS, due to concerns that the organization's political advocacy for drug reform might be a liability, highlighted ongoing worries about the lingering influence of Leary's controversial legacy at Harvard.[45]

Danielle Giffort's book *Acid Revival* describes a "respectability politics" that girds the new wave of psychedelic research.[46] The term originally referred to a code of conduct that minority communities followed to gain social acceptance, but Giffort's application to the world of psychedelics makes a lot of sense. Everyone involved in psychedelic research worries that politicians might take their gains away if something goes wrong, so they compensate by suppressing any sign of deviance. That is why most prominent scientists in the field have, at least until recently, refused to discuss whether they've tried the drugs themselves. (Halpern made an exception regarding peyote use since he'd taken it at the invitation of the Native American Church. As he told one journalist, "I would not be able to do the work if I had not."[47])

Sewell's article, ironically, had breached the basic norm within psychedelic research: the performance of sobriety and respectability. Halpern argued that everything Sewell did subsequently only proved Halpern's point: in emails to Wold he'd argue that the postdoc lacked "sufficient character to handle the firestorm that we will be passing through." This is respectability politics in action.

But as Giffort points out, it's hard to keep up appearances, given the political realities of the field. On the one hand, it's hard to seem objective about drugs if you come back from Burning Man with blue hair (as, apparently, Andrew Sewell later did—though I heard his colleagues at Yale weren't nearly as put out). On the other, fund-raising and material support for research relied on philanthropists who developed their interest in promoting psychedelics research because of their personal experiences with mind-expanding drugs. Holding the counterculture at arm's length while maintaining a strong relationship with the underground is a balancing act.

Sewell warned readers to keep up appearances, so why did he fail to take his own advice? Burning Man, I later learned, had been one of Sewell's many passionate interests. He adored—and, so far as I can tell, was adored by—the broader psychedelic community. If McLean wanted to distance itself from MAPS to signal "objectivity," is it possible that Sewell wanted to distance himself from Halpern to signal his "trustworthiness"?

● ● ●●●●●●●●●●●●●●●●●●● ● ●

John Halpern has always insisted in our conversations that Halperngate did not harm his career. He conducted science, which had nothing to do with (and this, he admitted, was a "rather sensational thing to say") "the Taliban wing of the psychedelic movement."

His conscience, he told me, was clear.

Pickard had given him money when he was in his twenties. (Only about a third of the amount that was reported, he says). The cash made him more confident that he could "afford" a career in academic research when clinical practice would have paid much more.

"So, a bunch of cretinous scumbags of the psychedelic underground who wished that they had been somehow involved directly in Pickard's conspiracy attacked me as if I'm some snitch. Which is bullshit," he told me.

The underground's concerns about him were misguided, he claimed. Halpern was there not to "infiltrate the system" but to be the best part of the system. And he had receipts to prove it: his advocacy and research on the long-term safety of peyote helped secure religious freedom for the Native American Church and its members. An amicus brief he'd written on behalf of the União do Vegetal, a small international church founded in Brazil that used ayahuasca as a sacrament, had helped convince the Supreme Court to issue a unanimous decision protecting the religious freedom of any recognized religious group—even newly formed groups—to use Schedule I substances. His research on the long-term safety of MDMA cleared the path for clinical trials testing its efficacy as a medicine.

He's right: John Halpern deserves more credit for the psychedelic "renaissance" than almost anyone is willing to grant him.

But I think he's wrong about the psychedelic underground. Halperngate made his work much harder to do. I could especially see the impact on his ability to fundraise. While most people likely believe a Harvard Medical School professor earns a large salary, research professors like Halpern rarely earn a guaranteed fixed salary, let alone receive funding from their employers for "overhead" like laboratory equipment and computers. They're much more like entrepreneurs, who must "earn" their income and overhead by either securing research funding or seeing patients.

In 2006, Halpern earned 60 percent of his salary from the National Institute on Drug Abuse grant that funded his study on Mormons using MDMA. He depended on philanthropists like Peter Lewis for the remaining 40 percent of his funding needs. However, by year's end, he could see that his access to private funds was drying up. Lewis's grant money was tied up in bureaucratic red tape. Halpern had been stretching that NIDA grant to cover all his projects, but the situation made him anxious.

MAPS could no longer donate their funds to McLean (at least, not openly), but Doblin was still trying to fundraise for Halpern. Doblin, however, struggled to find people willing to support Halpern. MAPS, in his words, had "paid a price" for supporting Halpern. Halperngate had turned the researcher into a pariah in the psychedelic community. MAPS, according to Doblin, not only received complaints about its decision to collaborate with Halpern, people specified this single issue in their decision *not* to become members of MAPS. Their wealthiest donors put riders on money they gave to MAPS, specifying that none of it be allocated to Halpern's research.

If Andrew Sewell exposed himself as too tightly allied to the underground, then John Halpern's error had been his reputed alliance with law enforcement.[48]

You can't be a psychedelic researcher if nobody trusts you.

I believed Halpern when he said that he was there to be the best part of the system—but the "system" is a network that connects those with credentials with both the underground and indigenous cultures. When restrictive regulations on psychedelic science force aboveground scientists to rely on underground knowledge, there is, at some point, no aboveground or underground—there is only dirt. The connections between the two cannot be so easily disentangled.

Rick Doblin's success has relied on his ability to navigate this network, strengthening his ties between underground and aboveground research. But the pressure of appearing "objective" all too often encourages scientists to present their research—the fruit of this work—as though it came from nowhere. Doing so runs the risk of biopiracy—the exploitation of knowledge and resources from those with less power. Indigenous communities have long faced the exploitation of their knowledge and resources, and now, as we broaden our perspective, we must also recognize and guard against similar thefts from underground patient communities and citizen scientists. Initiatives that promote respectful collaboration and equitable benefit sharing among all parties—researchers, companies, community groups, indigenous communities, and citizen scientists—could be key in addressing and alleviating these multifaceted tensions.

Obscuring outlaw innovation, however, doesn't make it irrelevant. In the same way that admiring only the mushroom emerging aboveground obscures the importance of the tangled threads of mycelium below, we can't allow our admiration for eminent scholars to blind us to their connections to the underground. One simply cannot exist without the other.

One can easily observe the irony in valuing the knowledge contributions of those who are "aboveground" more than those working "underground," which is to say, illegally and without credentials, by attending any Clusterbusters conference. At these events, physicians, residents, and pharmaceutical representatives listen to the passionate testimonies of Clusterheads who describe how psychedelic drugs saved them after medicine nearly ruined their lives. I've seen physicians, initially skeptical, transformed and transfixed by the experience—a room full of energized, optimistic cluster headache patients is very different from the typical clinical encounter with a single, struggling cluster headache patient, which is too often marked by medication failures.

And there's so much knowledge here. I've kept this story focused on mushrooms, but there have been a lot of innovations developed in this patient group, including a vitamin D supplementation protocol under study at the University of Texas Health Science Center at Houston. As one pharmaceutical representative in attendance at a conference told me, "There's nothing [these patients] can learn from us. They are the ones at the cutting edge of research." Humility like this is in short supply—but necessary for thriving in this field.

•  •  •••••••••••••••••••••  •  •

"Everything okay? I haven't heard from you in a while?" Halpern asked Wold in a message sent on Tuesday, January 2, 2007, at 6:54 a.m.

It had been a full two weeks since he'd gotten a reply to any of his emails.

Wold replied two days later. "All is well here, thanks for asking. Just needed to step back for a few days over the holidays. Get ready for some email replies LOL."

He'd gotten at least seven messages from Halpern over the previous two weeks—each one a new drama containing accusations about the theft of mail, allegations about integrity and ethics, meltdowns about Sewell's behavior, and instructions for Wold to review the "Free Leonard Pickard" website, because although there was a "segment of people that belong to MAPS and/or donate to MAPS [who] do have this agenda of destroying any research I am involved in," Wold would not find a "single comment [on the site] attacking me or trying to make me look like the devil. . . . The people that should count don't support this agenda."[49]

More of this was to come.

For years now, Wold had organized his entire life around helping people survive this awful disease. Quite a lot weighed on him over the psychedelic New Year. Had he made a mistake in choosing this path? Was Harvard up to the task? What was the alternative? Clusterbusters' Board of Directors tried to find a way out of the situation. But where else could they go? Limited funding and sunk costs kept them tied to Halpern. The only way forward, it appeared, was through. They'd made their bed; they were going to have to keep lying in it.

## Chapter Fifteen

# SKIP THE TRIP

TAKING A PSYCHEDELIC DRUG IS A BIT LIKE JUMPING INTO THE OCEAN at night. You can prepare, but even the most experienced psychonaut doesn't know what will happen once surrounded by the deep blue. Maybe the kaleidoscopic sea will offer smooth sailing. Maybe tendrils of anxiety— or even panic—will present threats along the way. But there are certain dependable qualities: Patterns unfold in geometric harmony. Distances warp, making something distant seem just a few feet away. The world, now animated, feels more alive, more real. Take a big-enough dose, and the world begins to feel—really feel—infused with a profound sense of unity. Ideas that had previously seemed trite now seem utterly brilliant; thoughts and ideas that were once blurry have sharpened into crystalline focus.

We are all one.

There is more beauty in the world than we can ever know.

The present moment is all there is.

This has happened before. It will happen again.

Change is the only constant.

That a psychedelic experience might have a spiritual dimension is no secret to indigenous communities that have used psychoactive plants and fungi as sacraments for millennia. That this same altered consciousness might find a place within the highly regimented corridors of Western medicine represents a significant departure from business as usual. Science— the epistemology of medicine—grounds its authority in opposition to the world of mysticism and spirituality. Knowledge based on meticulous experimentation, solid evidence, and air-tight logic allowed scientists to say, "The preacher can teach you how to live your life. We will teach you the truth."

Aldous Huxley, for one, found this reductionist approach to life lacking. For him, science and spirituality could—nay, should—coexist. Caring for his first wife, Maria, as she was dying of cancer led Huxley to foster a deep conviction about the potential of consciousness, and even spirituality, to mitigate the physical and existential agonies of death. He observed that the living could facilitate a gentler passage for the dying, elevating what is perhaps the most physiological act of human existence to a plane of awareness and spiritual resonance.

Huxley's 1962 utopian novel *Island*—the book that inspired Esalen's founders—described a land where a fictional psychedelic drug called moksha helped residents confront their mortality with serenity, acceptance, and relief. One of the characters, Lakshmi, an elderly woman grappling with cancer, explains how moksha detached her from her pain, stating, "It would be bad, if it were really my pain. But somehow it isn't. The pain's here; but I'm somewhere else. It's like what you discover with the moksha-medicine. Nothing really belongs to you. Not even your pain."[1]

The novel read like a sermon. The very next year, Huxley entrusted his second wife, Laura, with administering to him one hundred micrograms of LSD just before he died. Laura would later describe how he'd been in physical and psychic agony before the injection, but then the LSD had brought him peace, so that "like a music that becomes less and less audible, he faded away."[2]

● ● ●●●●●●●●●●●●●●●●●● ● ●

When, in November 2006, *New Scientist* magazine invited fifty "brilliant minds" to forecast the future, Halpern's entry could have been ghostwritten by Huxley. In it, he described how his psychedelic research might "lead to a new field of medicine in which spirituality is kindled to help us accept our mortality without fear, and where those with addiction problems, anxiety or cluster headache discover a path to genuine healing."[3]

Halpern, with the assistance of Rick Doblin and the Multidisciplinary Association for Psychedelic Studies (MAPS), came tantalizingly close to success. If all went as planned, he (and Doblin) would have empirical data demonstrating that MDMA was the real moksha medicine.

Huxley germinated one of the spores for this idea. But Halpern and Doblin's plan had been grounded in research in the 1960s and 1970s that had produced strong evidence that psychedelic therapy might ease existential suffering. Less known, however, is that this research had begun as a series of studies about pain.

* * ●●●●●●●●●●●●●●●●●●●●● ● ●

Aldous Huxley's writing about LSD and death was first put to the test by Dr. Eric C. Kast, a psychiatrist who held positions as assistant professor of medicine and psychiatry at Chicago Medical School and anesthesiologist at Chicago's Cook County Hospital in the early 1960s. Kast, however, had not been inspired by Huxley, but instead, by a pragmatic quest to address the limitations of opioids, which were the default treatment for severe pain.

Medicine, Kast observed, lacked an ideal analgesic. Opioids, the preferred painkiller, impaired patients' senses, undermined their interest in life, led to addiction, could cause overdoses, and often failed to provide relief. Kast hypothesized that LSD might be a viable alternative because pain wasn't just an objective mechanical process. It was an interaction between the cold, hard fact of our bodies and the complex narratives our minds spun around them. People in pain get tied up in a knot between a desire, he argued, to hold onto their bodily integrity and the contrasting urge to separate themselves from the painful parts.[4]

Opioid-based analgesics, he noted, worked not because they numbed sensation but because they induced a "feeling of removal of the self from emotional problems."[5] In other words, it wasn't that opioids dulled the pain; it was that they allowed patients to alter their mental perceptions of the pain. But opioids, as we in the twenty-first century are all too aware, created more problems than they solved. Kast wanted to find a drug that could alter the mind's perception of pain without leaving a trail of devastation behind.

The psychological component of LSD offered a potential substitute. Kast was particularly interested in how the drug made it difficult to pay attention to specific sensations. Perhaps this quality would help pain patients reduce their focus on what ailed them.[6]

Sandoz agreed. Kast was one of only seventeen investigators the company allowed to study LSD in the wake of new regulatory controls set in place by the Food and Drug Administration (FDA) after the thalidomide scandal frightened the public about the risk of medications.[7]

Between 1963 and 1967, Kast administered LSD to over 250 people with severe pain, most of whom had terminal cancer, at Chicago Medical School and Cook County Hospital. But unlike contemporary researchers who are now studying the psychospiritual healing capacity of psychedelics, Kast wasn't focused on end-of-life anxiety—he wanted to alleviate patients' physical pain. The results were astonishing: a single one-hundred-microgram dose of LSD provided longer-lasting pain relief than opioids like Demerol and hydromorphone. Immediate relief lasted up to twelve hours, with effects persisting for as long as three weeks. Furthermore, LSD appeared to be well tolerated, even by terminally ill patients.[8]

Kast hypothesized that a high dose of LSD distracted patients from their pain by making other, less distressing sensations more prominent in the person's awareness. Anticipation of events, he argued, might be an excellent evolutionary adaptation, but it offered few positive benefits for those who knew that death was their best chance at experiencing relief. Depriving a person of the ability to focus—even for a short time—offered a potent escape, a release from a hypervigilance to pain and fear of what's to come.

In a high-enough dose, the dissolution of ego offered patients the cognitive space to distance themselves from their pain.

As Lakshmi said, "The pain's here; but I'm somewhere else."

● ● ●●●●●●●●●●●●●●●●●●●● ● ●

Little in Kast's research suggested any real engagement with either Aldous Huxley or the psychospiritual. If Kast's interest in dying was psychospiritual, then he did a wonderful job keeping it undercover. But at a time when it was taboo to say the word *cancer*, Kast couldn't help but notice that patients who had taken LSD often spoke about their own deaths with a casual frankness.[9]

At first, he mentioned this as a side note. Patients in his first study expressed "a peculiar disregard for the gravity of their [serious medical] situations, and talked freely about their impending death with an affect considered inappropriate in our western civilization, but most beneficial to their own psychic states."[10] They'd sprinkle conversation with casual observations about their own mortality, then remark on the beauty of the moment or something seemingly mundane, highlighting a dramatic shift in perspective and a breaking down of societal norms concerning discussions of death.

Kast's insights into the therapeutic potential of LSD represent one of the missed opportunities in medical history. Part of the problem was simply timing. Scientific research on LSD declined sharply after the 1962 US Kefauver-Harris Act. Kast had been one of the lucky few scientists to receive permission from Sandoz to conduct his 1964 research on LSD. Medicine's newfound emphasis on distinguishing the therapeutic effect of drugs from placebo didn't bode well for LSD, either. Nor did Kast's findings interest his colleagues in anesthesiology, who sought analgesics they could control. Nevertheless, Kast's insight that LSD could ease the anguish of an impending death caught the eye of a few remaining researchers in the field.

Sidney Cohen noticed. Cohen, one of the first psychiatrists to embrace the therapeutic potential of LSD, had also been one of the first to warn of its dangers. In 1962, Cohen published an influential study warning that the drug could be dangerous if misused. Research on the drug, he worried, had become much too relaxed: LSD parties and fringe, pseudoscientific theories had no place in science.[11]

Kast's research, on the other hand, impressed him. In a 1965 essay published in *Harper's Magazine*, Cohen described how well Kast's findings resonated with the research he'd been doing over the previous decade, writing, "It would seem that LSD does not act directly on the part of the brain that receives pain impulses. Instead, it appears to alter the meaning of the pain, and in doing so, diminishes it."[12]

Take, for example, his patient Irene. "Attending to thoughts and feelings beyond herself, she was unconcerned about pain, which had been the main focus of her waking existence for months. No longer did it have ominous significance." Irene's perceptions shifted so dramatically that she twice needed to be reminded to take her pain medication. And the analgesic effect seemed to last. Irene, according to Cohen, put it this way: "The pain is back, but I think I can cope with it. What a day yesterday was. A sort of holiday from me."[13]

Kast's research was taken up by scientists at Spring Grove Hospital's psychedelic research program in Baltimore, Maryland, who designed a clinical trial that could cross-validate his key findings. LSD-assisted therapy would be administered to end-of-life cancer patients with two questions in mind: Would the intervention reduce the need for opioids to control pain? And would the intervention alleviate the anxiety and depression that so often accompanied impending death?

Evidence that LSD-assisted therapy could alleviate existential crises was strong. But the researchers struggled to understand their data on pain reduction. Patients reported a significant drop in how much pain they experienced, but their research question asked if LSD-assisted therapy reduced patients' reliance on narcotics. It did not. People still needed their pain meds.

Had they simply asked the wrong question? Opioids usually didn't fully control end-of-life pain. LSD-assisted therapy seemed to make their patients more comfortable.[14] The researchers at Silver Spring never had a chance to figure it out. Everything they had been doing came to a standstill when the federal government pulled the plug on their research.

That is, until 2006, when Bob Jesse's Council on Spiritual Practices and Roland Griffiths at Johns Hopkins brought the dream of spiritually inflected medical care one step closer to fruition. The year might have gone badly for Halpern, but elsewhere psychonauts were celebrating a publication in *Psychopharmacology* titled "Psilocybin Can Occasion Mystical-Type Experiences Having Substantial and Sustained Personal Meaning and Spiritual Significance."[15]

The study, a meticulously designed clinical trial, found that large doses of psilocybin, when administered in a comfortable, supportive setting, fostered the same kind of mystical experiences reported by spiritual seekers around the world. The "trip"—a frame of mind once considered so pathological that scientists believed it mimicked schizophrenia—created such a profound sense of interconnectedness with the world that 67 percent of participants described it as one of the top-five most meaningful experiences they'd ever had—comparable to the birth of a child or the death of a parent.[16] A follow-up study showcased the enduring impact of the experience: fourteen months later, 58 percent and 67 percent of volunteers, respectively, ranked the experience among the top five in terms of personal meaning and spiritual significance in their lives. The experience enhanced their well-being and life satisfaction—and the impact lasted.[17]

It would take half a dozen years before a clinical trial that applied this finding made it to print. But in 2011, UCLA psychiatrist Charles Grob and a team of researchers published a Heffter Research Institute–funded clinical trial exploring the potential therapeutic properties of psilocybin-assisted therapy for those facing the deep existential distress common in late-stage cancer patients.[18] The treatment seemed to work: a single dose of psilocybin lowered participants' anxiety and improved their mood, even as they grappled with their own demise.

In 2016, Roland Griffiths published a much larger clinical trial that confirmed Grob's findings. And then a second clinical trial published by Grob's former student Stephen Ross, a physician at New York University, would do the same. Meanwhile researchers in Basel, Switzerland, administering LSD to end-of-life patients in clinical trials were finding much the same: the psychedelic trip seemed to really help people deal with their existential struggles.[19]

But while each of these studies dutifully cited Eric Kast's foundational research, they gave physical discomfort almost no attention. It was almost as if pain didn't matter at all.

Halpern's clinical trial would not only have resuscitated the research at Spring Grove but might have also brought attention to the analgesic effects of psychedelics. At least, that was a goal of the study. Trial participants would be asked to complete a daily log recording their pain.[20] But by November 2009, a mere three years after the *New Scientist* article published Halpern's prediction, funding for this future had dried up. The only viable path for remaining at Harvard would be to skip the psychedelic trip. Bob Wold couldn't help but think that Clusterbusters was getting screwed in the process.

● ● ●●●●●●●●●●●●●●●●●●●● ● ●

People expected shenanigans when they worked in construction, but nothing in Wold's day job compared to the dysfunctional behavior he experienced at Harvard. It seemed like every day brought a new crisis to manage.

In early 2007, Halpern began sending Wold indications that the financial situation at Harvard had become precarious. Clusterbusters' board was beginning to find his requests for additional funding both odd and somewhat discomforting, given the cost overruns on their collaboration thus far. Wold and Weil had both been under the impression that a clinical trial would cost about as much as had been agreed upon in the original February 2004 memo of understanding that Doblin had provided them: $50,000 plus a matching grant, equaling $75,000 in total. Halpern was tossing around "guestimates" of $250,000, with the caveat that "much more will need to be raised if we have a neuroimaging component woven into the study."[21] An email in January 2007 casually tossed out $500,000 as a possibility.[22] This significant increase came without much observable progress on the protocol development.

But the pleas for funding were nothing compared to the epic feud between Halpern and Sewell, which was somehow still ongoing. Halpern wanted nothing to do with the man and hated that Clusterbusters still collaborated with him. That it had only taken weeks for Sewell to find a philanthropist willing to donate $10,000 to allow some of his cluster headache research to continue infuriated Halpern.[23] The money would be wasted, Halpern told Wold. That guy had no future in academic medicine. But by September 2007, Sewell had picked up a research job at Yale Medical School and a clinical position as an attending physician at the local Veterans Administration Hospital.[24]

For his part, Sewell couldn't stand being in the same room as Halpern, whom he often referred to as "criminal" in his emails. Halpern felt much the same about "Angry Swill." Both asked Wold to act as a mediator in their relationship so often that he thought the two Harvard-trained psychiatrists ought to pay *him* to be their therapist.

Did scientists treat other funders this way? Wold couldn't imagine that Halpern issued demands to any of the other philanthropists who sponsored his research. He'd sometimes send an email to Doblin and ask how it was possible that Peter Lewis had been able to place progress milestones in his grant while Clusterbusters felt squeezed for every penny. But who knows? Maybe Halpern was blowing up Lewis's phone. I don't have those records! In any case, a billionaire could afford to let Halpern fail. The leader of a patient community desperate for treatment didn't enjoy the same luxury.

Every request for funding felt like hubris, given the recent implosion of their collaboration with Andrew Sewell. The latest request involved a clinical trial costing $10,000. Halpern explained that this was a very reasonable fee, and quite necessary. The funding would support a small open-label trial testing a nonhallucinogenic analog of LSD called 2-bromolysergic acid diethylamide (BOL-148).

"Are there places where Clusterbusters might apply for grant money?" Wold asked.

Halpern didn't have many helpful suggestions. "There are other private foundations," he said, but he didn't think "hyper-conservative neurology foundations" or "headache foundations" would be interested. "I think you already know the score with them."

Federal grants, he added, might be a possibility once they had pilot data, but "funding [would] be an uphill battle all the way." Best bet would be "direct funding from famous people." Somebody he knew with a "mega-trust fund" had a brother with cluster headache. That's how they'd get funding. Friends with money.[25]

Wold wondered, *Did they need another study that they couldn't afford?*

Halpern insisted they did. McLean's Institutional Review Board (IRB) was already expressing skepticism about a research protocol testing LSD for cluster headache. So Halpern hatched a plan: They could demonstrate that the psychedelic effects of LSD played an essential role in its ability to treat cluster headache by giving cluster patients a nonhallucinogenic version of LSD. Then, when the treatment failed—whammo. They'd have rock-solid evidence that the magic ingredient in LSD was the trip itself.

Wold was skeptical—and pissed—but he'd found over the course of their collaboration that pushing back against Halpern never seemed to work. Halpern simply refused to take no for an answer. In this case, Halpern argued it didn't matter whether Clusterbusters *wanted* to pay for a study testing BOL-148. The politics at Harvard's McLean Hospital *required* them to pursue the study. Sometimes Halpern seemed downright incredulous that they even resisted the idea—why not, instead, just thank him for developing such a remarkable opportunity to receive so much return for a tiny investment?[26]

Clusterbusters' board didn't quite see the point of giving people in excruciating pain a drug that they thought wouldn't work. Worse, what if the drug *did* work? Wouldn't a case study demonstrating that a nonhallucinogenic version of LSD worked strengthen the hospital's opposition to their psilocybin clinical trial?

Halpern pushed back against their concerns. He couldn't see how the small study could derail Clusterbusters' mission. Even if the drug helped a bit, this study involved only five people. They had much stronger data that LSD and psilocybin were effective from the *Neurology* article that documented fifty-three case reports of people with cluster headache who had gained benefit from these drugs.[27] They should, instead, look at the big picture: the study would take place in Germany in collaboration with two prestigious physicians at Hannover Medical School. Clinical trials in Germany cost much less than they did in the United States (especially when Harvard hosted the study). Funding a study like this, Halpern argued, would help Clusterbusters solidify its reputation as a patient-centered organization that cared more about finding an effective treatment than getting high.

Nobody pushed back on this, despite how unsettling the premise. Of course, board members knew that they had to navigate that stigma, given they represented people in pain *and* a patient group seeking to legitimate the use of psychedelic medicine. They'd already been working on a broad range of other projects to patch up the holes left by the healthcare system: diagnosis, epidemiology, access to oxygen therapy.

After much discussion, the board decided in August 2007 that it would allow the study, so long as Halpern followed through with the psilocybin clinical trial submission. In the meantime, Wold did what he could to make sure the study ran smoothly.

●  ●  ●●●●●●●●●●●●●●●●●●  ●  ●

John Halpern announced that he had submitted a psilocybin clinical trial protocol to the IRB at the September 2008 Clusterbusters conference—four years after their $50,000 grant began and one year after they made it a condition of releasing more funds.

The IRB rejected the proposal soon after. Halpern, however, had no interest in revising and resubmitting a protocol. BOL-148 produced remarkable results—the effects were so powerful it might even work better than any other drug, including psilocybin *and* LSD.

Halpern insisted that the tremendous efficacy of BOL-148 made perfect sense, which is somewhat strange given that he'd pitched the study to Clusterbusters' board as a sure failure. But now he'd changed his tune. It was all so obvious: medicines work better when they're taken in a higher dose, but side effects limit the amount a person can take. This hadn't been a problem with BOL-148. In other words, from a dosing standpoint, they could go way beyond what they could ever dream of with hallucinogenic LSD. As far as he was concerned, proposing research on any other treatment for cluster headache at this point "verged" on unethical, never mind that Clusterbusters had always been very clear that the purpose of their grant had been to obtain an approved protocol for the study of psilocybin.

Clusterbusters' board was less enthusiastic than Halpern anticipated. Discovering a new medication for cluster headache ought to have been cause for celebration, but the board saw BOL-148 as just another stumbling block in a frustrating process. The obstacles to getting a psychedelic clinical trial were only getting higher four years into their collaboration. What good was a miracle drug they couldn't grow in their closet and that would take years to bring to the market? People needed a treatment now.

They had paid for a specific "deliverable": an IRB-approved clinical trial. Constant bickering, complaints, excuses, delays, and drama had worn them down. Learning that Halpern had already begun filing paperwork to patent BOL-148 only compounded their skepticism about his motivations. (Of course, they noted, Halpern had not bothered to include anyone from Clusterbusters on the patent. To which he would reply, *my invention? That you didn't want to fund?*)

Wold wasn't always sure what to do or whom to trust. Results from the small clinical trial had been impressive, but he'd spent a lifetime fighting to access *oxygen*. The best medicine is the one you can get. The best medicine is the one that people aren't frightened to take. Psilocybin could be accessed now, albeit illegally. Wold hoped that the Harvard label would help destigmatize its outlaw status as they moved through the process of medicalizing the drug. But he found it difficult to convince Halpern of the pragmatic politics of why Clusterbusters prioritized an "all of the above" solution.

But they wouldn't really have a choice. Rick Doblin, a true believer in the transformational healing powers of psychedelic medicine, supported Halpern's decision to pursue BOL-148. Doblin wrote to Wold, "Finding a non-psychedelic drug that is patented is the best thing that could have happened to Clusterbusters in helping to reach the goal of a legal, effective medicine for CH. . . . I don't think you appreciate the magnitude of that discovery."[28]

Wold was appreciative of this potentially monumental advance. But the thing that was most bothering him felt almost taboo to say out loud. Years of helping people with cluster headache had taught Wold that you couldn't just take away the pain of a disease this cruel and call it a day. Psychedelic medicine healed the entire person.

Cluster headache, everyone seemed to agree, could be treated by tweaking neurotransmitters. No need to muck around with messy things like a person's consciousness. Where was Dr. Eric Kast when he needed him?

● ● ●●●●●●●●●●●●●●●●●●●●●● ● ● ●

By the beginning of February 2009, John Halpern's funding problems had become dire. The biggest problem, of course, had to do with challenges of raising money for clinical trials testing drugs so transgressive. But the Great Recession hadn't helped—a potential funder had lost his money in the Bernie Madoff scheme. Halpern hadn't even managed to meet the next research milestone that would have unlocked the rest of the funding already allocated to his MDMA-assisted therapy study. Worse, the DEA had refused to grant Halpern a license for providing Schedule I drugs to research subjects—a slightly awkward situation for a professor trying to position himself as a leader in psychedelic research. Halpern would need to hire a physician with a Schedule I license or the study would be shut down.

Rick Doblin offered to send Wold a grant worth $26,000—the exact amount once earmarked for a psychedelic clinical trial—to fund Halpern's new hire: Dr. Pedro Huertas.

Wold didn't understand. "We don't need Pedro . . . MDMA needs Pedro."[29]

Without Pedro, there was no John. Without John, there was no Harvard. Huertas had experience developing therapeutics for inherited, rare, and orphan diseases, and he understood how to raise money from venture capitalists. Ask him to help you develop BOL-148, Doblin suggested. Have him crunch some numbers. Wold could think of other ways to spend that money, but Doblin left him no choice.

Huertas's prognosis, however, was not optimistic. It would cost them $30 million to $40 million just for FDA approval, according to Huertas's calculations. Their data on cluster headache was limited, and left significant gaps in understanding, particularly regarding the drug's safety profile in human subjects. The FDA would require animal studies before pursuing more clinical trial research in humans. Venture capitalists probably wouldn't be interested, given the limited return on investments in such a niche market. Breaking into the migraine market might give the group a chance at more success, but then they should anticipate a $100 million investment in drug development. While the potential for success exists, substantial financial, research, and clinical hurdles marked the road ahead. His final assessment: "BOL is the perfect molecule to be developed by a non-profit, foundation or patient interest group where revenue potential can offset the costs of development in the long term."[30]

Doblin, who had recommended Huertas, now argued that he had erred by a factor of ten in his calculations. "The income is 10x more than he first suggested." And for reasons Doblin declined to explain, Huertas "reduced his estimate of the cost of the research by $5–10 million."[31] Once they got the government to designate cluster headache as an orphan disease, they'd qualify for incentives offered by the FDA's Orphan Drug Act, like tax credits for suitable clinical trials and extended market exclusivity once a drug receives approval.

Halpern didn't think these numbers ought to stop them either. Anyway, Huertas had said the plan could work if nurtured by a nonprofit foundation, adding, "Ah . . . hello Clusterbusters."[32] How could they even dream of developing a psychedelic medicine if they couldn't interest investors in a nonpsychedelic substance?

But just months later, the lab had become so deeply in debt that Halpern was forced to recant. He could study psilocybin if that's what Clusterbusters' Board of Directors insisted he do before it would release additional funding. It was a bitter pill to swallow for a man staking his reputation and life's work on BOL-148. But he had to buy some time. Maybe one of his pleas for a donation would bear fruit. Halpern slashed his salary in half and began looking for side gigs in clinical psychiatry. Seeing real patients could help right the ship—at least for a while. In the meantime, the lab's financial lifeline kept thinning.

Clock ticking, Halpern sent a grave email to Clusterbusters' Board of Directors in September 2009: just six more weeks of operational funds. He wasn't sure what life after Harvard might look like, but a future somewhere else seemed imminent. He hadn't given up yet: he always believed that BOL-148 was the perfect drug for the Bill & Melinda Gates Foundation, and in an unbelievable twist of fate, Rick Doblin had just met someone in the organization! Some Swiss donors expressed interest . . . and in even better news, National Geographic was about to air a documentary called *Inside LSD* that would dedicate at least five minutes to Halpern's cluster headache research. Surely the media attention would attract a big pharmaceutical company?

Of course, none of these opportunities came to fruition, at least not in the way Halpern had hoped. Especially galling was how little interest the National Geographic episode generated. The segment was terrific. Halpern estimated it would have cost $10 million to $20 million to pay for that much advertising, and he was proud to get it for free.

Despite a media blitz worth millions, the phone stayed silent. That's when Ari Mello, a friend with a somewhat obscure background in finance, made an audacious proposal. "Why not found our own company? Develop BOL-148 ourselves?"

● ● ●●●●●●●●●●●●●●●●●●● ● ●

Entheogen Sciences Corp, Halpern's last-minute Hail Mary, claimed BOL-148 was the next big thing in headache treatment—a $3.6 billion market. And at first everything seemed like it was going great. Clusterbusters landed a few positions in the company's structure, including Marsha Weil as a founding member of its board of directors and Bob Wold as a member of the advisory board. Halpern even found a wealthy philanthropist willing to fund the company as a silent partner.

But this victory would be short-lived, and the company's prospects another casualty of the tiresome, never-ending war between Halpern and Sewell.

When Halpern discovered that Sewell had somehow beat him to the US Patent and Trademark Office by six months, Halpern exploded.[33] But Sewell insisted: he'd been thinking about the possibility that a nonhallucinogenic analog of LSD might benefit people with cluster headache ever since he'd read Federigo Sicuteri's landmark 1963 paper investigating the use of lysergic derivatives in headache treatment. BOL-148 seemed like the most likely candidate.

A protracted, expensive standoff resulted in a stalemate. When the dust settled, Sewell retained ownership of BOL-148 in the United States while Halpern and Passie held the rights everywhere else. Neither side showed any willingness to cooperate with the other. But John Halpern wouldn't need to deal with Andrew Sewell much longer.

● ● ●●●●●●●●●●●●●●●●●●●● ● ●

Dr. R. Andrew Sewell passed away on July 21, 2013, at the age of forty-one— just twelve days after undergoing what was supposed to be a routine surgery. He had multiple tumors removed, a standard procedure for a hereditary condition known as multiple endocrine neoplasia, a diagnosis he had lived with for half his life. Sewell and his medical team had expected a smooth and uneventful recovery.

The circumstances surrounding Sewell's departure from Harvard six years before his death had always been somewhat murky. Everyone knew the Halpern-Sewell rivalry consumed all the oxygen in the room, but so many allegations had been made across the aisle, it seemed impossible to sort out truth from fiction.

The root of Sewell's conflicts may have been a fundamental frustration with the system. His widow, Nikki Sewell, a psychotherapist who specializes in grief—"a legacy his death left me"—described him as a maverick, with a big personality, brilliant, passionate, indefatigable, and very, very bold. "He pushed the envelope. . . . So when you would say, 'Oh, you can't do that,' he'd want to know, 'Well, why can't I?'"

The idea that "bureaucratic red tape" might keep good medicine from patients enraged him.

After Harvard, she said, Sewell found a more accommodating atmosphere at Yale, where his maverick tendencies were not just tolerated but welcomed. Even so, his irreverence for academic formalities never completely faded. Maybe it was this very skepticism of established norms that allowed him to truly hear his patients, to listen to what improved their conditions.

In return, they adored him. After his death, messages poured in from around the globe. Patients referred to Dr. Sewell as their "hero," the man who had given them "hope" and "relief," the doctor who had "saved [their] life." The cruel irony was that the man who had extended so many lifelines could not save his own, cut short in a devastating twist of fate.

● ● ●●●●●●●●●●●●●●●●●●● ● ●

John Halpern's last visit to the annual Clusterbusters conference happened to coincide with my first, in September 2013. At the time, I didn't yet understand the full implications of his talk: an update on Entheogen Sciences Corp's efforts to seek corporate financing to develop BOL-148. But even as a conference newbie, I noted his frustration—it was palpable to everyone in the room. The ongoing patent battle with Sewell had made it impossible to interest potential buyers. And investors seemed to figure out what Pedro Huertas had told them all along: the size of the cluster headache market wouldn't offer enough return on their investment.

Rick Doblin's proposal to obtain orphan disease designation from the FDA hadn't yet worked out. An orphan disease, according to the FDA, affects fewer than two hundred thousand US adults per year. Cluster headache affects three hundred thousand in the United States, a figure that exceeds that definition of a rare disease by 50 percent. Too few individuals to grab the attention of medicine and pharmaceutical companies. Too big to qualify for government-funded incentives.

But the real problem, Halpern confided to the group of patients he cared so much, about had to do with the stinginess of investors. All they cared about was "who you know and how much money are you going to make. Not about patients and suffering."

At the close of that year's Clusterbusters conference, Wold asked Halpern not to return the next year. He didn't want people to lose hope. And Halpern has never felt like returning, saying, "I just haven't had the heart to go back yet. It just kills me that I don't have any way of moving forward with this anymore."

It must have stung Wold to watch Clusterbusters' relationship with Harvard dissolve. But it had run its course. Hopefully, the experience had taught them that their collective embodied knowledge had real worth. Going forward, Clusterbusters would need trustworthy partners, or they would have to go it alone.

Chapter Sixteen

● ● ●●●●●●●●●●●●●●●●●●● ● ●

# MAKING A MEDICINE

B OB WOLD LEFT HARVARD AS CYNICAL AS ANY HARDENED ACADEMIC.
If asked about a future clinical trial, he'd shake his head and mutter
something about a miracle.

But now that the social mycelium had taken root, Wold didn't know
everything that happened underfoot. Every time someone mentioned psychedelics and cluster headache—whether in an academic talk, a news story,
or online—a new thread unspooled. Sometimes that thread connected with
another like-minded hypha, their fibers strengthening underground.

This is the inherent grace of social networks: they operate beyond the
constraints of linearity and hierarchy, functioning without the need for centralized control. Their growth fuels an ever-evolving, boundless capacity for
change. You could never predict where the next mushroom—the next breakthrough, the next story, the next wellspring of optimism—might emerge.

● ● ●●●●●●●●●●●●●●●●●● ● ●

The 2014 Annual Clusterbusters Conference in Nashville, Tennessee, presented Bob Wold with a fresh challenge: finding speakers who were both
able and willing to fill slots once reserved for John Halpern and Andrew

Sewell. *Maybe*, Wold thought, *that young doctor who had worked with Sewell on one of their projects might agree to update Clusterbusters in his stead.*

Dr. Emmanuelle Schindler almost didn't accept the invitation. Would it be ethical to work on her mentor's research posthumously? She was still a resident—essential training to practice as a physician—so she thought she should check.

Wold reassured her. All they needed was a simple overview of the survey that she had helped Sewell analyze. Schindler had a PhD in neuroscience. She was more than capable. Her expertise and connection to the late Dr. Sewell made her an ideal candidate.

●  ●  ●●●●●●●●●●●●●●●●●●●  ●  ●

Schindler enjoyed her visit to Nashville. Just thinking about how much the organization had done for patients filled her with admiration. Her talk described a patient-led survey that she and Sewell had been analyzing. They weren't yet done with the study, but so far it looked like most people surveyed found real benefit from the use of psilocybin and that LSD really was exceptional as a treatment. She also shared a few details about the psilocybin cluster study that she'd been helping Sewell design. "I don't have any funding for it," she confessed, her voice tinged with regret. "It's an aspiration. But I'd like to help you."

She had no idea that the perfect funder was sitting right in the audience. Carey Turnbull, a philanthropist who had invested in psychedelic research, had flown to Nashville to hear a talk by James Fadiman, a psychedelic "elder," who'd recently published his influential book about microdosing.[1] Schindler's name didn't ring a bell, but he took notice of the woman saying, almost as an apology to the patients gathered in the audience, that she'd like to study psilocybin at Yale.

Was she serious? Turnbull sat on the board of the Heffter Research Institute, a psychedelic philanthropy that funded high-quality scientific research testing psilocybin at prestigious universities. But it was a tough mission: only a few universities in the entire country would approve a study like that.

Turnbull made sure to find Schindler after the talk, so he could ask if she really thought that Yale's Institutional Review Board (IRB) would approve human trials using psilocybin.

According to Turnbull, Schindler replied, "Yeah, that's a thing that'll help treat headaches. And we'd like to figure it out."

Her answer sounded so wonderfully hopeful that he presumed she must not understand the challenge ahead. But he figured that made sense: such a young psychiatrist wouldn't know how challenging universities made this work.

Turnbull would later discover that he'd been wrong. Schindler still had two years of medical training to go before she could call herself a *neurologist*. She could, however, already lay claim to the title "psychedelic researcher." She'd written an entire doctoral thesis in neuroscience based on laboratory work involving psychedelics and rabbit models.

"How much do you think you would need for a study?" Turnbull asked her.

"I estimate the protocols would be about $60,000."

Schindler, he decided, needn't know that he could get her three times that amount. "If you can get the Yale IRB to approve human trials using Schedule I classic psychedelics, I'm sure that I can get you the $60,000."

Clusterbusters' hope now lay with a naive neurology resident and the optimism of a quixotic billionaire.

●  ●  ●●●●●●●●●●●●●●●●●●●●  ●  ●

Carey Turnbull and his wife and investment partner, Claudia, make a striking pair—tall and slender, with matching silver hair, black wardrobes, and the radiant wellness that only the truly rich can achieve. They're both fascinated by psychedelic research and believe in its potential, but I got the sense that the headache stuff is all Carey. Claudia excused herself after our brief introduction and left Carey to do the talking.

Turnbull presents himself as a "sober" philanthropist, guided by a blend of altruism and strategic thinking, rather than personal experience, even though he's admitted in interviews to being a "child of the sixties."[2] The couple met while undergraduate students at Goddard College, a small liberal arts school in Vermont known for its experimental educational approach. As he told one journalist, "Where I went to college, LSD was washing down the walls of the dorm."[3]

After college, the Turnbulls chose transcendental meditation as their path to self-discovery and enlightenment. They were drawn to Fairfield, Iowa, a hub for followers of the Maharishi Mahesh Yogi, who had inspired figures like Ram Dass and the Beatles. There, they became part of an intentional community and university devoted to the Maharishi's teachings.

As the years passed, the Turnbulls' lives took an unexpected turn. The birth of a child led Turnbull to contemplate his career path and consider how to support his growing family without losing sight of his spiritual foundation. He never pictured himself as a suit in the business world, but he felt compelled to see how it felt to work a nine-to-five job when a business opportunity presented itself.

The transformation from dedicated meditation practitioner to business executive may appear contradictory, but within the context of Fairfield's community, it was a well-trodden path. The town had long cultivated a generation of CEOs and entrepreneurs. Transcendental meditation and capitalism were not opposing forces; they were complementary aspects of a broader philosophy embraced by the community. The Maharishi himself endorsed the pursuit of material wealth, not as a contradiction to spiritual growth but as an extension of it. Turnbull was good at business, and in 2006 he sold the interdealer energy market derivatives and futures brokerage firm he founded in 1983, Amerex, to the New York Stock Exchange–listed GFI Group.[4]

That same year, he stumbled upon Roland Griffiths's groundbreaking 2006 article in *Psychopharmacology* that demonstrated psilocybin could produce meaningful mystical experiences when administered under the right circumstances.[5]

Donating to psychedelic science made sense to the Turnbulls. They wondered how much science had missed in the years when moral panic made psychedelic research taboo. Psychedelic philanthropy offered a space in which their financial contributions might really make a difference. A contribution of $50,000 to cancer research would hardly "move the needle." The same amount in psychedelic research could be "leveraged"—a term often tossed around at psychedelic conferences—to attract attention and funding.

Their philanthropic journey started with a cautious step: a donation to Stephen Ross, an addiction psychiatrist at New York University (NYU), who was exploring the potential of psilocybin-assisted therapy to alleviate anxiety and depression in terminal cancer patients. That's how Turnbull learned about psychedelic treatment for cluster headache. The idea that psychedelics might have a physiological benefit, as opposed to a strictly psychiatric use, piqued his interest.

Turnbull also met John Halpern, and learned about his research on BOL-148, the nonhallucinogenic variant of LSD that was showing promising initial results. To Turnbull, Halpern's work had far-reaching political implications. The fledgling, stigmatized field of psychedelic medicine needed to break through the stigma that still had a stranglehold on the field. Here was a compound that could fundamentally change the narrative. BOL-148 was free from LSD's countercultural associations. It was the kind of investment he could openly discuss with his mother—a stepping-stone toward broader societal acceptance.

Halpern took Turnbull to a Clusterbusters conference so he could learn more about the people who would be benefiting from BOL-148. The experience shook him to his core. Money couldn't solve everything, but this might be something that Turnbull could fix.

Halpern and Clusterbusters didn't just identify an effective treatment; they landed on an appealing narrative. The serendipitous finding that BOL-148 treated cluster headache "proved" these patients had been telling the truth all along. They took psychedelics to manage unendurable pain, not because, as Turnbull put it, they "were looking for an excuse to get high." They just needed help developing it into an FDA-approved medicine.

In early 2010, Carey Turnbull invested $250,000 in Entheogen Sciences Corp, albeit as a silent investor. Turnbull knows business, but he seemed humbled by his first attempt at drug development. Trusting Halpern to captain the ship, he told me, had been naive. "It's a very different thing to be a drug development professional, very different from doing some, some science, inquisitive science, and, you know, doing a small study."

Turnbull decided that the next time he tried his hand at drug development—if there ever was a next time—he would collaborate with a biotech firm from the start. In the meantime, he was pleased with how well his philanthropic efforts were going. Stephen Ross, at NYU, had even managed to attract the spotlight in Michael Pollan's first article about psychedelic medicine, a 2015 *New Yorker* piece titled "The Trip Treatment."[6]

Entheogen Sciences Corp might not have worked out, but Carey Turnbull usually had an eye for opportunity. And he saw something big in Dr. Schindler.

● ● ●●●●●●●●●●●●●●●●●● ● ●

Schindler, who chooses her words carefully, often describes herself as "left-brained," by which she means hyperrational, systematic, and, above all else, "rule abiding." Like most psychedelic researchers, ensuring that people understand what can and can't be supported by evidence is a priority for her. But she's also not one of the psychedelic researchers just pretending to be "sober" during the day, while spending long nights out at psychedelic science conferences. She's usually game for a quiet dinner and a glass of wine, but given her druthers, she'd opt for the company of her cats. What you see is what you get: a Calvinist approach to life, in modest cardigans in neutral colors.

Her modesty is unwarranted. Physician-scientists like Schindler, who earned her PhD in neuroscience while attending medical school, boast far more comprehensive training than most physicians who lead clinical research. In a profession often overshadowed by male counterparts and media glitz, Schindler's name doesn't often make headlines. And that suits her just fine.

But her interest in psychedelics is a bit curious.

Schindler happened upon the topic somewhat accidentally. Her doctoral research had been part of a larger effort in the laboratory where she worked to understand how serotonin receptors influence learning and behavior. Experiments used psychoactive drugs as tools to manipulate specific receptor sites in animals to observe how doing so might alter their behavior. So, here rabbit—take this drug that we know will block a certain receptor—and then we can observe what happens.

She was initially using antipsychotic drugs (5-HT2A receptor antagonists) in her experiments, but—as often happens in research—the studies weren't panning out. When she changed course, she decided that serotonin 2 receptor *agonists* would make more sense: that the drugs happened to be psychedelics—LSD and DOI—seemed irrelevant.

Schindler, of course, downplayed the edginess and importance of this research with self-deprecating humor. "I injected rabbits with LSD and counted how often their heads bobbed. I mean, I mostly just watched their heads bob all day long."

But the pharmacology of the drugs had caught her interest. *Maybe*, she thought, *she could find a way to continue studying psychedelics as she continued her education in medical school?* But few physicians were studying psychedelics when she graduated from Drexel University College of Medicine in 2012, and the few who were working in the area were either psychiatrists or addiction doctors. Schindler wanted to become a neurologist.

She did, however, remember reading an intriguing 2006 *Neurology* article describing how people with cluster headache used psychedelic substances for acute and preventive treatment. She was struck by how unusual it was to see a paper suggesting that psychedelics might be helpful in a neurological, rather than a psychiatric, disorder. As she explained to one journalist, "Psilocybin and other psychedelics such as LSD are chemically and pharmacologically similar to existing headache medications. [To] think that they have effects in headache disorders is not a stretch, though they do have the unique ability to produce lasting effects after a single dose."[7]

A little sleuthing revealed that Dr. Sewell, the first author of the study, had moved to Yale Medical School, which had a terrific residency program in neurology, including a headache center that trained residents and research fellows. She also really liked the people there, which mattered a lot to her. Schindler ranked their residency training program high on her list. Yale must have liked her too.

Schindler moved to New Haven in the summer of 2012 to begin the work of a resident. It's a demanding schedule (eighty hours per week in the hospital and the clinic is the norm), but she found as much time as she could to help Sewell with his projects.

The first project—analyzing a medication-use survey asking patients around the world to rate their experiences using various treatments—had been initiated by Marsha Weil, who often wondered if there was another Flash out there, somewhere, sitting on the next novel treatment. Weil had wanted to conduct the survey, she told me, because she couldn't shake the feeling that "maybe there's something that we haven't heard." But she had no idea what to do with the data she collected. "Nobody," she told me, "was going to be interested in a bunch of people with cluster headache that did a study." But Sewell cared. More data meant more support for a psilocybin clinical trial.

The second project had been the same psilocybin clinical trial that Sewell had been pulling together since 2004. He had never given up that dream.

Schindler wanted to continue the work, but a medical resident was far too junior to become a principal investigator. She wasn't even qualified to treat patients on her own yet. Luckily, Dr. Deepak Cyril D'Souza, the same psychiatry professor who had hired Sewell after his falling-out with Halpern, offered to take on the job. Dr. Christopher Gottschalk, director of the Yale Headache and Facial Pain Center and a prominent neurologist, came on to help. But everybody understood who would do the work: Schindler.

● ● ●●●●●●●●●●●●●●●●●● ● ●

Designing the clinical trial could have been a nightmare, but Emmanuelle Schindler managed to avoid many of the problems that befell the research team at Harvard by presuming the clinical trial was the first step in a long process of drug development rather than a once-in-a-lifetime opportunity.

Of course Schindler didn't have the same pressures to manage as the Harvard McLean folks had. No need to incorporate an "LSD intervention" to make Rick Doblin happy, given that Carey Turnbull had already expressed interest in funding a psilocybin clinical trial. It must have also helped to work in a welcoming, friendly environment where colleagues found her research interesting. The big decision would just be dosage and regimen.

What if she got the dosage wrong, I wondered. The fear of a failed clinical trial had haunted the previous Harvard group. A poor outcome in the initial clinical trial could end future funding for psychedelic cluster headache research.

Schindler thought this was a nonissue. Drug development often required multiple iterations of early-stage experiments, she told me. The analysis of early results helped researchers refine the dosage and regimen for the next clinical trial.

Was she as naive as Turnbull thought? Or just unflappable? Neither, according to Schindler. Just look at the evidence—most of which, she always made sure to mention, came from patients. In medication-use surveys, people with cluster headache consistently reported that psychedelics were the most effective preventive drug they had ever used. Some people only needed one or two doses to tame their cycles. More conventional medications, like oxygen and sumatriptan, ranked higher in the abortive category, but psilocybin was a close third.[8]

More recently, Schindler had coauthored a review article evaluating every published study examining the efficacy of cluster headache treatments and had similarly concluded that LSD and psilocybin were the most effective preventives for cluster headache. The inverse was also true: none of the published studies suggested these drugs could *not* treat cluster headache.[9] But, once again, this was almost entirely based on anecdotal evidence.

Why, I asked Schindler, did she find this particular group of patients credible? Wasn't she worried that this might be one of those antiscience, conspiratorial movements leading patients to reject everything from vaccines to 5G technology?

But Schindler saw something different in Clusterbusters' community: a genuine desire for understanding, a rigor in self-reporting, and a pattern that aligned with emerging scientific insights. She also found it reassuring that, while psychedelics could be an outstanding treatment, they didn't work for everyone, and didn't work reliably. That's how headache medicine generally operates. "It would have been suspicious," she told me, "if every single Clusterbuster patient found profound therapeutic benefit from psychedelics."

Listening to patients made sense, but her interest in pursuing this research wasn't based on anecdotal evidence alone. She looked for the convergence of lived experiences with rigorous scientific inquiry—a nexus that could illuminate a new path forward in medicine and healing.

Schindler valued patient input, but credibility mattered. She needed evidence that aligned with existing biomedical knowledge. And the biomedical research literature supported Clusterbusters' conclusion: "The chemical structure of psychedelics is very, very close, nearly identical to migraine medications," she had pointed out.[10] It all added up. Psychedelics penetrate the blood-brain barrier, which—in theory—could make them a more potent therapy. And there's been some research leaving clues suggesting a variety of biological reasons why these drugs worked so well: psilocybin and LSD can increase neuroplasticity, which—in theory—could contribute to the long-lasting relief that patients were experiencing. Studies had shown that psychedelics altered functional connections to and from the hypothalamus—the part of the brain most likely implicated in cluster headache. Who knew? Maybe, she has suggested, the drugs were "flipping" whatever that switch was in the hypothalamus that turned cluster cycles "on" and "off."[11]

Patients had a lot of knowledge, Schindler explained. But she didn't think that necessarily made them experts on every treatment. Outlandish claims—she paused, perhaps thinking of her cats—like the healing power of "ground-up tiger ears," were easily dismissed.

Schindler is a clinician who shares her patients' joyful relief when they feel better, but she hasn't followed up every claim that every patient has made with a scientific study. She's a scientist—suggested treatments need to work within the realm of biomedical possibility.

The FDA spoke the language of randomized clinical trials. Schindler viewed her role as that of a translator who could transform Clusterbusters' wisdom into the kind of evidence that the federal agency might recognize.

* *  * * * * * * * * * * * * * * * * *  * *

Schindler decided that if the goal was to show that magic mushrooms could treat cluster headache, following Clusterbusters' protocol was logical. Bob Wold's protocol advised three one- to two-gram doses of *Psilocybe* mushrooms, spaced five days apart, and outlined certain medications to avoid that might hinder the treatment. Since mushrooms don't yield a standardized psilocybin dose, Schindler converted the protocol into clinical trial terms by calculating the psilocybin average in the *Psilocybe cubensis* variety and determining a weight-based dose. She chose a dosage of 0.143 mg/kg per subject—a third of the dose used in clinical trials focused on mental health and addiction.

From there, she designed a relatively straightforward study. Participants would be randomly assigned to either a psilocybin or a placebo group. Each would undergo three experimental dosing sessions in an outpatient lab, spaced about three to seven days apart depending on scheduling needs.

Schindler found it relatively easy to get approval from Yale and the Veterans Administration's IRB. Nor did she think getting permission from the FDA or registration with the DEA was difficult. Maybe, she laughed, it helped that she'd been so busy at the time. "If I hadn't been in [medical] residency, I would have thought, ugh, this is taking forever."

The FDA didn't even seem to mind that she based her protocol on the expertise of people who, from the government's perspective, were "misusing" illicit substances. Not a peep was said about the dosing advice she received via personal correspondence from a Mr. Robert Wold, a man with zero letters indicating credentials following his name.

● ● ●●●●●●●●●●●●●●●●●●● ● ●

Carey Turnbull was so surprised that Schindler had gotten approval from Yale Medical School that he visited Yale on behalf of Heffter and, in his words, "buttonholed the chair of the psychiatry department" to ask if maybe "Emmanuelle had kind of kept her head down, and you maybe don't notice what she's doing over here. I'd like to know, really, if we do this, is there going to be hostility, and are we going to be fighting our way uphill?"

Heffter wouldn't fund a research study unless they knew it had the backing of the institution—because they'd seen how a hospital could create a supportive working environment or could make research unsustainable. Would Yale, a conservative Ivy League university, want to take the reputational risk of studying psilocybin? Even as late as 2016, universities didn't want to host Heffter-funded research.

Turnbull received the assurance he needed. The department had a history of working with Schedule I drugs, and the medical school was enthusiastic about Schindler's research. D'Souza, the principal investigator on the study, had been administering Schedule I drugs, including cannabis and salvinorin A, a powerful hallucinogen, to human subjects since the 1990s. The medical school already had the infrastructure in place to do this work safely. Schindler had their full support.

Social scientists have long observed that institutional culture matters more than a single leader's opinion when it comes to decision-making. Following standard operating procedures—we call this "path dependence"—is far easier for an IRB than approving a protocol that signals a radical change. When it came to predicting the success of Schindler's study, the chair of psychiatry's endorsement was important but not nearly as significant as the infrastructure that Yale already had in place.

Heffter agreed to lend their expertise to the project and to offer scientific review, which would ensure that Schindler's clinical trial lined up with research on psilocybin that was already being done at Johns Hopkins and New York University. The Turnbulls would be the donors behind the project.

In 2017, Turnbull began to reevaluate his earlier stance on the need to partner with biotech companies for new medications. Entheogen Sciences Corp hadn't gone well, but the market for psychedelic medicines was developing much more quickly than he ever anticipated. "I thought [this] was a whole generation or two away," he told me.

Several efforts, Turnbull had noted, were underway to commercialize, and even patent, psilocybin. Working with Heffter allowed him to watch the process up close, and it seemed straightforward. "You go to the FDA, have a [pre–Investigational New Drug] meeting, present the molecule, discuss the work that Harvard had done. . . . And they sort of say yes, no, or maybe," he told me.

Clusterbusters deserved a real medicine, in his opinion, and Turnbull genuinely liked and admired Wold. "Bob," he told me, "has become a friend. . . . He's a great guy."

Turnbull decided to form a new corporation called CH-Tac (he would eventually change its name to Ceruvia) with the idea that a $1 million investment would "prime the pump" and attract "big pharma money" to develop BOL-148. That patent war between Halpern and Sewell? Turnbull settled the dispute like any other business venture: with financial resources and diplomacy. It helped that neither of the patent holders harbored a deep resentment toward Turnbull. That Carey Turnbull decided to expand his portfolio to include migraine came as a delightful surprise to the headache community.

Everything was on the up-and-up. Clusterbusters had a champion, and Schindler had funding. Turnbull's backing allowed her to run two clinical trials: a study testing psilocybin for cluster headache *and* a study testing psilocybin for migraine. The first-ever approved clinical trial testing psilocybin as a treatment for cluster headache opened its doors in November 2016.

●  ●  ●●●●●●●●●●●●●●●●●●●  ●  ●

Working with a supportive university, collegial colleagues, and sufficient funding boosted Bob Wold's confidence that something good might come of his efforts after all. They just faced one problem: finding eligible people to participate in the study.

Carey Turnbull found this so frustrating that he turned up to Clusterbusters' 2018 annual meeting in Denver to attempt to rally the troops. He underscored how critical it was for patients to take "a bullet for the team" and sacrifice their time, energy, and well-being. He couldn't help but choke up as he spoke with the attendees. They were so close! "It's not the DEA saying, *Don't touch that stuff or we'll arrest you.* It's not the FDA saying, *Don't study that unless you do it this way.* It's not the administration at an elite, academic institution. . . . The limiting factor is the efforts of Clusterbusters," he told them.

But drumming up interest in the study had never been the problem. Schindler's office received a steady stream of inquiries. Like all investigators she had to be careful to screen potential research subjects to minimize the risks of participation and to increase the validity of her findings. For example, as a safety measure Schindler's study excluded those with a serious psychiatric or medical disease, and anyone who took a medication that might interfere with the validity of the results, which unfortunately included several drugs that people in this patient population relied upon. She eventually allowed the limited use of sumatriptan when it became clear that asking cluster patients to go without would make recruitment nearly impossible.

There were other issues as well.

About 85 percent of people with cluster headache have the episodic form of the disease, which means they're usually "in cycle" once or twice a year. Studying people with an episodic disease that cycles on and off presented challenges. Most episodic cluster headache patients, Schindler told me, got better too quickly to get them enrolled in a study and test if a drug worked properly. "Their cycles were just not long enough. They would call us like halfway through the cycle, and then, you know, it's already too late. Then we say, okay, we can take you next year and . . . Oh, my God, forget it."

Not to mention, how many people could call out of work for ten to twelve days so they could travel (on their own dime) to Connecticut for the duration of the study? Most Americans struggle to pay unexpected medical expenses. Many people with cluster headache live precarious lives on the edge of employment.

Of 238 prospects, only 20 qualified for additional screening.[12]

Unlike most drugs under development by pharmaceutical companies, potential study participants can access psilocybin with relative ease. Not only was it easier to obtain magic mushrooms than to qualify for Schindler's clinical trial, the DIY method didn't require submitting oneself to a placebo.

Major global pharmaceutical companies also have trouble studying this disease. They can compensate somewhat with their deep pockets—by, for example, enrolling cluster headache patients in clinics around the world, in more convenient locations, rather than asking everyone to fly to one specific outpatient laboratory. But deep pockets only go so far. Cluster headache is such a difficult disease to study that the trials simply don't get done.

● ● ●●●●●●●●●●●●●●●●●●● ● ●

Even with Schindler's dogged persistence in tracking down potential study participants, she still needed a little luck. Ken Maxwell, a US veteran and successful entrepreneur, had been living with cluster headache for six years when, in 2019, he heard Yale University was conducting a clinical trial testing whether psychedelics worked as a treatment. "If a university like Yale—a prominent academic institution—is doing the research, I want a copy of their report. But I couldn't find a report," he told me.

He called the Department of Neurology and asked for a copy of the findings. Two weeks later, he received a phone call from Schindler's office recruiting him for the study. He couldn't believe his luck. He'd been reading about psychedelic treatment on Clusterbusters, but it sounded kind of out there to him. "That's just not my deal. Not my wheelhouse."

Maxwell, who wears a neatly cropped silver beard that matches a similarly clean-cut hair style, used to enjoy drinking a glass of red wine with his wife before it began triggering his attacks. "I mean, my only experience with recreational drugs is in high school. Literally, I smoked pot once on a church trip. Holy Rollers." He paused. "I didn't know you were supposed to inhale it. So, I've had the Bill Clinton exemption."

In short, he was a prime example of the kind of Clusterhead that Wold knew Schindler would need to reach. Maxwell had chronic cluster headache and experienced multiple attacks every day, nonstop. The US veteran turned executive prided himself on the success he'd achieved in both business and work for the community. But the cluster headache had gotten in the way of all of it.

"I was operating at a pretty high level there for a while. And since this diagnosis, it just got worse and worse—just relentless. There were no days without attacks. From August of 2020 until October of 2021, I had 415 consecutive days of attacks."

Despite his stance on drugs—and his skepticism about psychedelics—the idea that this study was taking place at Yale University changed everything. This was legit. Maxwell wanted in.

The study's medical screening process took two months to complete. Yale's study team consulted with his primary care physician, neurologist, hematologist, and neurosurgeon to evaluate his psychological health, family history, and personal background. They even contacted personal references. Maxwell found their meticulous screening process reassuring.

"They don't want you to get in there and have a bad psychological breakdown or something during trips and have to abort it because they've invested so much to get you there," he said.

Unfortunately, the timing couldn't have been worse. His clearance came through at the beginning of March 2020, just before COVID shut down the experiment. Schindler's monthly calls helped him manage that turbulent time. At that point, the attacks hadn't stopped for almost two years.

On the plus side, the shutdown gave Schindler the time to submit for publication the results of a clinical trial testing psilocybin on migraine.

It was a small study—just ten people—but the results, published in *Neu-rotherapeutics*, mirrored what people had been saying online for years: a single low dose of psilocybin (the same used in the cluster headache trial) reduced migraine frequency by an average of 50 percent for at least two weeks. The migraine attacks that remained were about 30 percent less painful and 60 percent less functionally impairing than people usually experienced.[13]

Other drugs on the market can effectively reduce the frequency of migraine attacks, but those need to be taken daily and/or remain in a person's system. Psilocybin, however, offered a long-lasting preventative effect on migraine after just one dose, even though it was metabolized and eliminated from the body within hours. Schindler wasn't quite sure how it worked, but nothing else on the market could do anything like it.

• • •••••••••••••••••••• • •

Schindler called Ken Maxwell in October 2020 with very good news. The clinical trial would be opening again in November, and she would love for him to join the study. There were still some COVID restrictions, however. Connecticut, for example, required all those entering the state to remain in quarantine for two weeks prior to entering the state. The study didn't have funding to cover this, but luckily Maxwell could stay with his daughter, who lived nearby.

Maxwell had to abide by other rules too. Two weeks before the study, he would be required to track every attack, and he'd have to limit his use of the sumatriptan injections he relied on as an abortive. To make sure he understood the full process, Schindler quizzed him on the protocol's requirements: The first day of the study involved a physical, blood tests, and a COVID test. He would receive a "dose" on day two, and then he'd return for two additional doses over the next ten days. But because it was a double-blind study, neither he nor the staff would know whether he received psilocybin or a placebo.

Maxwell thought it might be a good idea to read Michael Pollan's book *How to Change Your Mind* about psychedelic-assisted therapy, even though the Yale study used much lower doses of psilocybin than Pollan had described, and didn't aim to shift participants' cognitive perspective about their pain. But Maxwell didn't know anything about the psychedelic experience, and he figured it would help him better understand what would happen.

The more he read, the more he wondered if a transformative frame of mind might help him heal. Maybe it was desperation. Maybe it was arrogance. But he was determined to discover if something deeply rooted in his psyche had broken his brain and caused this disease.

Maxwell felt prepared on the morning of his first dose. The experiment took place on a hospital gurney in an area separated by a hospital curtain, which meant he could hear everybody milling around outside, and they could hear him. A blood pressure machine sat nearby so a nurse could take regular measurements, and oxygen tanks had been placed by the bed in case he needed to abort an attack. Unlike most psilocybin clinical trials, which pair participants with two therapists while they take the drug, Maxwell would be alone. But a trained nurse would be stationed outside the room and would check in on him if he so much as sneezed, and a camera fixed on the bed monitored everything that happened. Medicine could be administered quickly via an intravenous line in case of emergency. A nurse took his vitals and asked a few questions about how he felt, before handing him a blue gelatin capsule and a cup of water.

After reading Pollan's description of therapy rooms outfitted with plush sofas, Buddha sculptures, and stone mushrooms, Maxwell hadn't expected the spare medical aesthetic of the room.[14] The design decision hadn't been an explicit choice made by Schindler; it was merely the research laboratory that she had access to at Yale. But Maxwell signed up to participate in a hospital study to feel safe, and taking psilocybin in a setting filled with medical equipment offered him comfort. The process helped him feel cared for and secure.

His prayers that the pill contained "the high-end stuff" were soon answered. The bleak gray hospital room transformed into a "magic carpet ride" that expanded his mind and made everything bigger and more beautiful than he'd ever seen before. His body shook with laughter when he looked at a book that he'd brought to pass the time. He wouldn't need that at all.

When he decided that the time had come to search his unconscious mind to discover what was going on in there, "I started asking questions. . . . And, and that's when everything started happening. I wouldn't hear words as much as I *felt* words. I felt meaning. I understood intuitively what was going on, even though it wasn't obvious. It was an unbelievable experience in that regard."

There wasn't a cluster beast hidden in the depth of his subconscious memory, so far as he could tell. But he found something resembling peace and self-forgiveness.

Maxwell considered his participation a success, even though his pain only improved the tiniest bit. After the study, he still got hit three to four times per day, but the attacks didn't last as long or hurt quite as badly as before. Any relief was welcome, even if the effect eventually wore off two months later.

Schindler, for her part, was thrilled. A slight improvement in attack frequency wasn't quite enough to count him as a patient who responded to psilocybin according to the criteria outlined in her study, but she could see that the drug had shifted something—however small. Finding slivers of light mattered when treating a disease as stubborn as chronic cluster headache.

● ● ●●●●●●●●●●●●●●●●●●●●● ● ●

Results from the trial, published in a 2022 issue of the journal *Headache*, captured a good deal of Schindler's optimism about psilocybin as a treatment for cluster headache. The eight people in the psilocybin treatment group experienced an average 30 percent reduction in the number of attacks they experienced, relative to the six people in the placebo group. The six people in the placebo group didn't experience any reduction at all.[15]

The results weren't spectacular, but Schindler felt good about the outcome. The "30 percent reduction" in attacks, she likes to remind people, is an average of how well people did after the protocol. Some people experienced a sharp reduction in the number of attacks they experienced. Others, like Maxwell, did not. The study enrolled too few people for the outcome to produce statistically significant results, but she was encouraged by the reduction seen and was later pleased to see that her results lined up nicely with an open-label psilocybin cluster headache study completed at the University of Copenhagen.[16]

This Danish study caught me by surprise, largely because there'd been no Herculean struggle to make it happen. Clusterbusters and their social mycelium had inspired the project: Dr. Martin Madsen, the neuroscientist and psychiatrist who led the study, is a Clusterhead himself.

Madsen, who experienced his first attack at age twenty-four while a PhD student, described the pain to me as "out of this world." Luckily, regular prescription medicine works well on his episodic cycles, and he seemed to be doing fine health wise. His experience, however, had inspired his interest in the brain. Reading patient accounts on Clusterbusters' website led him to John Halpern and Schindler's body of work, which in turn led him to exchange several emails with Bob Wold.

Madsen's clinical trial tested the busting protocol in the most severe patient population: chronic cluster headache. Ten people with the diagnosis received three low doses of psilocybin, spaced about seven days apart; none received a placebo. Results offered good news on safety. Nobody experienced any serious side effects, and at least one person reported long-lasting psychological benefits. Attack frequency dropped by 30 percent on average, and one person experienced a twenty-one-week remission. Brain scans included in the protocol suggested that psilocybin helped reset the neural pathways connecting the parts of the brain most likely to be involved in cluster headache: the posterior hypothalamus and the diencephalic cluster. By altering these connections and increasing the brain's ability to form new pathways (a phenomenon known as *neuroplasticity*), psilocybin might be able to reduce the frequency of cluster headache. The idea is not that far from the theory that Flash and PinkSharkMark used to toss around back in the old CH.com forum, when they figured the shrooms must reset some broken switch.

Madsen has moved on to other research now—but it doesn't seem like the reason has to do with the political challenges involved in this research. Obtaining approvals for the study, he told me, hadn't been difficult. Denmark categorizes psilocybin as a "potential pharmaceutical," even though recreational use of the drug was criminalized.

Denmark's policy makes so much more sense than the Catch-22 embedded in the US regulatory scheme, which, in practice, prevents clinical research investigating therapeutic applications of Schedule I drugs because these drugs had already been assessed as having "no medical value."

●　●　●●●●●●●●●●●●●●●●●●●　●　●

Emmanuelle Schindler knew from clinical experience that headache treatments often took time to work. In fact, this was so often the case that she usually prescribed patience along with medications.

The reason was neurobiological: repeated headache attacks invoked a state of "central sensitization" in the nervous system that took time to reverse. Chronic pain has multiple causes, such as nerve damage that occurs when a disc in the spine herniates and presses on a nerve, which can be excruciating; neuropathic pain occurs when a nerve is injured, as can happen with diabetes-induced neuropathy; and, of course, because pain is processed in the consciousness, psychology can make pain more stubborn.

Central sensitization, a fourth contributor to chronic pain, occurs when the central nervous system undergoes a process of amplification, which makes the body process stimuli in a much more exaggerated fashion. Researchers believe that prolonged exposure to acute pain may be the culprit behind central sensitization. Keep applying pain to the nervous system and the body's processing pathways become exaggerated and perceive all stimuli as painful. It could take some time to undo the damage. I think of it as a bit like driving on a dirt road: the first time over the gravel is bumpy, but keep traveling down the same path, and the tires wear smoother tracks in the ground. Every headache attack works the same way, engraining pathways in the nervous system, making it prone to experience pain with less provocation each time. More pain leads to more pain—an oversimplification of a complicated process, but that's the general principle.

Schindler's funding from Turnbull's company, Ceruvia, included funding to bring people back for a second round of treatment. Everyone in the cluster headache trial would receive psilocybin this time, including the six people who initially took a placebo. Ten people, including Ken Maxwell, returned.

The second round didn't put Maxwell into full remission—alas, it didn't even give him a pain-free day. But he still maintains that the treatment changed his life. The "shadow pain" that had long haunted him between attacks nearly disappeared, leaving him with more energy and mental clarity than he'd had in a long time. He still had daily attacks, but for the first time in three years, he and his wife were able to hike the Great Smoky Mountains, the backdrop of their home in North Carolina.

A sign of hope.

But there are drawbacks to citizen science. How can they tell if the benefit comes from a placebo? How can they know the real dosage in a mushroom? What sort of bias might be built into the interpretation of the results?

● ● ●●●●●●●●●●●●●●●●●●● ● ●

Ken Maxwell wasn't the only person who benefited from a second round of dosing. Those, like Maxwell, who had received psilocybin during the first wave of the study had better results the second time they went through the protocol.

Schindler now had data to report that psilocybin had a *statistically significant* effect on the number of attacks that people with cluster headache experienced.

It's a great example, Schindler says, of why it's important to remember that it often takes more than one round of treatment before a difficult headache disorder yields to treatment. A so-called negative study must not be interpreted with too much pessimism.

After all, Clusterbusters had always gotten the best results by tweaking their doses to figure out what worked for them. Some people get lucky—a small dose goes a long way. Schindler sometimes wished she could tweak doses the same way that Wold did for those he helped. An RCT offered credible data on the efficacy of a drug on a fixed regimen, but the overall outcome for patients was less dramatic than the anecdotal evidence. "It is a fixed thing." A limitation. She wished she could do her research as quickly as Clusterbusters, but everything took time and money in the aboveground.

● ● ●●●●●●●●●●●●●●●●●●●● ● ●

Alas, one tiny study cannot achieve the dream Bob Wold has been working toward for years: definitive proof that a mushroom can heal the most painful disease that humans experience. Wold believes fungi can do a lot of good for not much money, but he's not a snake oil salesman selling an empty miracle. He's trying to patch a broken system and keep people alive. Teaching people how to grow their own medicine offers them immediate access to something that might ease their pain right away. And if it doesn't? It might just help them live with the pain.

That's what happened to Ken Maxwell.

Maxwell returned to Clusterbusters' website after he realized that psilocybin could offer him some relief. Its instructions explained that truly stubborn cases of chronic cluster headache sometimes required multiple rounds of psilocybin treatment before they responded. Some people said they had to dose *nine times* before experiencing remission—an exhausting proposition considering that each "trip" took six hours.

Still, he had to try. "I've still got to provide for a family, my wife and I have goals and dreams in our life. . . . All of this is in jeopardy. [If] I don't get this disease under control, I'm not any good to anybody," he told me.

Growing mushrooms himself looked far too complicated, so he found a source he trusted and tried his best to approximate the dose that he received in the hospital. Lo and behold, the pain ceased for three blissful days after he took his ninth dose. The remission didn't last, but he's continuing to tweak the busting protocol so that it works for him. His cluster headache attacks have dropped in frequency by about 48 percent, and he now has 80 percent fewer severe attacks. Some months, he only has one attack per day.

Psychedelics, he tells me, are the first treatment that has given him hope, which is vital to survival. "When you're having an attack, and it's a bad one," he tells me, "it's like a five-alarm fire. I mean, it's all hands-on deck. You got to get it under control. But the real damaged thinking occurs in between the attacks because your mind goes to all these places: Am I going to have another attack? If I go to a restaurant or a new place, what will I do when it hits? I have to scope it out and find the rest room. I've got to have my oxygen with me. You know you're constantly trying to manage what will happen next, or what could happen next."

But Maxwell is also careful not to let his optimism get out of hand. He doesn't want me to think it's defeatist, but a neurologist recently warned him that cluster headache medicines always stop working. And he wants to be prepared for that eventuality. Because that, he tells me, is when people are most vulnerable to suicide. A newfound ability to live in the present, he says, is where psychedelics have really helped. "I feel like I've got my life back. [But] I'm not euphoric. I appreciate it in the moment."

● ● ●●●●●●●●●●●●●●●●●●●● ● ●

Anyone who has worked—or suffered—in this field understands that treating headache diseases requires a heavily stocked toolkit and a considerable amount of trial and error. Nobody understood this better than Bob Wold— Clusterheads need treatment in any form they can get it.

So Wold sprang into action when he learned that multiple pharmaceutical companies were sponsoring clinical trials testing a new class of medication for migraine, which worked by inhibiting a protein called calcitonin gene-related peptide (CGRP). Since CGRP, according to research, played an important role in migraine, reducing its presence might stop the disease. Wold wondered if the same might be true for cluster headache.

It wasn't easy to convince a pharmaceutical company to test their product on cluster headache patients, given how difficult it was to study the disease. But Eli Lilly obliged. As a result, episodic cluster headache now has a new FDA-approved preventive drug called Emgality. (The clinical trial unfortunately didn't demonstrate benefits for chronic cluster headache.)

Clusterbusters also arranged a new research study to test the efficacy of oxygen to appease the US Center for Medicare Services, which had insisted—somewhat nonsensically—that they lacked sufficient evidence of the treatment's safety or efficacy to pay for the treatment.

None of these advances have been easy, but turning mushrooms into medicine will be the hardest thing by far. "Psychedelics," Martin Madsen told me, is an "unexplored field. . . . There's a lot we don't know."

●  ●  ●●●●●●●●●●●●●●●●●●●  ●  ●

Carey Turnbull was finding it extraordinarily difficult to attract a biotech company to partner with him on the development of migraine and cluster headache research. The tiny market for cluster headache remained a problem. And by 2023, he'd become a lot less bullish about the corporatization of psychedelics than he had been in 2017.

He just couldn't make the investment work. It's extraordinarily expensive, he explained, to develop a drug, "probably $100 million," he estimated.

His investments in psychedelic medicine will continue, as will his philanthropic engagement. But when it comes to headache medicine, he's going into hibernation mode again. He knows that what already exists out there—what has been shown in a variety of studies, both carefully orchestrated academic ones, like those at Harvard and Yale, and the slightly messier ones that the Clusterbusters had been running on themselves for years—are incredibly promising. "I've got some solid science from Harvard and from Yale that underlies the fact that this is useful."

Turnbull isn't the only person putting the brakes on psychedelic drug development. In 2023, almost none of the nearly fifty psychedelic companies that had gone public on the stock market in the previous few years were doing well. Wesana, the company that professional hockey player Daniel Carcillo founded to develop psychedelic treatments for traumatic brain injury and migraine, had already gone under. When the Silicon Valley Bank collapsed in March 2023, Turnbull realized that private biotech companies would also soon find their funding in a crunch. Investing in headache research had to stop.

"I haven't given up on this," he told me. But belief alone won't do it. He's not as naive as he'd once been about drug development. In its effort to encourage innovation and protect patient safety, the government had produced what he described as a "thicket full of problems." He believed that regulatory oversight was vital: people should have access to safe medications. But the system means there's a "$100 million wall between you and getting a medicine made into prescription medicine." The illegality of psychedelics only complicates the math. Maybe with the right partner—a network of support—he'd walk that road again.

# CONCLUSION

## From the Counterculture to the Medicine Counter

HE AFTERNOON SUN WAS STILL BRIGHT IN THE MILE HIGH CITY WHEN we broke down Clusterbusters' informational booth at Psychedelic Science 2023, a conference produced by the Multidisciplinary Association for Psychedelic Studies (MAPS). Everything, including their table and displays, could easily be carried in a single trip. Eileen Brewer, longtime president of the Clusterbusters' board and the group's event organizer, gestured back at the exhibit hall as we left. "Time to invest in a bigger display, huh?"

I've rarely seen so many yurts in one space, let alone indoors.

A block and a bit and we made it to Bob Wold's hotel room, where we could rehash the event. Over twelve thousand people had preregistered to hear more than five hundred speakers talk about the healing potential of substances that, for over half a century, have been treated as some of the most dangerous drugs in the world.

But there was little sign that anyone here felt the need to suppress their authentic psychedelic selves or feign sobriety in Denver, Colorado, the heart of the nation's movement to decriminalize what are now euphemistically called "plant medicines." By 2023, Coloradoans and their visitors enjoyed the most relaxed laws on the cultivation, distribution (so long as it's "sharing"), and consumption of psychedelic substances in the country. Reflecting this open spirit, Colorado governor Jared Polis welcomed the crowd during the opening ceremony.

The convivial vibe spilled into the city itself. Everywhere I looked, people wore their badges atop the suggested attire for the conference, "psychedelic business casual." My novelty mushroom socks looked tame next to all the mushroom-inspired hats, animal print jumpsuits, denim overalls on top of bare chests, baggy vintage dresses, and cowboy hats combined with outfits far too chic for a ranch. One of the booths in the exhibit hall offered therapy dogs to help people calm themselves when things too intense— maybe getting lost in *Deep Space*, a giant immersive interactive art installation, or a frightening encounter with one's Jungian shadow self.

To launch the conference, Rick Doblin meandered onstage to an upbeat bossa nova tune, looking every bit the guru in a white suit paired with an unbuttoned collared linen shirt. He was ready: he'd been preaching the gospel of ecstatic experience for decades. He giggled a bit while peering out onto the audience. Five thousand had gathered in the auditorium.

"Amazing!" he gushed.

How much had things changed? Doblin listed the advances that had happened in just the past few years: MAPS's Public Benefit Corporation, the organization's pharmaceutical arm founded in December 2014, had just completed the last Phase III study required by the Food and Drug Administration prior to applying for the approval of MDMA-assisted therapy for PTSD. Compass Therapeutics had almost completed Phase III clinical trials testing psilocybin for treatment-resistant depression, and Usona Institute, a nonprofit medical research organization, was making good progress with clinical trials testing psilocybin for major depression.

Everything was thrumming along nicely. The growth in research publications over the last twenty years showed a dramatic increase, resembling the steep rise of a hockey stick's blade, a clear indication of a booming field. The market had even expanded to the development of novel psychedelic substances, which Doblin half-joked that he "look[ed] forward to trying." And he was encouraged by the American Medical Association's recent decision to create a billing code for "long therapy sessions."[1] Doing so was a necessary, but not sufficient, requirement for insurance coverage for lengthy MDMA sessions.

Evidence of a real culture shift emerged when Doblin, who exited stage right, was replaced by former Republican governor of Texas Rick Perry, a career politician better known for conservative stances, like vehement opposition to the legalization of same-sex marriage, than resisting the War on Drugs.

Perry, whose cadence sounded far more like that of a southern preacher than Doblin's, addressed the elephant in the room right away. He gestured toward the backstage area.

"So you got to see the light and the white with Rick Doblin. I'm the dark, knuckle-dragging, right-wing, Republican former governor of the state of Texas. I love Rick Doblin."

The crowd responded with resounding laughter and cheers. If those in the room were closely aligned with the progressive left wing, as one might assume about people who attend psychedelic events, it didn't take much for them to forgive Perry for his right-wing political positions.

It's hard to remain a cynic when hearing testimonies as powerful as the story that the governor shared. He and his wife had befriended a veteran who struggled with complex PTSD for years. For over a decade, the Perrys had done everything in their power to help him find a treatment. They initially rejected psychedelic therapy as ridiculous. But in the end, psychedelic-assisted therapy was the only treatment that worked. Witnessing this healing had made a convert out of Perry. And now, he stood before us to testify. We all had to have the courage of our convictions and stand up for what was right. People's lives were on the line.

Veterans, the latest constituency to join Doblin's psychedelic "big tent," offered the movement a potent narrative for the "political science" that MAPS practices. The suicide rate among veterans is 57 percent higher than for US adults who never served in the military—with a loss of seventeen vets every single day in 2020.[2] The nation, Perry reminded the audience, had a responsibility to help the people protecting its citizens' freedoms.

Like the Clusterheads before them, a stream of veterans have either turned to the underground or begun traveling to psychedelic retreats for relief.[3] Decorated soldiers—many of whom served in the most prestigious units of the military—have been telling the media captivating stories of redemptive healing. Former Navy Seals, Top Gun pilots, and Green Berets—heroes of Middle America—fortified the movement's credibility while also adding a layer of poignant urgency to the call for more research.[4] MAPS even hired a former US Army sergeant to help convince conservatives that MDMA-assisted therapy was the solution they so desperately needed.[5]

The gambit worked so well that psychedelic research is one of the few bipartisan issues in the nation. Rick Perry has now been joined by some of the most hard-right conservatives in the Republican Party, including Rep. Matt Gaetz (R-FL) and army veteran Rep. Dan Crenshaw (R-TX).[6]

Testimonies that psychedelics offered remarkable, near-miraculous healing filled every hour of every day that week. Each story was as powerful as the last, and they came so fast that the moment a story receded, the next took hold. I sometimes felt I might get carried away in a secular reawakening.

Rick Doblin—at least to my eye—enjoyed basking in the afterglow. I'd occasionally see him, his infectious laughter a beacon alerting everyone to his presence as he rushed across the convention center surrounded by a small, affectionate entourage. Lest anyone forget who had brought us all to the event, MAPS had papered the place with FREE RICK DOBLIN slogans surrounding his image. I couldn't help but wonder how many people here thought it was a bit too cute.

Halpern hadn't attended the meeting. After Entheogen Sciences went bust, he accepted a position as the medical director of a swanky, private rehab hospital in the suburbs of Boston. When, in August 2017, the Boston Globe and STAT magazine ran an exposé about "shoddy care" at the hospital, reporters couldn't help but note that Halpern had "a sterling resume, but a past that includes a role in allegedly helping to launder money for a massive LSD-trafficking operation."[7] Leonard Pickard haunts Halpern far more than Timothy Leary.

But Halpern says he's happy now that he's in private practice. Seeing patients gives him great joy. He's also the president of the American Association for Social Psychiatry, a professional organization oriented toward social issues that affect psychological well-being. Every year, they bestow the Abraham L. Halpern Humanitarian Award to someone who has demonstrated extraordinary achievement in advancing human rights. Which reminds me of one last piece of news.

In summer 2020, Leonard Pickard was granted compassionate release from prison because of the threat of COVID-19. He works at a psychedelic venture capitalist firm and has made it back to Harvard as an affiliated researcher in their Project on Psychedelics Law and Regulation. John Halpern, he told me, had called him to apologize, which he appreciated, but that had been the last he heard from him.

Plenty of others have offered Pickard a hero's welcome, describing him as a "prisoner of war" who deserves the deepest respect.

•  •  ••••••••••••••••••••  •  •

We were chatting about these optics back at the Hilton when Bob Wold entered the room. "You mean, Rick Goblin?"

He was just repeating a nickname that he'd overheard earlier, but Wold's laugh carried an edge. There was comfort in knowing that others felt cynical in a space seemingly sprinkled with rainbow unicorn joy. Doblin's choices—especially when it came to the size and shape of his alliances—had rubbed plenty of people the wrong way over the years.

Doblin's tightrope dance between mainstream medicine and alternative wellness has raised tensions in various underground worlds. Who stands to gain financially from the knowledge unearthed in indigenous and subterranean circles? How will medicalization affect access to these substances? How will the Western world reciprocate the benefits reaped from indigenous communities that continue to be exploited? How can a movement that promises to bring about world peace partner with the military, let alone accept money from right-wing zealots? If psychedelics reduce racism, why are so few people of color at the convention? Will the successes of the psychedelic movement help or harm efforts to dismantle the most harmful drug policies?

Advocates and skeptics alike fear that the overzealous promotion of psychedelic science may be overshadowing its actual merits. In an ironic twist, psychedelic medicine's paranoia that the government might stop research meant that, until very recently, there's been little assessment of potential harms associated with psychedelics. However, these findings never seem to make the news, eclipsed as they are by the radiant promise of mental health breakthroughs and transformative experiences. A person could easily walk away from a Psychedelic Science conference with the impression that every bad trip was merely a "challenging experience"—difficult, yes, but ultimately serving to build resilience. The fact that these substances occasionally broke people too often went unsaid.

And the ethical quandaries continue to stack up. In one of the most shocking examples, a participant in a clinical trial administered by MAPS came forward with allegations of sexual assault by one of her therapists. The therapist, according to reports, did not deny having sex with the participant, instead arguing that they "were fellow participants in a study." MAPS faced a backlash for its inadequate response.[8]

Psychedelic studies have several mechanisms in place to prevent this kind of abuse—including video cameras that record dosing sessions. But the incident sparked multiple debates about the ethics involved in psychedelic therapy: inducing so much suggestibility in people undergoing a therapeutic process creates a whole host of new dilemmas that still require a great deal of careful thought and discussion.

And that really leads to the big question underlying so much of the tension: Who will make the rules?

Everyone wants a seat at the table.

●  ●  ●●●●●●●●●●●●●●●●●●●  ●  ●

In an alternate universe, Bob Wold and Rick Doblin might have been raising a toast in Denver to two decades of fruitful collaboration, a reminder of a time when Doblin saw people with cluster headache as vital players in his daring plan to transform the public's perception of psychedelic therapy and catapult LSD back into the academic mainstream, with Harvard as the ultimate prize.

Their alliance faltered when Doblin's vision didn't manifest as planned. John Halpern's plummet from grace, McLean Hospital's refusal to work with MAPS, and the bureaucratic challenges of recruiting participants for the MDMA-assisted therapy trial at Harvard threw a wrench into everything. Doblin, who already faced the Herculean task of fund-raising for drug development, struggled to find donors willing to keep a much-despised alleged informant afloat. Halpern's discovery of a nonhallucinogenic treatment for cluster headache seemed like the best possible solution for everyone involved. Doblin didn't see how Clusterbusters could be unhappy. Sure, they didn't get the project they funded, but they got something so much better. A veritable "cure" with an unscheduled drug!

That a patient group might reject a seemingly "perfect" drug seemed nonsensical, but cluster headache patients had a demonstrated ability to articulate their needs far better than any credentialed expert. Even if BOL-148 proved to be as safe and effective as everyone hoped, a drug was only as helpful as a patient's ability to access it. And accessing BOL-148 would require resources that the headache community might never have. Wold could get magic mushrooms to people now. What he really wanted was Harvard's stamp of approval, which would be a huge boost to gain access to the same donors funding the broader psychedelic renaissance.

But a shift in research focus would devastate the already fragile alliance between the two entities. Clusterbusters, rooted in a pragmatic use of psychedelics for symptom relief, found itself sidelined in favor of Doblin's broader mission to explore the spiritual and transformative aspects of psychedelic therapy. If cluster headache (and, by extension, pain) could be treated without the psychedelic effect, then there was little point in Doblin's expending resources to keep Clusterbusters within his widening circle of alliances.

The Clusterbusters needed more than a medication; they needed a movement. Success required a strong network of support—much stronger than headache had ever produced. Psychedelic medicine was still small back in 2010, but its advocates had the ability to tap into wealthy preexisting networks via its links to New Age spirituality and Silicon Valley tech workers, who were already inclined to support a movement that challenged old dogmas.

By June 2023, Clusterbusters' relationship with MAPS had eroded so far that the conference organizers rejected the group's application to hold a workshop. Meanwhile, it seemed like every other OG in the psychedelic world had their own keynote.

Still, signs of hope kept making their appearance. Clusterbusters, in coordination with cofounders REMAP Therapeutics and Psychedelics Today, and with funding from the RiverStyx Foundation, announced the formation of the Psychedelic and Pain Association, an organization dedicated to advancing research, understanding, awareness, and access to psychedelic medicine for the treatment of chronic pain. A new crop of researchers presenting on the final morning of the conference offered updates on clinical trials testing psilocybin as a treatment for phantom limb pain, fibromyalgia, and chronic low-back pain. And in a quite optimistic development, psychiatrist Stephen Ross at New York University's Center for Psychedelic Medicine, where Carey Turnbull is a founding donor and the chair of the Advisory Board, announced plans to revisit Dr. Eric C. Kast's classic end-of-life LSD research, in a large multihospital clinical trial investigating whether the drug can ease the pain associated with metastatic bone cancer. The National Institutes of Health seemed interested in funding their research. In this context, even a *might* is significant news.

●  ● ●●●●●●●●●●●●●●●●●●●●  ● ●

Listening to young researchers speak so enthusiastically about the future of psychedelic research for pain on the last morning of the conference felt refreshing after so many years spent mucking around in depressing archives. They spoke with frankness and optimism unjaded by persistent bureaucratic hurdles and misleading narratives. However, the zest of the young sometimes lacks the seasoned wisdom of those who've trod these paths before.

What might this renewed aboveground learn from a patient-led group like Clusterbusters? How do we bring the best of what the underground does to the surface—even, or perhaps especially, if it's not profitable?

Bob Wold had some thoughts.

"I know that the number one rule is always 'do no harm.' . . . But there's been harm—a system that is actually deciding who will live and who's gonna end up taking their life."

Medicines only worked as well as the system that delivered them. And the system was pockmarked with injustice. He'd spent a lifetime battling a system that made it nearly impossible for patients to get oxygen, let alone psychedelic drugs.

Even growing your own wasn't enough. How many people had needed help figuring out the right dose? Or working out the best way to wean themselves off other medications? And when the medicine didn't work—and, yes, it doesn't always work—what then? Who will catch the patients when they fall?

The biggest mistake? Believing that a magic mushroom might be a magic bullet.

Communities rooted in empathy and understanding bridge this gap. As psychedelic medicine emerges from quiescence, government authorities and physicians alike will continually insist these drugs are only safe when administered within "controlled medical settings." But isn't there merit in recognizing the therapeutic potential outside these confines?

Wold's no doctor, but so far as he can tell, clearing the path to heaven from hell starts with hope. Start small. Listen. Create an environment where it's okay for someone to share their vulnerabilities. Pain isolates, but knowing you are not alone can make all the difference.

# CODA

BOB WOLD HAS COME A LONG WAY IN THE DECADES SINCE HIS FIRST mushroom trip. I'm still not sure what he saw in those fireworks, but his audacious mission is paying off. Clusterbusters, now the go-to patient advocacy organization for cluster headache, does everything it can to ensure that those with cluster headache receive care in all its forms.

There was just one last thing on Wold's bucket list.

Ainslie Course joined Clusterbusters' Board of Directors in 2020 with the aim of raising the group's profile in the United Kingdom and Europe. Hosting a conference on the continent was a must. Holding it in Glasgow—a city just hours from Aberdeen—meant that Flash would be able to join them. He'd always wanted to go, but traveling any farther than a few hours' drive, he assured me, was out of the question. Flying scared the bejesus out of him; plus he was the only person who could properly care for Chilli, his green-winged macaw.

If Flash wouldn't come to the United States, then Clusterbusters would come to him.

● ● ●●●●●●●●●●●●●●●●●●● ● ●

A small group of Clusterheads and staff members arranged a quiet room off the hotel lobby where they could film Flash and Bob's first in-person interaction. The plan, however, was thwarted when Flash arrived and saw Wold in his usual spot—standing with a group of Busters, drinking coffee, smoking cigarettes. They stood there for a moment, too overwhelmed to say much more than hello before a board member spotted the logistical error and maneuvered Wold back inside where he was meant to be waiting.

Flash strode in a moment later, wearing a newer-than-usual volcanic tiki-bar T-shirt and blue jeans, and hugged his old friend. "Finally."

Laughter diffused the absurdity of the entire scenario—a decades-long digital friendship materializing in analog form.

"Amazing." Flash sighed. "When I first went on that message board, I felt lost in the noise. . . . But you were one of the original ones." Not everyone appreciated what Flash had on offer. Wold's support had meant something back then. He chuckled. "There were so many wacky ideas on that site, and this was the wackiest one of all!"

Wold grinned, proud of what they'd accomplished. "And now tens of thousands of people all over the world are being helped."

"So surreal. I can't believe this is happening." Flash shook his head.

Wold agreed. He still couldn't get over the fact he was in Scotland—a place he always dreamed of visiting—now his reality.

And so there they were, two outlaws who had dared to tread where many had feared to go, now standing in the same room—a rendezvous years in the making that felt right on time.

Not everyone had made it. PinkSharkMark, the enigmatic third pioneer of the patient movement, had passed away nearly a decade before. Neither Flash nor Wold had ever met Pinky, but they'd spoken to him on the phone. He once even considered traveling to Aberdeen to check out Flash's bar, but he backed out when he realized how shite the weather would be.

Wold rummaged through his computer and found a picture of him. "He was a handsome looking guy."

Flash added, "He looked like an actor. He reminded me a bit of Sam Elliot, you know, the older bouncer from *Road House*?"

Flash, now a family man, successful in business, and devoted to his children, laughed when he thought about the acid trip that launched a movement. "Just imagine, I was on the brink of this discovery that was going to affect so many people, and all I was really interested in was getting off my tits!"

Did he realize that the real innovation was never about illicit drugs but about the refusal to isolate and the insistence on sharing what he knew might help? That's the real magic: humanity, in all its beautiful, flawed glory, forever reaching for relief and connection.

# ACKNOWLEDGMENTS

WHAT IS AN AUTHOR, IF NOT THE FRUIT OF A COLLECTIVE EFFORT, A WEB of dialogues, comments traded on paper drafts, late-night pep talks, work meetings at coffee shops, thousands of texts, and an untold number of favors? I am endlessly grateful to the social mycelium that nourished me these past few years.

Thank you, Clusterbusters, for inviting me into your world. You've taught me so much about the true meaning of community. My heartfelt gratitude to all the "helpers" that Mr. Rogers encouraged each of us to see when trouble was afoot: Bob and Mary Wold, Eileen Brewer, Kevin Lenaburg, Ainslie Course, Craig "Flash" Adams, Marsha Weil, and Joe McKay. You inspire me to be a better person.

I owe a great deal to the support of the headache advocacy community, with special mention to Shirley Kessel, Jill Dehlin, Katie Golden, Katie MacDonald, Alan Kaplan, Catherine Charrett-Dykes, Tammy Rose, Paula K. Dumas, Angie Glaser, Anna Williams, and Drs. Robert E. Shapiro, William B. Young, Stephanie Nahas-Geiger, Christopher Gottschalk, Mark Weatherall, Emmanuelle Schindler, Dawn Buse, Elizabeth Loder, and Brian McGeeney. You have always been so generous with your time, knowledge, and constructive feedback. Thank you also for your extraordinary support in my own effort to control chronic migraine. Dr. Young, Jen Cho, and Carla Alizzo go above and beyond to keep me on my feet.

So much of my sensibility as a researcher comes from my dear friend, the late, great Chuck Bosk. His eyes lit up when I told him about Clusterbusters over lunch at his favorite Chinese restaurant in Narberth. I learned quite a bit over the next hour about the supply closet in Spring Grove, Maryland, before he leaned back in his chair and said, "You have to do this."

Chuck had great instincts, which I suspect were rooted in his deep conviction about the vital importance of witnessing pain. But he also knew that a conscientious ethnographer would struggle to keep themselves at arm's distance when they witnessed suffering. I could use his advice, however cryptic it could be. Thank goodness I have Emily Bosk and Betsy Armstrong to step in when needed. Thank you, dear Emily and Betsy. I couldn't do any of this without you.

I have a whole network of people who give me superpowers: my A-Team writing group, Rene Almeling, Laura Carpenter, and Jen Reich; local scholar Anastasia Hudgins; Catherine Lee and Norah MacKendrick, my virtual water cooler; bioethicists and dear friends Jon Merz and Dominic Sisti; my own OGs, Olga Shevchenko and Chloe Silverman; Shelby Siegel, the best film editor I've ever worked with on a book; artist and designer Lizzy Hindman-Harvey; and the best men Jules Evans, Jonty Claypole, and Ben Smith.

Thank you, John Bailey, for bringing your sharp insights to our collaborations. Chapter 10 is based on our work together. And many thanks to Gabriel Varela for getting these data into workable condition.

I've had the good fortune to meet so many wonderful scholars while writing this book. Thank you to everyone in the Outlaw Bio crew, especially Anna Wexler, Christi Guerrini, Alex Pearlman, and Lisa Rasmussen. I owe immeasurable thanks to historians Nancy Campbell, Jonathan Moreno, and Lucas Richert for their generous help navigating this new territory. It's been terrific having scholars like Danielle Giffort, Nicolas Langlitz, Tehseen Noorani, Ksenia Cassidy, and Jarrett Rose to chat with about all things psychedelic. Many thanks to William Russell for wordsmithing, Ben Gambuzza for research assistance, editing, and fact-checking and to Sheena Raja for her assistance with references. Thanks to Barbara Di Gennaro Splendore, a historian of medicine, for helping me track down archival evidence of Frederico Sicuteri's research in Italy, which led to a fascinating interview with Sicuteri's widow and former collaborator, Dr. Maria Nicolodi.

Thank you, Gretchen Bakke, for gifting me with "social mycelium." Many thanks to Brendan Burns for gamely serving as a sounding board, Holly Lynch-Fernandez for astute policy advice, Dan Menchik for deep sociological insights, Anna Mueller for helping make this manuscript as respectful and useful as possible, Hannah Glassman for lessons in profound empathy and holding space, and Court Wing at REMAP Therapeutics for his brilliant help decoding the science of psychedelics and pain.

My gratitude to Dr. Ethan Russo for sharing his correspondence with Dr. Albert Hofmann. I am grateful to Daren Johnson, owner of Web Vision Enterprises LLC, for permitting the reproduction of excerpts from the online forum Clusterheadaches.com. That doctors still don't understand how much they owe DJ for transforming their understanding of cluster headache in the new millennium underscores a significant gap between patient-driven initiatives and traditional medical recognition.

Wrangling these stories into a book that did them justice terrified me. Bridget Wagner Matzie, literary agent and occasional therapist, believed in this project—and me—from day one. She steered me in the direction of Lauren Marino, whose editorial direction and vision made this a far stronger book. Thank you to the entire team at Hachette Book Group: Niyati Patel, Cisca Schreefel, Carolyn Levin, and Jennifer Kelland. Jane Franken Franssen's kindness, experience, and ingenious editing kept this project afloat.

I lucked into a job that lets me follow my curiosity wherever it goes. I've received generous support from several institutions dedicated to academic freedom and inquiry, the most vital being my home Department of Sociology at Rutgers University. Special thanks to Julie Phillips, Paul McLean, and Lisa Iorillo, the fearless leaders who have made sure I have everything I need to succeed.

I've benefited from the ability to present this work to audiences around the world, thanks to invitations from the University of Edinburgh, the University of Pennsylvania, Montclair State University, the University of Wisconsin, Thomas Jefferson University, the Qualitative Analysis Conference in Canada, Williams College, the Student Psychedelic Conference, PhilaDelic, and, of course, Clusterbusters. I'm so thankful for Martyn Pickersgill, who sponsored a public panel featuring Ainslie Course and Craig "Flash" Adams.

I'm the grateful benefactor of several visiting scholar programs, including Princeton University's Center for Health and Wellbeing, the University of Pennsylvania's Department of Bioethics, and Rutgers University's Center for Cultural Analysis and its Institute for Research on Women. Portions of this research were supported by generous grants made by Rutgers University's Department of Sociology and Porta Sophia Psychedelic Prior Art Library. My heartfelt thanks to AAUP-Rutgers for ensuring that New Jersey has the university it deserves.

You don't get to choose your family, which makes me the luckiest girl in the world. Jim and Ruth Kempner loved me into their world of curiosity, justice, endless debate, piles of books, and wry humor. Dad, you are an extraordinary writer. Thank you for your edits, your advice, and your patient listening. Mom, you are the reason I write.

I hate being the middle child, but thank goodness I'm sandwiched between Evan and Michelle, two funny, beautiful geniuses. And now my family includes Supriya, Sona, and Thara. I am a proud Bua. The Stone family keeps my cup filled. Melissa, thank you for coaching me through another book.

The Drury family is wonderful too. Martin and Liz have adopted me into their family these last twenty years, and I'm just so grateful to spend time with these two brilliant, wise souls. Matt, Kate, Daisy, James, Sam, Nancy, Tommy, Frankie, Billie, and Freddie make every holiday a joy.

Only the best of friends could get me through the one-two punch of pandemic parenting and book writing. Thinking of you, Mara Cooper, Shelby Siegel, Erica Benjamin, Lisa Katzer, Amy Chao, and the Hollace Detwiler experience. Special love for all the friends and extended kin in my beloved West Philly neighborhood. Thank you for helping our family navigate these last few years, with special love to Pete, Sugirtha, Zoe, and Kalin.

That Joe Drury has chosen to live with me is proof in the power of manifestation. Thank you for being a true partner. Thank you for believing in the power of this story. And thank you for reading every word of this manuscript.

Noah and Tessa: My favorite creations and the best companions.

# APPENDIX

ALBERT HOFMANN
DR. PHIL. II, DR. H.C. MULT.
CH-4117 BURG I.L.
RITTIMATTE TEL. 061 731 14 33

19 May, 1997.


Ethan B. Russo, M.D.
The Western Montana Clinic
515 West Front Street
Missoula,  Montana 59802

Dear Dr. Russo,

I beg to apologize for the long delay in responding to your
letter of February 28 and the very interesting reprints.

Your idea, that LSD in low doses may be effective in migraine
prophylaxis, seems to me very reasonable. I am glad that MAPS
will support a study in this direction. I do hope that the
Health Authority will allow use of LSD for this kind of investigation.

In addition to the suspected effect on migraine, I could imma-
gine that other valuable therapeutic observations could be
made during a chronical application of such very low doses of
LSD.

I had always planned to investigate in self-experiments the
effects of daily use of low, no hallucinations producing
doses of LSD, but came only to very preliminary studies. I
am therefore very interested in your approaching investigation.

I thank you for the information about your work for which
I wish you much success.

Sincerely,

*Albert Hofmann*

Please convey kind regards to Rick Doblin.

# REFERENCES

"About Clusterbusters." Clusterbusters. Accessed September 24, 2023. https://cluster busters.org/about.

"About ICEERS." International Center for Ethnobotanical Education, Research, and Service. Accessed May 12, 2023. https://www.iceers.org/about-us.

Ahlman, Austin. "House Moves to Expand Psychedelic Therapy Research." The Intercept, July 26, 2022. https://theintercept.com/2022/07/14/ptsd-psychedelic -therapy-research-congress/.

Allen, Scott. "A Doctor's Downfall, Mclean's Fallout: Sex Secret Kept Quiet for a Year." *Boston Globe*. October 14, 2007.

Allena, Marta, Roberto De Icco, Grazia Sances, Lara Ahmad, Alessia Putortì, Ennio Pucci, Rosaria Greco, and Cristina Tassorelli. "Gender Differences in the Clinical Presentation of Cluster Headache: A Role for Sexual Hormones?" *Frontiers in Neurology* 10 (2019). https://doi.org/10.3389/fneur.2019.01220.

Andersson, Martin, Mari Persson, and Anette Kjellgren. "Psychoactive Substances as a Last Resort: A Qualitative Study of Self-Treatment of Migraine and Cluster Headaches." *Harm Reduction Journal* 14, no. 60 (2017).

Andre, Laura, and Debbie Cavers. "'A Cry in the Dark': A Qualitative Exploration of Living with Cluster Headache." *British Journal of Pain* 15, no. 4 (2021): 420–428.

Armstrong, David, and Evan Allen. "Behind the Luxury: Turmoil and Shoddy Care Inside Five-Star Addiction Treatment Centers." *STAT*, July 25, 2023. https://www .statnews.com/2017/08/25/recovery-centers-of-america-addiction/.

Bailey, John, and Joanna Kempner. "Standards Without Labs: Drug Development in the Psychedelic Underground." *Citizen Science Theory and Practice* 7, no. 1 (2022): 41. https://doi.org/10.5334/cstp.527.

Bebergal, Peter. "Will Harvard Drop Acid Again?" *Boston Phoenix*. May 28, 2008.

Begasse de Dhaem, O., R. Burch, N. Rosen, K. Shubin Stein, E. Loder, and R. E. Shapiro. "Workforce Gap Analysis in the Field of Headache Medicine in the United States." *Headache* 60, no. 2 (2020): 478–481.

Bender, George A. "Rough and Ready Research—1887 Style." *Journal of the History of Medicine and Allied Sciences* 23, no. 2 (1968): 159–166.

Benkli, B., S. Y. Kim, N. Koike, C. Han, C. K. Tran, E. Silva, Y. Yan, K. Yagita, Z. Chen, S. H. Yoo, and M. Burish. "Circadian Features of Cluster Headache and Migraine:

A Systematic Review, Meta-Analysis, and Genetic Analysis." *Neurology* 100, no. 22 (2023): e2224–e2236.

Blau, J. N. "Behaviour During a Cluster Headache." *The Lancet* 342, no. 8873 (1993): 723–725.

Bonnelle, Valerie, Will J. Smith, Natasha L. Mason, Mauro Cavarra, Pamela Kryskow, Kim P. C. Kuypers, Johannes G. Ramaekers, and Amanda Feilding. "Analgesic Potential of Macrodoses and Microdoses of Classical Psychedelics in Chronic Pain Sufferers: A Population Survey." *British Journal of Pain* 16, no. 6 (2022): 619–631.

Bothwell, Laura E., Jeremy A. Greene, Scott H. Podolsky, and David S. Jones. "Assessing the Gold Standard—Lessons from the History of RCTs." *New England Journal of Medicine* 374, no. 22 (2016): 2175–2181.

Bowler, Kate. "When Your Child Is Diagnosed." *Everything Happens*, May 14, 2019. https://katebowler.com/when-your-child-is-diagnosed.

Breen, Benjamin. *The Age of Intoxication: Origins of the Global Drug Trade.* Philadelphia: University of Pennsylvania Press, 2019.

Brown, Phil. "Popular Epidemiology and Toxic Waste Contamination: Lay and Professional Ways of Knowing." *Journal of Health and Social Behavior* 33, no. 3 (1992): 267–281.

Burch, Rebecca, Paul Rizzoli, and Elizabeth Loder. "The Prevalence and Impact of Migraine and Severe Headache in the United States: Updated Age, Sex, and Socioeconomic-Specific Estimates from Government Health Surveys." *Headache* 61, no. 1 (2021): 60–68.

Burish, Mark J., Stuart M. Pearson, Robert E. Shapiro, Wei Zhang, and Larry I. Schor. "Cluster Headache Is One of the Most Intensely Painful Human Conditions: Results from the International Cluster Headache Questionnaire." *Headache* 61, no. 1 (2021): 117–124.

———. "Oxygen as the Optimal Acute Medication for Cluster Headache: A Comment and Additional Validation Step from the Cluster Headache Questionnaire." *Headache* 60, no. 10 (2020): 2592–2593.

Buture, Alina, Fayyaz Ahmed, Lisa Dikomitis, and Jason W. Boland. "Systematic Literature Review on the Delays in the Diagnosis and Misdiagnosis of Cluster Headache." *Neurological Sciences* 40 (2019): 25–39.

Carbonaro, Theresa M., Matthew P. Bradstreet, Frederick S. Barrett, Katherine A. MacLean, Robert Jesse, Matthew W. Johnson, and Roland R. Griffiths. "Survey Study of Challenging Experiences After Ingesting Psilocybin Mushrooms: Acute and Enduring Positive and Negative Consequences." *Journal of Psychopharmacology* 30, no. 12 (2016): 1268–1278.

Carey, Benedict. "Tim Ferriss, the Man Who Put His Money Behind Psychedelic Medicine." *New York Times.* September 6, 2019. https://www.nytimes.com/2019/09/06/health/ferriss-psychedelic-drugs-depression.html.

Carhart-Harris, Robin L. "The Entropic Brain-Revisited." *Neuropharmacology* 142 (2018): 167–178.

Carpenter, Daniel. *Reputation and Power: Organizational Image and Pharmaceutical Regulation at the FDA.* Princeton, NJ: Princeton University Press, 2014.

Carrell, Severin. "Trump Golf Course Staff Photographed Urinating Woman 'to Detect' Crime." *The Guardian*. April 4, 2017. https://www.theguardian.com/uk-news/2017/apr/04/donald-trump-golf-course-aberdeenshire-staff-photographed-urinating-woman.

Castellanos, Joel P., Chris Woolley, Kelly Amanda Bruno, Fadel Zeidan, Adam Halberstadt, and Timothy Furnish. "Chronic Pain and Psychedelics: A Review and Proposed Mechanism of Action." *Regional Anesthesia and Pain Medicine* 45, no. 7 (2020): 486–494.

Centers for Disease Control and Prevention. "U.S. State Opioid Dispensing Rates, 2021." Accessed September 24, 2023. https://www.cdc.gov/drugoverdose/rxrate-maps/index.html.

Cetina, Karin Knorr. *Epistemic Cultures: How the Sciences Make Knowledge*. Cambridge, MA: Harvard University Press, 1999.

Christie, Devon, Berra Yazar-Klosinski, Ekaterina Nosova, Pam Kryskow, Danielle Lessor, and Elena Maria Argento. "MDMA-Assisted Therapy Is Associated with a Reduction in Chronic Pain Among People with Post-Traumatic Stress Disorder." *Frontiers in Psychiatry* 13 (November 2022): 1–10.

Chrysanthos, Natassia, and Aisha Dow. "Australia Becomes First Country to Recognise Psychedelics as Medicines." *Sydney Morning Herald*. February 3, 2023. https://www.smh.com.au/politics/federal/australia-becomes-first-country-to-recognise-psychedelics-as-medicines-20230203-p5chs6.html.

Cohen, Sidney. "The Anguish of the Dying." *Harper's Magazine* 231 (September 1965): 69–78.

———. "Complications Associated with Lysergic Acid Diethylamide (LSD-25)." *JAMA* 181, no. 2 (July 14, 1962): 161.

Courtwright, David T. *Dark Paradise: A History of Opiate Addiction in America*. Cambridge, MA: Harvard University Press, 2001.

———. *Forces of Habit: Drugs and the Making of the Modern World*. Cambridge, MA: Harvard University Press, 2001.

Danforth, Alicia L., Charles S. Grob, Christopher Struble, Allison A. Feduccia, Nick Walker, Lisa Jerome, Berra Klosinski, and Amy Emerson. "Reduction in Social Anxiety After MDMA-Assisted Psychotherapy with Autistic Adults: A Randomized, Double-Blind, Placebo-Controlled Pilot Study." *Psychopharmacology* 235, no. 11 (2018): 3137–3148.

Davis, Erik. "The Bad Shaman Meets the Wayward Doc." *Tripzine*. February 10, 2006. https://www.tripzine.com/listing.php?id=650.

Deleuze, Gilles, and Felix Guattari. *A Thousand Plateaus: Capitalism and Schizophrenia*. Translated by Brian Massumi. Minneapolis: University of Minnesota Press, 1987.

DiMasi, Joseph A., Henry G. Grabowski, and Ronald W. Hansen. "Innovation in the Pharmaceutical Industry: New Estimates of R&D Costs." *Journal of Health Economics* 47 (2016): 20–33.

Doblin, Richard Elliot. "Regulation of the Medical Use of Psychedelics and Marijuana." PhD diss., Harvard University, 2000. https://search.proquest.com/openview/c8680fcf5e470c0470d9fe8cfedc9917/1?pq-origsite=gscholar&cbl=18750&diss=y.

Doblin, Rick. "The Future of Psychedelic-Assisted Psychotherapy." TED. April 2019. https://www.ted.com/talks/rick_doblin_the_future_of_psychedelic_assisted_psychotherapy?language=en

———. "Pahnke's 'Good Friday Experiment': A Long-Term Follow-Up and Methodological Critique." *Journal of Transpersonal Psychology* 23, no. 1 (1991): 1–28.

Dworkin, Robert H., Brian T. Anderson, Nick Andrews, Robert R. Edwards, Charles S. Grob, Stephen Ross, Theodore D. Satterthwaite, and Eric C. Strain. "If the Doors of Perception Were Cleansed, Would Chronic Pain Be Relieved? Evaluating the Benefits and Risks of Psychedelics." *Journal of Pain* 23, no. 10 (2022): 1666–1679.

Dyck, Erika. *Psychedelic Psychiatry: LSD from Clinic to Campus.* Baltimore: Johns Hopkins University Press, 2008.

Eadie, M. J. "Ergot of Rye—the First Specific for Migraine." *Journal of Clinical Neuroscience* 11, no. 1 (2004): 4–7.

Edmond, Andrew. "Pioneers of the Virtual Underground: A History of Our Culture." *Resonance Project* 1 (1997). https://erowid.org/psychoactives/history/references/other/1997_edmond_resproject_1.shtml.

Edwards, Ezekiel, Emily Greytak, Brooke Madubuonwu, Thania Sanchez, Sophia Beiers, Charlotte Resing, Paige Fernandez, and Sagiv Galai Galai. *A Tale of Two Countries: Racially Targeted Arrests in the Era of Marijuana Reform.* New York: ACLU, 2020.

Elliott, Matt. "Ex-Informant in Tulsa Jail." *Tulsa World.* September 3, 2004. https://tulsaworld.com/archive/ex-informant-in-tulsa-jail/article_f172d57b-257d-532c-9a16-19b4c5ad0ca1.html.

———. "Life Term Given in Torture Case." *Tulsa World.* July 21, 2006. https://tulsaworld.com/archive/life-term-given-in-torture-case/article_986c46a7-6a53-54ea-817d-54449be51fd1.html.

Ellis, Havelock. "Mescal—the Divine Plant." *Popular Science Monthly* 61 (1902): 52–71.

Ellison, Katherine. "A New Treatment May Halt Cluster Headaches. But Some Say Psychedelic Drugs Are the Real Answer." *Washington Post.* April 4, 2021. https://www.washingtonpost.com/health/cluster-headaches/2021/04/02/66ac73f0-8cdc-11eb-9423-04079921c915_story.html.

Epstein, Steven. *Impure Science: AIDS, Activism, and the Politics of Knowledge.* Berkeley: University of California Press, 1996.

"Erowid Character Vaults: R. Andrew Sewell." Erowid. Updated August 15, 2013. Accessed September 18, 2023. https://erowid.org/culture/characters/sewell_andrew/sewell_andrew.shtml.

Erowid, Earth, and Fire Erowid, "The State of the Stone: Science from the Underground." PowerPoint presentation, Psychedelic Science 2023, Denver, Colorado. June 21, 2023. https://2023.psychedelicscience.org/sessions/the-state-of-the-stone-science-from-the-underground.

Estrada, Alvaro. *María Sabina: Her Life and Chants.* Translated by Henry Munn. 1st Eng. ed. Santa Barbara, CA: Ross-Erikson, 1981.

Fadiman, James. *The Psychedelic Explorer's Guide: Safe, Therapeutic, and Sacred Journeys.* New York: Simon and Schuster, 2011.

Fanciullacci, M., G. Granchi, and F. Sicuteri. "Ergotamine and Methysergide as Serotonin Partial Agonists in Migraine." *Headache* 16, no. 5 (1976): 226–231.

Feinberg, Benjamin. *The Devil's Book of Culture: History, Mushrooms, and Caves in Southern Mexico.* Austin: University of Texas Press, 2003. doi:https://doi.org/10.7560/705500.

Floyd, L. J., P. K. Alexandre, S. L. Hedden, A. L. Lawson, W. W. Latimer, and N. Giles. "Adolescent Drug Dealing and Race/Ethnicity: A Population-Based Study of the Differential Impact of Substance Use on Involvement in Drug Trade." *American Journal of Drug and Alcohol Abuse* 36, no. 2 (2010): 87–91.

Ford, Janet H., Damion Nero, Gilwan Kim, Bong Chul Chu, Robert Fowler, Jonna Ahl, and James M. Martinez. "Societal Burden of Cluster Headache in the United States: A Descriptive Economic Analysis." *Journal of Medical Economics* 21, no. 1 (2018): 107–111.

Foucault, Michel. *The Birth of the Clinic: An Archaeology of Medical Perception.* New York: Vintage, 1994.

Frauenfelder, Mark. "Interview with Marc Franklin, Photographer of Psychedelic Explorers and High Frontiers' Art Director." *Boing Boing.* December 5, 2011. https://boingboing.net/2011/12/05/interview-with-marc-franklin.html.

Frood, Arran. "Cluster Busters." *Nature Medicine* 13, no. 1 (December 28, 2006): 10–11.

Gasser, P., K. Kirchner, and T. Passie. "LSD-Assisted Psychotherapy for Anxiety Associated with a Life-Threatening Disease: A Qualitative Study of Acute and Sustained Subjective Effects." *Journal of Psychopharmacology* 29, no. 1 (2015): 57–68.

George, Jamilah R., Timothy I. Michaels, Jae Sevelius, and Monnica T. Williams. "The Psychedelic Renaissance and the Limitations of a White-Dominant Medical Framework: A Call for Indigenous and Ethnic Minority Inclusion." *Journal of Psychedelic Studies* 4, no. 1 (2019): 4–15.

Gerard, Francis. "Pain, Death and LSD: A Retrospective of the Work of Dr. Eric Kast." *Psychedelic Monographs and Essays*, no. 5 (autumn–winter 1990): 114–121.

Gerber, Konstantin, Inti García Flores, Angela Christina Ruiz, Ismail Ali, Natalie Lyla Ginsberg, and Eduardo E. Schenberg. "Ethical Concerns About Psilocybin Intellectual Property." *ACS Pharmacology & Translational Science* 4, no. 2 (2021): 573–577.

Giffort, Danielle. *Acid Revival: The Psychedelic Renaissance and the Quest for Legitimacy.* Minneapolis: University of Minnesota Press, 2020.

Gillespie, Nick. "People Should Have the Fundamental Human Right to Change Their Consciousness." *Reason* 52 (July 2020). https://reason.com/2020/06/21/people-should-have-the-fundamental-right-to-change-their-consciousness.

Gill-Peterson, Jules. "Doctors Who? Radical Lessons from the History of DIY Transition." *The Baffler*, no. 65 (September–October 2022): 7–15. https://thebaffler.com/salvos/doctors-who-gill-peterson.

Goadsby, Peter J. "Pathophysiology of Cluster Headache: A Trigeminal Autonomic Cephalgia." *Lancet Neurology* 1, no. 4 (2002): 251–257.

Goldhill, Olivia. "Psychedelic Medicine Group Investigating a Board Member Accused of Financial Elder Abuse." *STAT News.* May 18, 2022. https://www.statnews.com/2022/05/18/maps-psychedelics-group-investigating-board-member-accused-of-financial-elder-abuse.

318 References

Gottlieb, Adam. *A Concise Encyclopedia of Legal Herbs and Chemicals with Psychoactive Properties*. Manhattan Beach, CA: 20th Century Alchemist, 1973.

Graham, John. "Cluster Headache." *Headache* 11 (1972): 175–185.

Graham, J. R., and H. G. Wolff. "Mechanism of Migraine Headache and Action of Ergotamine Tartrate." *Archives of Neurology & Psychiatry* 39, no. 4 (1938): 737–763.

Great Britain. Drugs Act 2005. c. 17, s. 21. http://www.legislation.gov.uk/ukpga/2005/17/section/21.

Greco, Allison. "Yale's Pioneering Research on Psychedelics Gives Hope to Headache Disorder Community." Yale School of Medicine. Updated March 13, 2023, accessed July 12, 2023.

Green, C. R., K. O. Anderson, T. A. Baker, L. C. Campbell, S. Decker, R. B. Fillingim, D. A. Kalauokalani, et al. "The Unequal Burden of Pain: Confronting Racial and Ethnic Disparities in Pain." *Pain Medicine* 4, no. 3 (2003): 277–294.

Greene, Jeremy A., and Scott H. Podolsky. "Reform, Regulation, and Pharmaceuticals—the Kefauver-Harris Amendments at 50." *New England Journal of Medicine* 367, no. 16 (2012): 1481–1483.

Greer, George R. "Using MDMA in Psychotherapy." *Advances* 2, no. 2 (1985): 57–59.

Griffiths, Roland R., M. W. Johnson, M. A. Carducci, A. Umbricht, W. A. Richards, B. D. Richards, M. P. Cosimano, and M. A. Klinedinst. "Psilocybin Produces Substantial and Sustained Decreases in Depression and Anxiety in Patients with Life-Threatening Cancer: A Randomized Double-Blind Trial." *Journal of Psychopharmacology* 30, no. 12 (2016): 1181–1197.

Griffiths, Roland R., William A. Richards, Matthew W. Johnson, Una D. McCann, and Robert Jesse. "Mystical-Type Experiences Occasioned by Psilocybin Mediate the Attribution of Personal Meaning and Spiritual Significance 14 Months Later." *Journal of Psychopharmacology* 22, no. 6 (2008): 621–632.

Griffiths, Roland R., William A. Richards, Una McCann, and Robert Jesse. "Psilocybin Can Occasion Mystical-Type Experiences Having Substantial and Sustained Personal Meaning and Spiritual Significance." *Psychopharmacology* 30, no. 12 (2006): 1181–1197.

Grob, Charles S., Alicia L. Danforth, Gurpreet S. Chopra, Marycie Hagerty, Charles R. McKay, Adam L. Halberstadt, and George R. Greer. "Pilot Study of Psilocybin Treatment for Anxiety in Patients with Advanced-Stage Cancer." *Archives of General Psychiatry* 68, no. 1 (2011): 71–78.

Gunther, Marc. "Carey Turnbull Wears Many Hats as a Donor and Investor." *Lucid News*. October 27, 2022.

Guzmán, Gastón. "Hallucinogenic Mushrooms in Mexico: An Overview." *Economic Botany* 62, no. 3 (2008): 404–412.

Haane, Danielle Y. P., Thijs H. T. Dirkx, and Peter J. Koehler. "The History of Oxygen Inhalation as a Treatment for Cluster Headache." *Cephalalgia* 32, no. 12 (2012): 932–939. https://doi.org/10.1177/0333102412452044.

Hagan, John. *Who Are the Criminals? The Politics of Crime Policy from the Age of Roosevelt to the Age of Reagan*. Princeton, NJ: Princeton University Press, 2010.

Hagenbach, Dieter, and Lucius Werthmüller. *Mystic Chemist*. Santa Fe, NM: Synergetic Press, 2013.

Haichin, Michael. "The Top 5 Psychedelic Clinical Trials of 2022." *Psychedelic Alpha*. https://psychedelicalpha.com/news/the-top-5-psychedelic-clinical-trials-of-2022.

Halpern, John H. "Cognitive Effects of Substance Use in Native Americans." 5K23DA000494. McLean Hospital. National Institutes of Health. https://reporter.nih.gov/search/c70FJ9QEzEeKxJoFLIMBlQ/projects.

———. "John Halpern Forecasts the Future." *New Scientist*. November 16, 2006.

———. "Neurocognitive Consequences of Long-Term Ecstasy Use." Grant No. 5R01DA017953. McLean Hospital. National Institutes of Health. https://reporter.nih.gov/search/c70FJ9QEzEeKxJoFLIMBlQ/project-details/7488415.

———. "The Use of Hallucinogens in the Treatment of Addiction." *Addiction Research & Theory* 4, no. 2 (1996): 177–189.

Halpern, John H., and Harrison G. Pope Jr. "Hallucinogens on the Internet: A Vast New Source of Underground Drug Information." *American Journal of Psychiatry* 158, no. 3 (2001): 481–483.

Halpern, John H., Andrea R. Sherwood, James I. Hudson, Deborah Yurgelun-Todd, and Harrison G. Pope Jr. "Psychological and Cognitive Effects of Long-Term Peyote Use Among Native Americans." *Biological Psychiatry* 58, no. 8 (2005): 624–631.

Hanna, Jon. "Halperngate." *Entheogen Review* 15, no. 1 (2006): 9–16.

Hansen, Helena, Julie Netherland, and David L. Herzberg. *Whiteout: How Racial Capitalism Changed the Color of Opioids in America*. Oakland: University of California Press, 2023.

Harris, Rachel. *Swimming in the Sacred: Wisdom from the Psychedelic Underground*. Novato, CA: New World Library, 2023.

Harris, W. "Ciliary (Migrainous) Neuralgia and Its Treatment." *British Medical Journal* 1 (1936): 457–460.

Harry, Prince, Duke of Sussex. *Spare*. New York: Random House Publishing Group, 2023.

Hart, Carl L. *Drug Use for Grown-ups: Chasing Liberty in the Land of Fear*. New York: Penguin, 2021.

Hartogsohn, Ido. *American Trip: Set, Setting, and the Psychedelic Experience in the Twentieth Century*. Boston: MIT Press, 2020.

Hattle, Ashley S. *Cluster Headaches: A Guide to Surviving One of the Most Painful Conditions Known to Man: For Patients, Supporters, and Health Care Professionals*. Pennsauken, NJ: BookBaby, 2017.

Heinrichs, R. Walter. *In Search of Madness: Schizophrenia and Neuroscience*. Oxford: Oxford University Press, 2001.

Heise, Kenan. "Dr. Eric C. Kast. 73. Ran Free Health Clinic." *Chicago Tribune*. December 1, 1988. https://www.chicagotribune.com/news/ct-xpm-1988-12-01-8802210024-story.html.

Herzberg, David. *White Market Drugs: Big Pharma and the Hidden History of Addiction in America*. Chicago: University of Chicago Press, 2020.

Herzig, Rebecca M. *Suffering for Science: Reason and Sacrifice in Modern America*. New Brunswick, NJ: Rutgers University Press, 2005.

Hettler, Brian, and Mark Plotkin. "The Amazonian Travels of Richard Evans Schultes." Amazon Conservation Team. April 8, 2019. https://www.amazonteam.org/maps /schultes/en.

Hevisi, Dennis. "Howard Lotsof Dies at 66; Saw Drug Cure in a Plant." *New York Times*. February 18, 2010. https://www.nytimes.com/2010/02/17/us/17lotsof.html.

Hoffman, K. M., S. Trawalter, J. R. Axt, and M. N. Oliver. "Racial Bias in Pain Assessment and Treatment Recommendations, and False Beliefs About Biological Differences Between Blacks and Whites." *Proceedings of the National Academy of Sciences* 113, no. 16 (2016): 4296–4301.

Hofman, Albert. *LSD: My Problem Child*. New York: McGraw-Hill Book Company, 1980.

Holbein, M. "Understanding FDA Regulatory Requirements for Investigational New Drug Applications for Sponsor-Investigators." *Journal of Investigative Medicine* 57, no. 6 (2009): 688–694.

Holze, F., P. Gasser, F. Muller, P. C. Dolder, and M. E. Liechti. "Lysergic Acid Diethylamide–Assisted Therapy in Patients with Anxiety with and Without a Life-Threatening Illness: A Randomized, Double-Blind, Placebo-Controlled Phase II Study." *Biological Psychiatry* 93, no. 3 (2023): 215–223.

Hooyer, Katinka, Kalman Applbaum, and Daniel Kasza. "Altered States of Combat: Veteran Trauma and the Quest for Novel Therapeutics in Psychedelic Substances." *Journal of Humanistic Psychology* 63, no. 6 (February 6, 2020): 744–763.

Horton, Bayard T., A. R. MacLean, and W. M. Craig. "A New Syndrome of Vascular Headache: Results of Treatment with Histamine: Preliminary Report." *Mayo Clinic Proceedings* 14 (1939): 257–260.

Huxley, Aldous. *The Doors of Perception*. London: Chatto and Windus, 1954.

———. *Island, a Novel*. 1st ed. New York: Harper, 1962.

Isler, H. "Episodic Cluster Headache from a Textbook of 1745: Van Swieten's Classic Description." *Cephalalgia* 13, no. 3 (1993): 172–174.

Jacobs, Andrew. "Psychedelic Revolution Is Coming. Psychiatry May Never Be the Same." *New York Times*. May 9, 2021. https://www.nytimes.com/2021/05/09/health /psychedelics-mdma-psilocybin-molly-mental-health.html.

Janevic, M. R., S. J. McLaughlin, A. A. Heapy, C. Thacker, and J. D. Piette. "Racial and Socioeconomic Disparities in Disabling Chronic Pain: Findings from the Health and Retirement Study." *Journal of Pain* 18, no. 12 (2017): 1459–1467.

Johnson, Matthew W., Roland R. Griffiths, Peter S. Hendricks, and Jack E. Henningfield. "The Abuse Potential of Medical Psilocybin According to the 8 Factors of the Controlled Substances Act." *Neuropharmacology* 142 (2018): 143–166.

Johnson, Matthew W., Peter S. Hendricks, Frederick S. Barrett, and Roland R. Griffiths. "Classic Psychedelics: An Integrative Review of Epidemiology, Therapeutics, Mystical Experience, and Brain Network Function." *Pharmacology & Therapeutics* 197 (2019): 83–102.

Johnson, Matthew W., R. Andrew Sewell, and Roland R. Griffiths. "Psilocybin Dose-Dependently Causes Delayed, Transient Headaches in Healthy Volunteers." *Drug and Alcohol Dependence* 123, no. 1–3 (2012): 132–140.

Jones, Wilfred F., Jr., Maxwell Finland, Clare Wilcox, and Ann Najarian. "Antibiotic Combinations: Antistreptococcal and Antistaphylococcal Activity of Plasma of Normal Subjects After Ingestion of Erythromycin or Penicillin or Both." *New England Journal of Medicine* 255, no. 22 (1956): 1019–1024.

Kandell, Jonathan. "Richard E. Schultes, 86, Dies; Trailblazing Authority on Hallucinogenic Plants." *New York Times*, April 13, 2001. https://www.nytimes.com/2001/04/13 /us/richard-e-schultes-86-dies-trailblazing-authority-on-hallucinogenic-plants.html.

———. "LSD and the Dying Patient." *Chicago Medical School Quarterly* 26, no. 2 (1966): 80–87.

———. "The Measurement of Pain: A New Approach to an Old Problem." *Journal of New Drugs* 2, no. 6 (1962): 344–351.

Kast, Eric C. "Attenuation of Anticipation: A Therapeutic Use of Lysergic Acid Diethylamide." *Psychiatric Quarterly* 41, no. 4 (1967): 646–657.

Kast, Eric C., and Vincent J. Collins. "Study of Lysergic Acid Diethylamide as an Analgesic Agent." *Anesthesia and Analgesics* 43, no. 3 (1964): 285–291.

Kempner, Joanna. "The Chilling Effect: How Do Researchers React to Controversy?" *PLOS Medicine* 5, no. 11 (2008): e222.

———. *Not Tonight: Migraine and the Politics of Gender and Health*. Chicago: University of Chicago Press, 2014.

Kempner, Joanna, and John Bailey. "Collective Self-Experimentation in Patient-Led Research: How Online Health Communities Foster Innovation." *Social Science & Medicine* 238 (October 2019): 112366.

Kempner, Joanna, Jon F. Merz, and Charles L. Bosk. "Forbidden Knowledge: Public Controversy and the Production of Nonknowledge." *Sociological Forum* 26, no. 3 (2011): 475–500.

Kinzer, Stephen. *Poisoner in Chief: Sidney Gottlieb and the CIA Search for Mind Control*. 1st ed. New York: Henry Holt and Company, 2019.

"The Kip Scale." Clusterheadaches. 1999. Accessed July 12, 2023. https://www.cluster headaches.com/scale.html.

Klein, Joe. "The New Drug They Call 'Ecstasy.'" *New York Magazine*. May 20, 1985.

Koehler, P. J. "Prevalence of Headache in Tulp's Observationes Medicae (1641) with a Description of Cluster Headache." *Cephalalgia* 13, no. 5 (1993): 318–320.

Koehler, P. J., and P. C. Tfelt-Hansen. "History of Methysergide in Migraine." *Cephalalgia* 28, no. 11 (2008): 1126–1135.

Koo, Brian B., Ahmed Bayoumi, Abdalla Albanna, Mohammed Abusuliman, Laura Burrone, Jason J. Sico, and Emmanuelle A. D. Schindler. "Demoralization Predicts Suicidality in Patients with Cluster Headache." *Journal of Headache and Pain* 22, no. 28 (2021): 1–10.

Kooijman, Nina I., Tim Willegers, Anke Reuser, Wim M. Mulleners, Cornelis Kramers, Kris C. P. Vissers, and Selina E. I. van der Wal. "Are Psychedelics the Answer to Chronic Pain: A Review of Current Literature." *Pain Practice* 23, no. 4 (2023): 447–458.

Langlitz, Nicolas. *Neuropsychedelia: The Revival of Hallucinogen Research Since the Decade of the Brain.* Berkeley: University of California Press, 2013.

Leary, Timothy. *Flashbacks, an Autobiography.* Los Angeles: Tarcher, 1983.

———. *High Priest.* New York: World Publishing Company, 1968.

Lekhtman, Alexander. "Why Indigenous Protesters Stopped a Global Psychedelic Conference." *Filter Magazine.* August 17, 2023. https://filtermag.org/indigenous-psychedelic-protest.

Letcher, Andy. *Shroom: A Cultural History of the Magic Mushroom.* 1st US ed. New York: Ecco, 2007.

Lindsay, Bethany. "'Corrective' Measures Ordered, but Health Canada Says 2nd MDMA Trial Can Continue." *CBC News.* July 22, 2022. https://www.cbc.ca/news/canada/british-columbia/health-canada-mdma-trial-compliant-1.6528137.

Ling, Thomas Mortimer, and John Buckman. *Lysergic Acid (LSD 25) and Ritalin in the Treatment of Neurosis.* London: Lambarde Press, 1963.

Lipton, Richard B., Dawn C. Buse, Benjamin W. Friedman, Lisa Feder, Aubrey Manack Adams, Kristina M. Fanning, Michael L. Reed, and Todd J. Schwedt. "Characterizing Opioid Use in a US Population with Migraine: Results from the CaMEO Study." *Neurology* 95, no. 5 (2020): e457–e468.

Loder, Elizabeth, and John Loder. "Medicolegal Issues in Cluster Headache." *Current Pain and Headache Reports* 8, no. 2 (2004): 147–156.

Lubecky, Jonathan M. "From the Personal to the Political: Why Psychedelic Therapy Is a Bipartisan Issue." *MAPS Bulletin* 28, no. 1 (2018): 30–31.

Lund, N. L. T., A. S. Petersen, R. Fronczek, J. Tfelt-Hansen, A. C. Belin, T. Meisingset, E. Tronvik, A. Steinberg, C. Gaul, and R. H. Jensen. "Current Treatment Options for Cluster Headache: Limitations and the Unmet Need for Better and Specific Treatments—a Consensus Article." *Journal of Headache and Pain* 24, no. 121 (2023).

MacIntosh, Jeane. "City Jet-Setter's Bizarre LSD Trip." *New York Post.* February 18, 2008. https://nypost.com/2008/02/18/city-jet-setters-bizarre-lsd-trip.

Madsen, Martin K., Anja Sofie Petersen, Dea S. Stenbæk, Inger Marie Sørensen, Harald Schiønning, Tobias Fjeld, Charlotte H. Nykjær, Sara M. U. Larsen, Maria Grzywacz, Tobais Mathiesen, Ida L. Klausen, Oliver Overgaard-Hansen, Kristoffer Brendstrup-Brix, Kristian Linnet, Sys S. Johansen, Patrick M. Fisher, Rigmor H. Jensen, and Gitte M. Knudsen. "Psilocybin-Induced Reduction in Chronic Cluster Headache Attack Frequency Correlates with Changes in Hypothalamic Functional Connectivity." *medRxiv.* July 10, 2022. https://www.medrxiv.org/content/10.1101/2022.07.10.22277414v1.

Magnuson, Mary, H. J. C. Swan, and Lucas Richert. "The Introduction of Peyote into Pharmaceutical and Pharmacological Frameworks." *History of Pharmacy and Pharmaceuticals* 65, no. 1 (October 1, 2023): 169–177.

"Maharishi School Makes Business Gurus." *Los Angeles Times.* May 15, 1997. https://www.latimes.com/archives/la-xpm-1997-05-15-fi-58842-story.html.

"MAPS, MPP and Dr. Ethan Russo Filed an Updated Version." Multidisciplinary Association for Psychedelic Studies. May 1, 2003. https://maps.org/2003/05/01/mmj-news-id1429.

Marks, Harry M. *The Progress of Experiment: Science and Therapeutic Reform in the United States, 1900–1990.* Cambridge: Cambridge University Press, 2000.

Marks, Mason, and I. Glenn Cohen. "Patents on Psychedelics: The Next Legal Battlefront of Drug Development." *Harvard Law Review* 135, no. 212 (March 24, 2023). https://harvardlawreview.org/forum/no-volume/patents-on-psychedelics-the-next-legal-battlefront-of-drug-development.

May, Arne, Anish Bahra, Christian Büchel, Richard S. J. Frackowiak, and Peter J. Goadsby. "Hypothalamic Activation in Cluster Headache Attacks." *The Lancet* 352, no. 9124 (1998): 275–278.

McDougal, Dennis. *Operation White Rabbit: LSD, the DEA, and the Fate of the Acid King.* New York: Simon & Schuster, 2020.

Metzl, Jonathan M. *The Protest Psychosis: How Schizophrenia Became a Black Disease.* Boston: Beacon Press, 2010.

———. *Prozac on the Couch: Prescribing Gender in the Era of Wonder Drugs.* Durham: Duke University Press, 2003.

Miech, Richard A., Lloyd D. Johnston, Megan E. Patrick, Patrick M. O'Malley, Jerald G. Bachman, and John E. Schulenberg. "Monitoring the Future National Survey Results on Drug Use, 1975–2022: Secondary School Students." ERIC No. ED627366. June 2023. https://files.eric.ed.gov/fulltext/ED627366.pdf.

Mitchell, Jennifer M., Michael Bogenschutz, Alia Lilienstein, Charlotte Harrison, Sarah Kleiman, Kelly Parker-Guilbert, Marcela Ot'alora, Wael Garas, et al. "MDMA-Assisted Therapy for Severe PTSD: A Randomized, Double-Blind, Placebo-Controlled Phase 3 Study." *Nature Medicine* 27, no. 6 (2021): 1025–1033.

Mitchell, S. W. "Remarks on the Effects of Anhelonium Lewinii (the Mescal Button)." *British Medical Journal* 2, no. 1875 (1896): 1625–1629.

Mojeiko, Valerie. "Interview with Dr. John Halpern." *MAPS* 11, no. 2 (2001): 10–11.

Moreno, F. A., and P. L. Delgado. "Hallucinogen-Induced Relief of Obsessions and Compulsions." *American Journal of Psychiatry* 154, no. 7 (1997): 1037–1038.

Mulligan, Jessee. "Using Psychedelics to Treat PTSD and Depression." *Radio New Zealand.* January 15, 2020. https://www.rnz.co.nz/national/programmes/afternoons/audio/2018729959/using-psychedelics-to-treat-ptsd-and-depression.

National Vital Statistics System. "Provisional Drug Overdose Death Counts." National Center for Health Statistics. Last modified February 15, 2023. https://www.cdc.gov/nchs/nvss/vsrr/drug-overdose-data.htm.

Newberry, Laura. "MDMA-Assisted Therapy Could Soon Be Approved by the FDA. Will Insurance Cover It?" *Los Angeles Times,* September 19, 2023.

Nichols, David E. "The Heffter Research Institute: Past and Hopeful Future." *Journal of Psychoactive Drugs* 46, no. 1 (2014): 20–26.

Nickles, David. "Mark McCloud Calls Out DEA Snitch & MAPS Researcher John Halpern January 13th, 2006." YouTube. July 22, 2020. https://www.youtube.com/watch?v=ZsoeQDHkjyQ.

Nilsson Remahl, A. I. M., E. Laudon Meyer, C. Cordonnier, and P. J. Goadsby. "Placebo Response in Cluster Headache Trials: A Review." *Cephalalgia* 23, no. 7 (2003): 504–510.

Novak, Steven J. "LSD Before Leary: Sidney Cohen's Critique of 1950s Psychedelic Drug Research." *Isis* 88, no. 1 (1997): 87–110.

Nutt, David J., Leslie A. King, and Lawrence D. Phillips. "Drug Harms in the UK: A Multicriteria Decision Analysis." *The Lancet* 376, no. 9752 (2010): 1558–1565.

Nuwar, Rachel. "A Psychedelic Drug Passes a Big Test for PTSD Treatment." *New York Times*, May 3, 2021. https://www.nytimes.com/2021/05/03/health/mdma-approval.html.

"Opinions, Facts & Observations—Expanded Psychedelic Section Volume Two Psychedelic and Other Alternative Treatment Manual." Clusterbusters. 2021. Accessed June 17, 2023. https://clusterbusters.org/resource/psychedelic-treatments.

Oram, Matthew. *The Trials of Psychedelic Therapy: LSD Psychotherapy in America*. Baltimore: Johns Hopkins University Press, 2018.

Oss, O. T., and O. N. Oeric. *Psilocybin, Magic Mushroom Grower's Guide: A Handbook for Psilocybin Enthusiasts*. Berkeley: And/Or Press, 1976.

Ott, Jonathan. *Pharmacotheon: Entheogenic Drugs, Their Plant Sources and History*. Kennewick, WA: Natural Products Company, 1993.

Pace, Brian, and Neşe Devenot. "Right-Wing Psychedelia: Case Studies in Cultural Plasticity and Political Pluripotency." *Frontiers of Psychology* 12 (2021): 4915.

Petersen, A. S., N. Lund, A. Snoer, R. H. Jensen, and M. Barloese. "The Economic and Personal Burden of Cluster Headache: A Controlled Cross-Sectional Study." *Journal of Headache and Pain* 23, no. 58 (2022).

Peterson, Melody. "Madison Ave. Has Growing Role in the Business of Drug Research." *New York Times*. November 22, 2002. https://www.nytimes.com/2002/11/22/business/madison-ave-has-growing-role-in-the-business-of-drug-research.html.

Pickard, Leonard. "Underground Histories and Overground Futures." Paper presented at the annual Horizons: Perspectives on Psychedelics conference, New York, 2021.

Pollan, Michael. *How to Change Your Mind: What the New Science of Psychedelics Teaches Us About Consciousness, Dying, Addiction, Depression, and Transcendence*. New York: Penguin, 2018.

———. "The Trip Treatment." *New Yorker*, February 2, 2015. https://www.newyorker.com/magazine/2015/02/09/trip-treatment.

Pollan, Michael, Imran Khan, and Taylor West. "UC Berkeley Center for the Science of Psychedelics Unveils Results of the First-Ever Berkeley Psychedelics Survey." UC Berkeley Center for the Science of Psychedelics. July 12, 2023. https://psychedelics.berkeley.edu/bcsp-first-study-results.

Pope, Harrison. *Voices from the Drug Culture*. Boston: Beacon Press, 1971.

Porter, Theodore M. *Trust in Numbers: The Pursuit of Objectivity in Science and Public Life*. Princeton, NJ: Princeton University Press, 1996.

Power, Mike. *Drugs Unlimited: The Web Revolution That's Changing How the World Gets High*. 1st US ed. New York: Thomas Dunne Books, 2013.

Prentiss, D. W., and Francis P. Morgan. *Mescal Buttons*. New York: Publishers' Printing Company, 1896.

"Psilocybin and Psilocin (Magic Mushrooms)." Government of Canada. February 2, 2023. https://www.canada.ca/en/health-canada/services/substance-use/controlled-illegal-drugs/magic-mushrooms.html.

Raudenbush, Danielle T. *Health Care Off the Books: Poverty, Illness, and Strategies for Survival in Urban America.* Berkeley: University of California Press, 2020.

"Reviews and Impressions from the 2006 LSD Symposium." Erowid. Accessed September 24, 2023. https://www.erowid.org/general/conferences/2006_lsd_symposium.

Richards, William, Stanislav Grof, Louis Goodman, and Albert Kurland. "LSD-Assisted Psychotherapy and the Human Encounter with Death." *Journal of Transpersonal Psychology* 4, no. 2 (1972): 121–150.

Rikard, S. Michaela, Andrea E. Strahan, Kristine M. Schmit, and Gery P. Guy Jr. "Chronic Pain Among Adults—United States, 2019–2021." *Morbidity and Mortality Weekly Report* 72, no. 15 (2023): 379–385.

Robbins, Matthew S., Amaal J. Starling, Tamara Pringsheim, Werner J. Becker, and Todd J. Schwedt. "Treatment of Cluster Headache: The American Headache Society Evidence Based Guidelines." *Headache: The Journal of Head and Face Pain* 56, no. 7 (July 1, 2016): 1093–1106.

Romero, Simon. "Demand for This Toad's Psychedelic Toxin Is Booming. Some Warn That's Bad for the Toad." *New York Times.* March 30, 2022. https://www.nytimes.com/2022/03/20/us/toad-venom-psychedelic.html.

Rosenfeld, Seth. "LSD Trafficking Suspect Has Intriguing Backers: D.A. Terence Hallinan and British Aristocrats." *San Francisco Gate.* December 19, 2000.

———. "William Pickard's Long, Strange Trip." *San Francisco Gate.* June 10, 2001. https://www.sfgate.com/crime/article/William-Pickard-s-long-strange-trip-Suspected-2910096.php.

Rosenthal, Phil. "Daniel Carcillo, the Former Chicago Blackhawks Enforcer, Tells HBO's 'Real Sports' That Psychedelic Drugs Helped Him Battle Post-Concussion Effects." *Chicago Tribune.* November 24, 2020.

Ross, Lily Kay, and Dave Nickels. "Who Am I Fooling?" *Cover Story: Power Trip* (podcast). March 15, 2022. https://www.thecut.com/2022/03/cover-story-podcast-who-am-i-fooling-episode-8.html.

Ross, Lily Kay, and David Nickles. "The Trials of Rick Doblin." *New York Magazine.* May 11, 2022.

Ross, Stephen, Anthony Bossis, Jeffrey Guss, Gabrielle Agin-Liebes, Tara Malone, Barry Cohen, Sarah E. Mennenga, Alexander Belser, Krystallia Kalliontzi, and James Babb. "Rapid and Sustained Symptom Reduction Following Psilocybin Treatment for Anxiety and Depression in Patients with Life-Threatening Cancer: A Randomized Controlled Trial." *Journal of Psychopharmacology* 30, no. 12 (2016): 1165–1180.

Rossi, Paolo, P. Little, E. R. de la Torre, and A. Palmaro. "If You Want to Understand What It Really Means to Live with Cluster Headache, Imagine . . . Fostering Empathy Through European Patients' Own Stories of Their Experiences." *Functional Neurology* 33, no. 1 (2018): 57–59.

Rothrock, John. "Cluster: A Potentially Lethal Headache Disorder." *Headache* 46, no. 2 (2006): 327.

Rozen, Todd D. "Cluster Headache Clinical Phenotypes: Tobacco Nonexposed (Never Smoker and No Parental Secondary Smoke Exposure as a Child) Versus Tobacco-Exposed: Results from the United States Cluster Headache Survey." *Headache* 58, no. 5 (2018): 688–699.

Rozen, Todd D., and Royce S. Fishman. "Cluster Headache in the United States of America: Demographics, Clinical Characteristics, Triggers, Suicidality and Personal Burden." *Headache* 52, no. 1 (2012): 99–113.

Rusanen, Sakari Santeri, Suchetana De, Emmanuelle Andree Danielle Schindler, Ville Aleksi Artto, and Markus Storvik. "Self-Reported Efficacy of Treatments in Cluster Headache: A Systematic Review of Survey Studies." *Current Pain and Headache Reports* 26, no. 8 (2022): 623–637.

Russell, Michael Bjørn. "Epidemiology of Cluster Headache." In *Cluster Headache and Other Trigeminal Autonomic Cephalgias*, edited by Massimo Leone and Arne May, 7–10. Cham, Switzerland: Springer, 2020.

Russo, Ethan B. "Headache Treatments by Native Peoples of the Ecuadorian Amazon: A Preliminary Cross-Disciplinary Assessment." *Journal of Ethnopharmacology* 36, no. 3 (June 1, 1992): 193–206. https://doi.org/10.1016/0378-8741(92)90044-r.

———. "Machiguenga: Peruvian Hunter-Gatherers." Weston A. Price Foundation. September 7, 2002. https://www.westonaprice.org/health-topics/in-his-footsteps /machiguenga-peruvian-hunter-gatherers/#gsc.tab=0.

Russo, Ethan B., Mary Lynn Mathre, Al Byrne, Robert A. Velin, Paul J. Bach, Juan Sanchez Ramos, and Kristin A. Kirlin. "Chronic Cannabis Use in the Compassionate Investigational New Drug Program." *Journal of Cannabis Therapeutics* 2, no. 1 (2002): 3–57. https://doi.org/10.1300/j175v02n01_02.

Sabina, María. *María Sabina: Selections*. Edited by Jerome Rothenberg. Berkeley: University of California Press, 2003.

Schindler, Emmanuelle A. D. "Psychedelics as Preventive Treatment in Headache and Chronic Pain Disorders." *Neuropharmacology* 215 (2022): 109166. https://doi .org/10.1016/j.neuropharm.2022.109166.

Schindler, Emmanuelle A. D., and Mark J. Burish. "Recent Advances in the Diagnosis and Management of Cluster Headache." *British Medical Journal* 376 (2022): e059577.

Schindler, Emmanuelle A. D., Vanessa Cooper, Douglas B. Quine, Brenda T. Fenton, Douglas A. Wright, Marsha J. Weil, and Jason J. Sico. "'You Will Eat Shoe Polish If You Think It Would Help'—Familiar and Lesser-Known Themes Identified from Mixed-Methods Analysis of a Cluster Headache Survey." *Headache: The Journal of Head and Face Pain* 61, no. 2 (2021): 318–328.

Schindler, Emmanuelle A. D., Christopher H. Gottschalk, Marsha J. Weil, Robert E. Shapiro, Douglas A. Wright, and Richard Andrew Sewell. "Indoleamine Hallucinogens in Cluster Headache: Results of the Clusterbusters Medication Use Survey." *Journal of Psychoactive Drugs* 47, no. 5 (2015): 372–381.

Schindler, Emmanuelle A. D., R. Andrew Sewell, Christopher H. Gottschalk, Christina Luddy, L. Taylor Flynn, Hayley Lindsey, Brian P. Pittman, Nicholas V. Cozzi, and Deepak C. D'Souza. "Exploratory Controlled Study of the Migraine-Suppressing Effects of Psilocybin." *Neurotherapeutics* 18, no. 1 (2020): 534–543.

Schindler, Emmanuelle A. D., R. Andrew Sewell, Christopher H. Gottschalk, Christina Luddy, L. Taylor Flynn, Yutong Zhu, Hayley Lindsey, P. Pittman, Hayley Cozzi, and Deepak D'Souza. "Exploratory Investigation of a Patient Informed Low Dose Psilocybin Pulse Regimen in the Suppression of Cluster Headache: Results from a Randomized, Double-Blind, Placebo-Controlled Trial." *Headache* 62, no. 10 (2022): 1383–1394.

Schultes, Richard Evans. "The Appeal of Peyote (Lophophora Williamsii) as a Medicine." *American Anthropologist* 40, no. 4 (1938): 698–715.

———. "Ethnopharmacological Conservation: A Key to Progress in Medicine." *Acta Amazonica* 18, no. 1–2 (suppl.) (1988): 393–406.

Schultes, Richard Evans, and Robert F. Raffauf. *The Healing Forest: Medicinal and Toxic Plants of the Northwest Amazonia*. Portland, OR: Dioscorides Press, 1990.

Schumaker, Erin, and Katherine Ellen Foley. "We're on the Cusp of Another Psychedelic Era. But This Time Washington Is Along for the Ride." *Politico*. August 12, 2023. https://www.politico.com/news/2023/08/12/medical-psychedelic-drugs-congress-00110851.

Semley, John. "Psychedelic Drugs Have Lost Their Cool. Blame Gwyneth Paltrow and Her Goop." *The Guardian*. February 17, 2020. https://www.theguardian.com/commentisfree/2020/feb/17/psychedelic-drugs-have-lost-their-cool-blame-gwyneth-paltrow-and-her-goop.

Sequiera, Luis. "Richard Evans Schultes, 1915–2001." In *Biographical Memoirs*, 1–15. National Academies Press, 2006. https://doi.org/10.17226/11807.

Sewell, R. Andrew. "Compositions and Methods for Preventing and/or Treating Disorders Associated with Cephalic Pain." Patent 8859579, filed October 14, 2014, and issued March 20, 2009.

———. "LSD and Psilocybin in the Treatment of Cluster Headaches: A Report on Proposed Research at Harvard Medical School." *MAPS Bulletin* 15, no. 1 (spring 2005): 20–25.

———. "Response of Cluster Headache to Kudzu." *Headache: The Journal of Head and Face Pain* 49, no. 1 (2009): 98–105.

———. "So You Want to Be a Psychedelic Researcher?" *Entheogen Review* 15, no. 2 (2006): 42–48.

———. "So You Want to Be a Psychedelic Researcher?" *MAPS Bulletin* 16, no. 2 (autumn 2006): 20–25.

———. "Unauthorized Research on Cluster Headache." *Entheogen Review* 16, no. 4 (2008): 117–125.

Sewell, R. Andrew, John H. Halpern, and Harrison G. Pope Jr. "Response of Cluster Headache to Psilocybin and LSD." *Neurology* 66, no. 12 (2006): 1920–1922.

Shakhnazarova, Nika. "Aaron Rodgers Says Psychedelic Drugs Led to 'Best Season of My Career.'" *New York Post*. August 4, 2022. https://nypost.com/2022/08/04/aaron-rodgers-says-psychedelic-drugs-led-to-best-season-of-my-career.

Sheldrake, Melvin. *Entangled Life: How Fungi Make Our Worlds, Change Our Minds and Shape Our Futures*. New York: Penguin Random House, 2021.

Short, April M. "Meet Rick Doblin, Psychedelic Pioneer Who Has Expanded the Boundaries of Medicine." *Alternet*. March 25, 2016. https://www.alternet.org/2016/03/meet-rick-doblin-psychedelic-who-has-expanded-boundaries-medicine.

Shroder, Tom. *Acid Test: How a Daring Group of Psychonauts Rediscovered the Power of LSD, MDMA, and Other Psychedelic Drugs to Heal Addiction, Depression, Anxiety, and Trauma.* New York: Plume, 2014.

Sicuteri, Federigo. "The Enrico Greppi International Headache Award: A Tribute to the Memory of One of Medicine's Pioneers." *Cephalalgia* 3, no. 1 (1983): 11–13.

———. "L'emicrania: Motivi di Fisiopatogenisi e di Terapia." Paper presented at the Relazione al 65th Congresso della Societá Italiana di Medicina Interna Rome, Italy, 1964.

———. "Prophylactic Treatment of Migraine by Means of Lysergic Acid Derivatives." *PubMed* 6 (October 1, 1963): 116–125.

Siff, Stephen. *Acid Hype: American News Media and the Psychedelic Experience.* Champaign: University of Illinois Press, 2015.

Silberstein, Stephen D., and Douglas C. McCrory. "Ergotamine and Dihydroergotamine: History, Pharmacology, and Efficacy." *Headache* 43, no. 2 (2003): 144–166.

Silberstein, Stephen D., Stephen B. Shrewsbury, and John Hoekman. "Dihydroergotamine (DHE)—Then and Now: A Narrative Review." *Headache* 60, no. 1 (2020): 40–57.

Smirnova, Michelle X. *The Prescription-to-Prison Pipeline: The Medicalization and Criminalization of Pain.* Durham, NC: Duke University Press, 2023.

Smith, Will. *Will.* New York: Penguin, 2021.

Sobo, Elisa J. "Parent Use of Cannabis for Intractable Pediatric Epilepsy: Everyday Empiricism and the Boundaries of Scientific Medicine." *Social Science & Medicine* 190 (October 2017): 190–198.

Stamets, Paul. *Mycelium Running: How Mushrooms Can Help Save the World.* Berkeley, CA: Ten Speed Press, 2005.

Stark, Laura, and Nancy D. Campbell. "The Ineffable: A Framework for the Study of Methods Through the Case of Mid-Century Mind-Brain Sciences." *Social Studies of Science* 48, no. 6 (2018): 789–820.

Starr, Paul. *The Social Transformation of American Medicine: The Rise of a Sovereign Profession and the Making of a Vast Industry.* New York: Basic Books, 2003.

Stevens, Jay. *Storming Heaven: LSD and the American Dream.* 1st ed. New York: Atlantic Monthly Press, 1987.

Strassman, Rick J. *DMT: The Spirit Molecule: A Doctor's Revolutionary Research into the Biology of Near-Death and Mystical Experiences.* New York: Park Street Press, 2000.

Substance Abuse and Mental Health Services Administration. Key substance use and mental health indicators in the United States: Results from the 2022 National Survey on Drug Use and Health (HHS Publication No. PEP23-07-01-006, NSDUH Series H-58). Center for Behavioral Health Statistics and Quality, Substance Abuse and Mental Health Services Administration, 2023.

Substance Abuse and Mental Health Services Administration. *Racial/Ethnic Differences in Substance Use, Substance Use Disorders, and Substance Use Treatment Utilization Among People Aged 12 or Older (2015–2019).* Rockville, MD: Center for Behavioral Health Statistics and Quality, 2021.

Taylor, Verta. "Social Movement Continuity: The Women's Movement in Abeyance." *American Sociological Review* 54, no. 5 (1989): 761–775.

Tfelt-Hansen, P. C., and P. J. Koehler. "History of the Use of Ergotamine and Dihy-droergotamine in Migraine from 1906 and Onward." *Cephalalgia* 28, no. 8 (2008): 877–886.

Timmermans, Stefan, and Steven Epstein. "A World of Standards but Not a Standard World: Toward a Sociology of Standards and Standardization." *Annual Review of Sociology* 36 (2010): 69–89.

Tobbell, Dominique. *Pills, Power, and Policy: The Struggle for Drug Reform in Cold War America and Its Consequences.* Berkeley: University of California Press, 2011.

US Congress. "Administered Prices in the Drug Industry." *Congressional Record*, 106th Cong., 2nd sess., vol. 106, pt. 5–6 (1960): 6228.

U.S. Department of Veterans Affairs, Office of Mental Health and Suicide Prevention. 2022 National Veteran Suicide Prevention Annual Report. 2022. Retrieved June 3, 2023, from https://www.mentalhealth.va.gov/suicide_prevention/data.asp.

Van der Gronde, Toon, and Toine Pieters. "Assessing Pharmaceutical Research and Development Costs." *JAMA Internal Medicine* 178, no. 4 (2018): 587–588.

Voiticovschi-Iosob, Cristina, Marta Allena, Ilaria De Cillis, Giuseppe Nappi, Ottar Sjaastad, and Fabio Antonaci. "Diagnostic and Therapeutic Errors in Cluster Head-ache: A Hospital-Based Study." *Journal of Headache and Pain* 15, no. 56 (2014).

Wasson, R. Gordon, and Valentina Pavlovna Wasson. *Mushrooms, Russia and History.* New York: Pantheon Press, 1957.

Wasson, Richard Gordon. "Seeking the Magic Mushroom." *Life Magazine.* May 13, 1957.

Wasson, Valentina P. "I Ate the Sacred Mushroom." *This Week.* May 19, 1957.

Wilkinson, Peter. "The Acid King." *Rolling Stone* 872 (July 2001): 113–123.

Williams, M. T., A. K. Davis, Y. Xin, N. D. Sepeda, P. C. Grigas, S. Sinnott, and A. M. Haeny. "People of Color in North America Report Improvements in Racial Trauma and Mental Health Symptoms Following Psychedelic Experiences." *Drugs* 28, no. 3 (2021): 215–226.

Williams, Monnica T., Amy Bartlett, Tim Michaels, Jae Sevelius, and Jamilah R. George. "Dr. Valentina Wasson: Questioning What We Think We Know About the Founda-tions of Psychedelic Science." *Journal of Psychedelic Studies* 4, no. 3 (2021): 146–148.

Williams, Monnica T., Sara Reed, and Ritika Aggarwal. "Culturally-Informed Research Design Issues in a Study for MDMA-Assisted Psychotherapy for Posttraumatic Stress Disorder." *Journal of Psychedelic Studies* 4, no. 1 (2020): 40–50.

Winsvold, Bendik S., Aster V. E. Harder, Caroline Ran, Mona A. Chalmer, Maria Car-olina Dalmasso, Egil Ferkingstad, Kumar Parijat Tripathi, Elena Bacchelli, Sigrid Børte, and Carmen Fourier. "Cluster Headache Genome Wide Association Study and Meta Analysis Identifies Eight Loci and Implicates Smoking as Causal Risk Factor." *Annals of Neurology* 94, no. 4 (October 2023): 713–726.

WIRED Staff. "LSD: The Geek's Wonder Drug?" *Wired.* January 16, 2006. https://www.wired.com/2006/01/lsd-the-geeks-wonder-drug.

Witt, Emily. "Diary: Burning Man." *London Review of Books* 36, no. 14 (2014): https://www.lrb.co.uk/the-paper/v36/n14/emily-witt/diary.

———. "A Field Guide to Psychedelics." *New Yorker.* November 15, 2015. https://www.newyorker.com/magazine/2015/11/23/the-trip-planners.

Wold, Robert. Memoir draft. Lombard, Illinois.

Wolff, Harold G. *Headache and Other Head Pain*. 2nd ed. New York: Oxford University Press, 1963.

Yakowicz, Will. "Why Toms Shoes Founder Blake Mycoskie Is Committing $100 Million to Psychedelic Research." *Forbes Magazine*. June 24, 2023. https://www.forbes.com/sites/willyakowicz/2023/06/24/why-toms-shoes-founder-blake-mycoskie-is-committing-100-million-to-psychedelic-research.

# SOURCES

## Author's Note

1. Many of the insights in this book come from over twenty years of research projects spanning the politics of headache medicine and the suppression of science. Data collection for this project began at a Clusterbusters conference in September 2013 and continued for the next ten years. I've attended nine Clusterbusters conferences (two of which were held online), five conferences about psychedelic substances (including MAPS Psychedelic Science, Horizons Perspectives on Psychedelics in New York, and Wonderland hosted by Microdose), and at least fifteen headache advocacy events, each of which offered an opportunity to have wide-ranging conversations with physicians, researchers, advocates, patients, caretakers, psychedelic enthusiasts, investors, and policymakers about the potential use of psychedelics for headache disorders and/or pain. But that just represents my systematic fieldwork. I've also been following how this conversation unfolds in the media and online as well.

Historical research tracking how the patient-led movement grew into Clusterbusters primarily relies on the digital traces left along the way. Three online archives served as my primary form of evidence in telling this story: (1) Clusterheadaches.com (CH.com), a public electronic support group forum, which provided the history between 1998 and 2002; (2) Clusterbusters, a private Yahoo! group founded by Robert "Bob" Wold, which provided a history from August 2002 onward (this analysis ends at the end of 2005); and (3) email correspondence between Wold and Richard Doblin, John H. Halpern, R. Andrew Sewell, and Marsha Weil between November 2003 and November 2011.

I'm grateful to Daren "DJ" Johnson, the owner of CH.com, and to Bob Wold, the founder of Clusterbusters, for providing me with permission and access to the forums they founded. Neither the Clusterbusters Yahoo! group nor the email correspondence is publicly accessible. Bob Wold and I both maintain digital copies of these archives for those who have questions about source material.

The amount of information held in these forums is overwhelming. The small slice of posts I examined in CH.com (between 1998 and 2002) includes hundreds of thousands of posts. Between August 2002 and 2005, the Clusterbusters Yahoo! forum produced 12,618 messages. I analyzed these archives using two approaches: (1) as a searchable historical archive documenting the group's activities and thought processes, and (2) as a dynamic reflection of the community's collective decision-making, where patterns of interaction, decision-making, and problem-solving emerged organically from the forum discussions. Details about this analysis can be found in peer-reviewed articles that I've written with my collaborator, John Bailey: "Collective Self-Experimentation" and "Standards Without Labs." Like any researcher, I had to consider what I could— and more importantly, what I couldn't—learn from these archives. I might have had *a lot* of messages, but plenty is missing: knowledge about people's offline lives; transcripts of their phone calls with each other; documentation of their in-person interactions, and private emails. How could I be sure that I understood what people meant, since I couldn't follow up? Almost everyone has had the experience of having an email or text misinterpreted. Then there was the issue of verification: as they say, "Nobody knows you're a dog on the internet."

The relative strength and weaknesses of these archives depend on the research question that I'm asking. Am I, for example, drawing on these data to ask about the experience of having cluster headache or to ask how an online group conducts self-experimentation? Or am I drawing on these archives as historical documents to say that an event happened? Online data are better at answering certain kinds of questions.

These archives provide very strong of evidence to describe *experience* because they haven't been tainted by my presence, and they don't rely on anyone's memory. There are, however, important limitations to consider. Learning about the experience of cluster headache from quite old internet forums created a strong "selection bias." I also couldn't assess the demographics of those who took part in these forums, but the content of the conversations, combined with my fieldwork, led me to believe that most contributors were white adults from the United States, Canada, and the United Kingdom, who had more severe forms of the disease than the rest of the population. Fieldwork, interviews, and informal conversations with dozens of people in the headache community helped me fill in these gaps.

Using these archives as a form of *historical evidence* has a different set of strengths and weaknesses. Sometimes an email is the smoking gun that proves an event occurred, especially if the event in question is "He sent an email. . . ."

Other sorts of claims required more documentary evidence: interviews (both on the record and confidential), fact-checks, court records, and other forms of public records. People's interviews about their past actions did not always align with public documents or their correspondence. Nor did people agree with one another about what happened. Memory can play funny tricks on all of us. I tried to triangulate with additional data when possible. I relied on the historical record to settle discrepancies.

As I stitched together this story, I began to realize that it sometimes didn't matter whether an event *happened* or people *believed* it happened. For example, in 1999, someone told the CH.com forum that a scientist had told them that a clinical trial testing psilocybin as a treatment for cluster headache would cost about $30,000. Over the next few years, I saw this claim repeated in various forms, and although the scientist's name was never mentioned, I deduced that the original poster must have spoken to Dr. Francisco Moreno, a professor of psychiatry at the University of Arizona.

At the time, Dr. Moreno had obtained funding from the Multidisciplinary Association of Psychedelic Studies and the Heffter Research Institute to conduct a small pilot study testing psilocybin as a treatment for obsessive-compulsive disorder. In a recent email, Dr. Moreno told me that he doesn't recall speaking to anyone from this group; nor would he—as a psychiatrist—"anticipate leading" a study on cluster headache, as it had been rumored he might on the forum. He also emphasized that the clinical trial he conducted in 2000 had cost $54,030, so the estimate provided in the forum struck him as too low.

I presume no malice intended by the person who shared the original information. We often lose information in translation. (And apologies if I inferred the wrong scientist.) However, as a *historical artifact*, it's vital to understand that Clusterbusters *believed* a scientist *could* and *would* conduct a clinical trial for $30,000. I do my best to distinguish between what *happened* and what people *believed* happened.

Does all this evidence support my sociological arguments? Readers will have to decide this for themselves.

All data collected for this book was approved by Rutgers University's Institutional Review Board.

One last, important admission: There's no use pretending that I have some sort of objective position toward the people in this patient community. I totally get what Carey Turnbull meant when he said, "I made the fatal mistake of becoming emotionally involved."

Me too.

## Introduction

1. "About Clusterbusters."
2. Ellison, "A New Treatment May Halt Cluster Headaches."
3. Carhart-Harris, "Entropic Brain-Revisited"; Johnson et al., "Classic Psychedelics."
4. Chrysanthos and Dow, "Australia Becomes First Country to Recognise Psychedelics as Medicines"; Schumaker and Foley, "We're on the Cusp of Another Psychedelic Era"; "Psilocybin and Psilocin."
5. Yakowicz, "Why Toms Shoes Founder Blake Mycoskie Is Committing $100 Million to Psychedelic Research."
6. Carey, "Tim Ferriss."
7. Shakhnazarova, "Aaron Rodgers Says Psychedelic Drugs Led to 'Best Season of My Career.'"
8. Romero, "Demand for This Toad's Psychedelic Toxin Is Booming."
9. Prince Harry, *Spare*; Semley, "Psychedelic Drugs Have Lost Their Cool"; Smith, *Will.*
10. Marks and Cohen, "Patents on Psychedelics."
11. Pollan, Khan, and West, "UC Berkeley Center for the Science of Psychedelics Unveils Results of the First-Ever Berkeley Psychedelics Survey."
12. Over a third of people with migraine (36.3 percent) reported that they currently used or kept on hand opioid medications to treat headaches, even though opioids often make head pain worse. Lipton et al., "Characterizing Opioid Use in a US Population with Migraine."
13. This survey doesn't include nursing home patients or active military members, which suggests this figure is an underestimate. See Rikard et al., "Chronic Pain Among Adults."

14. Burch, Rizzoli, and Loder, "Prevalence and Impact of Migraine and Severe Headache in the United States."

15. Bonnelle et al., "Analgesic Potential of Macrodoses and Microdoses"; Castellanos et al., "Chronic Pain and Psychedelics"; Kooijman et al., "Are Psychedelics the Answer to Chronic Pain."

16. Christie et al., "MDMA-Assisted Therapy Is Associated with a Reduction in Chronic Pain Among People with Post-Traumatic Stress Disorder."

17. Williams, Reed, and Aggarwal, "Culturally-Informed Research Design Issues in a Study for MDMA-Assisted Psychotherapy for Posttraumatic Stress Disorder"; Gerber et al., "Ethical Concerns About Psilocybin Intellectual Property"; Hart, *Drug Use for Grown-ups*.

## Chapter One

1. In a 2021 report prepared by SAMHSA, Black people reported a past-year illicit-drug-use rate of 20.8 percent versus a past-year use rate of 19.6 percent for white people. Substance Abuse and Mental Health Services Administration, *Racial/Ethnic Differences in Substance Use, Substance Use Disorders, and Substance Use Treatment Utilization Among People Aged 12 or Older* (2015–2019). For research on race, drug use, and drug selling, see Floyd et al., "Adolescent Drug Dealing and Race/Ethnicity."

2. Substance Abuse and Mental Health Services Administration, 2023.

3. Edwards et al., *A Tale of Two Countries*.

4. Racism has also shaped US federal response to the opioid epidemic; see Hansen, Netherland, and Herzberg, *Whiteout*.

5. Ibid.

6. Miech et al., "Monitoring the Future National Survey Results on Drug Use, 1975–2022."

7. National Vital Statistics System, "Provisional Drug Overdose Death Counts."

8. Kinzer, *Poisoner in Chief*.

9. Hagan, *Who Are the Criminals?*

10. Harris, *Swimming in the Sacred*; Williams et al., "People of Color in North America Report Improvements in Racial Trauma and Mental Health Symptoms Following Psychedelic Experiences."

## Chapter Two

1. Burch, Rizzoli, and Loder, "Prevalence and Impact of Migraine and Severe Headache in the United States"; Russell, "Epidemiology of Cluster Headache"; Rozen and Fishman, "Cluster Headache in the United States."

2. Burch, Rizzoli, and Loder, "Prevalence and Impact of Migraine and Severe Headache in the United States."

3. Schindler and Burish, "Recent Advances in the Diagnosis and Management of Cluster Headache."

4. Ibid.

5. Benkli et al., "Circadian Features of Cluster Headache and Migraine."

6. Goadsby, "Pathophysiology of Cluster Headache"; May et al., "Hypothalamic Activation in Cluster Headache"; Madsen et al., "Psilocybin-Induced Reduction on Chronic Cluster Headache Attack Frequency Correlates."

7. Burish et al., "Cluster Headache Is One of the Most Intensely Painful Human Conditions."

8. Ibid.

9. "The Kip Scale."

10. See, for example, Andre and Cavers, "A Cry in the Dark"; Rossi et al., "If You Want to Understand What It Really Means to Live with Cluster Headache"; Schindler et al., "Mixed-Methods Analysis of a Cluster Headache Survey."

11. For the case report, see Rothrock, "Cluster." Similarly awful case studies have been reported in Blau, "Behaviour During a Cluster Headache"; Loder and Loder, "Medicolegal Issues in Cluster Headache."

12. Rozen and Fishman, "Cluster Headache in the United States of America"; Koo et al., "Demoralization Predicts Suicidality in Patients with Cluster Headache."

13. Historians note that several physicians had described cluster headache prior to this date, but none of these authors appears to have recognized the phenomenon they described as a novel diagnosis. Horton, MacLean, and Craig, "A New Syndrome of Vascular Headache"; Koehler, "Prevalence of Headache in Tulp's Observationes Medicae (1641) with a Description of Cluster Headache"; Isler, "Episodic Cluster Headache from a Textbook of 1745"; Harris, "Ciliary (Migrainous) Neuralgia and Its Treatment."

14. My search for "cluster headache" in PubMed between 1939 and 1969 produced seventy-one articles.

15. Haane, Dirkx, and Koehler, "History of Oxygen Inhalation as a Treatment for Cluster Headache."

16. Graham, "Cluster Headache."

17. Ibid.

18. Allena et al., "Gender Differences in the Clinical Presentation of Cluster Headache?"

19. Foucault, *The Birth of the Clinic*.

20. Graham and Wolff, "Mechanism of Migraine Headache and Action of Ergotamine Tartrate."

21. Kempner, *Not Tonight*, 58.

22. Buture et al., "Systematic Literature Review on the Delays in the Diagnosis and Misdiagnosis of Cluster Headache"; Voiticovschi-Iosob et al., "Diagnostic and Therapeutic Errors in Cluster Headache"; Begasse de Dhaem et al., "Workforce Gap Analysis in the Field of Headache Medicine in the United States."

23. Ford et al., "Societal Burden of Cluster Headache in the United States of America"; Petersen et al., "The Economic and Personal Burden of Cluster Headache."

24. Lund et al., "Current Treatment Options for Cluster Headache."

25. Robbins et al., "Treatment of Cluster Headache"; Schindler and Burish, "Recent Advances in the Diagnosis and Management of Cluster Headache."

## Chapter Three

1. Stamets, *Mycelium Running.*

2. Sheldrake, *Entangled Life.*

3. Other well-known examples of classic psychedelics include mescaline (the active compound in peyote), N, N-dimethyltryptamine (DMT) (a key ingredient in aya-huasca), and 5-MeO-DMT (which is secreted by at least one toad species).

4. "Opinions, Facts & Observations—Expanded Psychedelic Section."

5. Nutt, King, and Phillips, "Drug Harms in the UK."

6. The social mycelium is, of course, a variation of Deleuze and Guattari's rhizome, albeit one that more explicitly acknowledges the invisibility and marginalization of uncredentialed and unauthorized scientists. See Deleuze and Guattari, *A Thousand Plateaus.*

7. Emily Witt's profile in the *New Yorker* of Erowid's founders, "A Field Guide to Psy-chedelics," offers detailed insight into how the internet offers (and continues to offer) an important unregulated space to produce illicit knowledge.

8. Halpern and Pope, "Hallucinogens on the Internet," reported finding eighty-one websites by searching Yahoo! in 2001.

9. Giffort, *Acid Revival*; Taylor, "Social Movement Continuity."

10. Huxley, *Island.*

11. Giffort, *Acid Revival.*

12. For more on Leo Zeff, the psychotherapist who developed MDMA-assisted ther-apy, see Stolaroff, *The Secret Chief Revealed.* For a broad historical overview of the use of MDMA prior to its criminalization, see Passie, "The Early Use of MDMA ('Ecstasy') in Psychotherapy (1977–1985)"; Passie and Benzenhöfer, "The History of MDMA as an Underground Drug in the United States, 1960–1979." Doblin assured me that I would find the account of his efforts to reschedule MDMA accurately portrayed in Shroder, *Acid Test.*

13. In 2010, the United Kingdom's Independent Scientific Committee on Drugs ranked MDMA as the fourth least harmful of twenty commonly used recreational drugs. The only drugs that scored less harmful were LSD, Buprenorphine (suboxone), and *Psilocybe* mushrooms. Alcohol is by far the most dangerous drug, followed by her-oin and crack cocaine. Nutt, King, and Phillips, "Drug Harms in the UK."

14. Shroder, *Acid Test.*

15. Greer, "Using MDMA in Psychotherapy."

16. Shroder, *Acid Test.*

17. Multidisciplinary Association of Psychedelic Studies (MAPS), https://www maps.org (accessed September 15, 2023).

18. Nichols's experience at Esalen led to multiple collaborations that would become foundational to the burgeoning psychedelic movement. For example, Nichols produced two kilograms of MDMA that met FDA requirements for purity for the low cost of $4,000 so that Rick Doblin would have the material to conduct all the preclinical tox-icology studies required by federal regulators. Since the toxicology tests only required 250 mg of material, Nichols was able to donate the remainder to researchers testing MDMA in clinical trials. See Nichols, "Heffter Research Institute."

19. Details about the founding of Heffter are captured in Nichols, "Heffter Research Institute."

20. Pollan, *How to Change Your Mind*.

21. Ibid.

22. The podcast *Cover Story: Power Trip* is an important exception. Ross and Nickels, "Who Am I Fooling?"

23. Danforth et al., "Reduction in Social Anxiety After MDMA-Assisted Psychotherapy with Autistic Adults"; Hevisi, "Howard Lotsof Dies at 66"; Rosenthal, "Daniel Carcillo, the Former Chicago Blackhawks Enforcer, Tells HBO's 'Real Sports' That Psychedelic Drugs Helped Him Battle Post-Concussion Effects."

24. Epstein, *Impure Science*; Gill-Peterson, "Doctors Who?"; Sobo, "Parent Use of Cannabis for Intractable Pediatric Epilepsy."

25. Raudenbush, *Health Care off the Books*; Smirnova, *Prescription-to-Prison Pipeline*.

## Chapter Four

1. Bowler, "When Your Child Is Diagnosed."

2. Witt, "Diary."

3. Research consistently demonstrates that people with cluster headache smoke cigarettes more often than controls; however, the causal relationship between smoking and cluster headache is not well understood. It seems likely that the relationship is epigenetic. In other words, a history of smoking—or even simply just being exposed to enough secondhand smoke—might "turn on" a genetic predisposition for cluster headache. Unfortunately, quitting cigarette smoking doesn't seem to stop the pain, and smoking can be a salve for those in the middle of a bout. Rozen, "Cluster Headache Clinical Phenotypes"; Winsvold et al., "Cluster Headache Genome-Wide Association Study and Meta-Analysis Identifies Eight Loci and Implicates Smoking as Causal Risk Factor."

4. Witt, "Diary."

5. Hattle, *Cluster Headaches*.

6. Green et al., "The Unequal Burden of Pain"; Hoffman et al., "Racial Bias in Pain Assessment and Treatment Recommendations, and False Beliefs About Biological Differences Between Blacks and Whites"; Janevic et al., "Racial and Socioeconomic Disparities in Disabling Chronic Pain."

7. Frood, "Cluster Busters."

## Chapter Five

1. Adams self-identifies as an "anarcho-syndicalist."

2. For a description of Craig Adams's case, see Sewell, "Unauthorized Research on Cluster Headache."

3. Hofmann, *LSD*.

4. Stamets, *Mycelium Running*.

5. Carrell, "Trump Golf Course Staff Photographed Urinating Woman 'to Detect' Crime."

## Chapter Six

1. I used two primary sources for biographical details about Hofmann: his memoir and a biography. Hagenbach and Werthmüller, *Mystic Chemist*; Hofmann, *LSD*.
2. Breen, *The Age of Intoxication*.
3. Courtwright, *Dark Paradise*; Courtwright, *Forces of Habit*.
4. Bender, "Rough and Ready Research—1887 Style"; Magnuson, Swan, and Richert, "The Introduction of Peyote into Pharmaceutical and Pharmacological Frameworks."
5. Prentiss and Morgan, *Mescal Buttons*.
6. Ellis, "Mescal"; Mitchell, "Remarks on the Effects of Anhelonium Lewinii (the Mescal Button)"; Prentiss and Morgan, *Mescal Buttons*.
7. Eadie, "Ergot of Rye."
8. Graham and Wolff, "Mechanism of Migraine Headache and Action of Ergotamine Tartrate."
9. Silberstein and McCrory, "Ergotamine and Dihydroergotamine"; Silberstein, Shrewsbury, and Hoekman, "Dihydroergotamine (DHE)"; Tfelt-Hansen and Koehler, "History of the Use of Ergotamine and Dihydroergotamine."
10. Hofmann, *LSD*.
11. Ibid., 11.
12. Ibid., 36.
13. Ibid., 26–27.
14. Heinrichs, *In Search of Madness*; Metzl, *The Protest Psychosis*.
15. Hartogsohn offers a fascinating overview of this shift in psychedelic research in his book *American Trip*. Research reported that LSD helps patients become more responsive, expressive, and self-aware as early as 1950. Huxley's writing in 1954 was very influential in moving researchers away from the psychomimetic model.
16. Dyck, *Psychedelic Psychiatry*.
17. Huxley, *Doors of Perception*.
18. Dyck, *Psychedelic Psychiatry*.
19. Stevens, *Storming Heaven*.
20. Ling and Buckman, *Lysergic Acid (LSD 25) and Ritalin in the Treatment of Neurosis*.
21. Sicuteri, "L'emicrania."
22. Sicuteri, "Enrico Greppi International Headache Award."
23. Fanciullacci, Granchi, and Sicuteri, "Ergotamine and Methysergide as Serotonin Partial Agonists in Migraine"; Koehler and Tfelt-Hansen, "History of Methysergide in Migraine."
24. Sicuteri, "L'emicrania."
25. Sicuteri, "Prophylactic Treatment of Migraine by Means of Lysergic Acid Derivatives."
26. Kempner, *Not Tonight*.

## Chapter Seven

1. Hart, *Drug Use for Grown-ups*.
2. Breen, *The Age of Intoxication*.

3. Letcher, *Shroom*.

4. Schultes, "Appeal of Peyote (Lophophora Williamsii) as a Medicine"; for a history of the debate, see Guzmán, "Hallucinogenic Mushrooms in Mexico."

5. Russo, "Headache Treatments by Native Peoples of the Ecuadorian Amazon."

6. Russo, "Machiguenga."

7. "MAPS, MPP and Dr. Ethan Russo Filed an Updated Version"; Russo et al., "Chronic Cannabis Use in the Compassionate Investigational New Drug Program."

## Chapter Eight

1. Nilsson Remahl et al., "Placebo Response."

2. Drugs Act 2005, c. 17, s. 21 (UK).

3. Gottlieb, *Concise Encyclopedia of Legal Herbs*; Ott, *Pharmacotheon*.

4. Oss and Oeric, *Psilocybin, Magic Mushroom Grower's Guide*.

5. Power, *Drugs Unlimited*.

6. Edmond, "Pioneers of the Virtual Underground."

7. Leary, *High Priest*.

## Chapter Nine

1. Dyck, *Psychedelic Psychiatry*; Herzberg, *White Market Drugs*; Oram, *Trials of Psychedelic Therapy*.

2. The slogan "Better Living Through Chemistry" was introduced by DuPont in 1935 to capture the belief that scientific advancements could improve American life. The phrase lives on because of its ability to capture the zeitgeist of each era, be it a drug-using counterculture or pessimism about the problems of corporate industrial science.

3. Metzl, *Prozac on the Couch*.

4. I've drawn on the work of several historians to describe the regulatory politics leading up to the 1962 Kefauver-Harris Act, including Carpenter, *Reputation and Power*; Greene and Podolsky, *Reform, Regulation, and Pharmaceuticals*; Herzberg, *White Market Drugs*; and Tobbell, *Pills, Power, and Policy*.

5. Herzberg, *White Market Drugs*.

6. Carpenter, *Reputation and Power*.

7. Tobbell, *Pills, Power, and Policy*.

8. Jones et al., "Antibiotic Combinations," 1057–1059.

9. Carpenter, *Reputation and Power*; Tobbell, *Pills, Power, and Policy*.

10. US Congress, "Administered Prices in the Drug Industry," 6228.

11. Kennedy's speech, originally covered in the May 1961 issue of *Drug Trade News*, is cited in Herzberg, *White Market Drugs*, 188.

12. Ibid.

13. Ibid., 188.

14. Oram, *Trials of Psychedelic Therapy*.

15. Tobbell, *Pills, Power, and Policy*.

16. The IND required information like the drug's chemical structure, the composition of the preparation, manufacturing and quality control standards, and details

on preclinical investigations, including toxicology reports from animal studies. Oram, *Trials of Psychedelic Therapy*.

17. Ibid.

18. Hofmann, *LSD*.

19. Novak, "LSD Before Leary."

20. Herzig, *Suffering for Science*.

21. Stark and Campbell, "Ineffable."

22. Oram, *Trials of Psychedelic Therapy*.

23. Leary, *High Priest*.

24. Leary, *Flashbacks*.

25. Oram, *Trials of Psychedelic Therapy*.

26. Novak, "LSD Before Leary."

27. The FDA maintained an informal expectation that drug companies would use RCTs to demonstrate the efficacy of new drugs. When asked what data they would require, the FDA often demurred with a "We know good evidence when we see it." RCTs became a codified rule in 1969. Oram, *Trials of Psychedelic Therapy*.

28. Marks, *Progress of Experiment*.

29. My use of the word *man* is intentional. Allopathic medicine became much more exclusionary in its bid for professional power. See Starr, *Social Transformation of American Medicine*.

30. Greene and Podolsky, "Reform, Regulation, and Pharmaceuticals."

31. Epstein, *Impure Science*.

32. Siff, *Acid Hype*.

33. Dyck, *Psychedelic Psychiatry*.

34. Oram, *Trials of Psychedelic Therapy*.

35. Bothwell et al., "Assessing the Gold Standard"; Greene and Podolsky, "Reform, Regulation, and Pharmaceuticals."

## Chapter Ten

1. Wold's welcome email inspired a lengthy discussion. Wold (psiloscribe), "Welcome and Mission Statement."

2. DiMasi, Grabowski, and Hansen, "Innovation in the Pharmaceutical Industry"; Van der Gronde and Pieters, "Assessing Pharmaceutical Research and Development Costs."

3. Cetina, *Epistemic Cultures*; Timmermans and Epstein, "World of Standards but Not a Standard World."

4. Brown, "Popular Epidemiology and Toxic Waste Contamination"; Porter, *Trust in Numbers*.

5. Holbein, "Understanding FDA Regulatory Requirements for Investigational New Drug Applications for Sponsor-Investigators."

6. Dworkin et al., "If the Doors of Perception Were Cleansed, Would Chronic Pain Be Relieved?"

## Chapter Eleven

1. A survey that the University of California, Berkeley's Center for Psychedelic Science conducted in 2023 suggests that Wold considerably overestimated how many people think these substances are safe. Most (61 percent) did not agree that psychedelics were "good for society," and 69 percent did not think psychedelics were "something for people like me." Most medicines, however, aren't expected to be accepted by the broad public as "something" for them.

2. GeorgieT, "long ramble on legalization."

3. Wold (psiloscribe), "long ramble on legalization."

4. Ibid.

5. Ibid.

6. Ibid.

7. Klein, "New Drug They Call 'Ecstasy.'"

8. Pollan, *How to Change Your Mind*.

9. Doblin, "Future of Psychedelic-Assisted Psychotherapy."

10. Mitchell et al., "MDMA-Assisted Therapy for Severe PTSD."

11. Nuwar, "A Psychedelic Drug Passes a Big Test for PTSD Treatment."

12. Jacobs, "Psychedelic Revolution Is Coming."

13. Klein, "New Drug They Call 'Ecstasy.'"

14. Doblin, "Future of Psychedelic-Assisted Psychotherapy."

15. Afternoons, "Using Psychedelics to Treat PTSD and Depression."

16. Shroder, *Acid Test*.

17. Ibid.

18. Doblin, "Future of Psychedelic-Assisted Psychotherapy."

19. Shroder, *Acid Test*, 226.

20. Doblin told Shroder that he created his own major, "an independent study program leading to a degree in a transpersonal psychology," in *Acid Test*, 231.

21. Ibid.

22. Short, "Meet Rick Doblin."

23. Rick Doblin often refers to "the bridge" or the concept of "being the bridge." The metaphor, according to Doblin, refers to a comment made by Timothy Leary at a 1990 fund-raiser for MAPS. "If you want to be a bridge, you have to get used to being stepped on." Doblin, personal communication to Ben Gambuzza, forwarded to author, September 19, 2023. The phrase also appears in an email that Doblin sent to Wold, "[re: albert's prints]," December 8, 2006.

24. Shroder, *Acid Test*, p. 352.

25. Doblin, "Pahnke's Good Friday Experiment."

26. Leonard Pickard, one of Mark Kleiman's former mentees and employees, identified him as an unsung hero of the psychedelic renaissance in "Underground Histories and Overground Futures."

27. Doblin, "Regulation of the Medical Use of Psychedelics and Marijuana."

28. Ross and Nickles, "Trials of Rick Doblin."

29. Gillespie, "People Should Have the Fundamental Human Right to Change Their Consciousness."

30. Doblin, email to Wold, November 12, 2003.

31. Ibid.

32. The description of this conversation and all quotes are pulled from Wold (psilo-scribe), "MAPS."

33. Ibid.

34. Harvard Medical School does not own a hospital but instead maintains agree-ments and partnerships with affiliate hospitals, which provide patient care and clinical training. John Halpern, like many of the physicians who work in these hospitals, also had a faculty position at Harvard Medical School. For clarity, I usually refer to McLean Hospital as Harvard, since this shorthand best captures the language people in my research used when discussing McLean and the hospital's symbolic status. However, I use McLean Hospital when describing the hospital's independent operational and gov-ernance structures.

35. Doblin, "research," December 6, 2003.

36. Weil, "re: research," December 22, 2003.

37. Sewell, Wold, and Doblin, "Re: FW: research," December 8–9, 2003.

38. Doblin, letter to Wold on February 9, 2004, to confirm agreement to conduct FDA-approved research into the use of psilocybin and LSD for cluster headaches.

39. Memorandum of understanding between MAPS, Dr. John Halpern, Dr. Andrew Sewell, Bob Wold, and David and Marsha Weil, April 12, 2004 (drafted on MAPS letterhead).

40. Wold, "re: cluster headache research," December 19, 2003.

## Chapter Twelve

1. Dyck, *Psychedelic Psychiatry*.

2. Strassman, *DMT*.

3. Halpern, "Use of Hallucinogens in the Treatment of Addiction."

4. Dyck, *Psychiatric Psychiatry*.

5. Wasson, "Seeking the Magic Mushroom."

6. Dr. Wasson's role in this "discovery" is too often overlooked. Wasson, "I Ate the Sacred Mushroom"; Williams et al., "Dr. Valentina Wasson."

7. Letcher, *Shroom*, 82.

8. Estrada, *María Sabina*.

9. Ibid., 39.

10. Ibid., 39.

11. Ibid., 40.

12. Ibid., 40.

13. Ibid., 46.

14. Wasson used the pseudonym Eva Mendez to disguise Sabina's identity, but a sharp-eyed reader observed from the photographs that she wore a *huipil* made in Huautla de Jiménez. The Wassons also used her real name in the book about mush-rooms that they had just published. Feinberg, *Devil's Book of Culture*.

15. Wasson, "I Ate the Sacred Mushroom."

16. Ibid.

17. Wasson and Wasson, *Mushrooms, Russia and History*.

18. Feinberg, *Devil's Book of Culture*, 131.

19. Estrada, *María Sabina*, 91.

20. Ibid., 10.

21. Wasson's actions are often held up as a prototypical case of extraction and appropriation in psychedelic research. See Gerber et al., "Ethical Concerns About Psilocybin Intellectual Property."

22. Kandell, "Richard E. Schultes, 86, Dies."

23. Sequiera, "Richard Evans Schultes, 1915–2001," 9.

24. Schultes and Raffauf, *Healing Forest*.

25. Schultes, "Ethnopharmacological Conservation."

26. Hettler and Plotkin, "Amazonian Travels of Richard Evans Schultes."

27. People from the global majority have spoken about these injustices for centuries. Additional information can be found from organizations like the International Center for Ethnobotanical Education, Research, and Service (ICEERS) and the Chacruna Institute of Plant Medicine. Dr. Monnica T. Campbell's research and advocacy have been particularly important in revealing the white supremacist logic underlying psychedelic science. MAPS sponsored Dr. Campbell's Phase 2 clinical trial at the University of Connecticut Health Center to study the safety and efficacy of MDMA-assisted psychotherapy as a treatment for PTSD in an ethnoracially diverse population. Unfortunately, the study was terminated prematurely due to bureaucratic hurdles and institutional racism and sexism. "About ICEERS"; George et al., "Psychedelic Renaissance and the Limitations of a White-Dominant Medical Framework"; Williams, Reed, and Aggarwal, "Culturally-Informed Research Design Issues in a Study for MDMA-Assisted Psychotherapy for Posttraumatic Stress Disorder."

28. Pope, *Voices from Drug Culture*.

29. Mojeiko, "Interview with Dr. John Halpern."

30. Halpern et al., "Peyote Use Among Native Americans."

31. Shroder, *Acid Test*.

32. Halpern, "Neurocognitive Consequences of Long-Term Ecstasy Use"; Halpern, "Cognitive Effects of Substance Use in Native Americans."

33. Halpern and Pope, "Hallucinogens on the Internet."

## Chapter Thirteen

1. Wold, Memoir draft.

2. Halpern, "couldn't send the attached mp3 file," October 27, 2004.

3. Ibid.

4. Halpern, "Letter #2 review," April 1, 2004.

5. Halpern, Doblin, and Wold, "Cluster headache research," February 22 and March 29, 2004; Sewell, "Cluster headache research at Harvard," October 15, 2004.

6. Sewell, "Psilocybin and LSD data," September 30, 2004.

7. Wold (psiloscribe), "Research Update."

8. Wold (psiloscribe), "Important."

9. Ibid.

10. Halpern, "Psilocybin and LSD Data," October 4, 2004.

11. Sewell, "FWD. Psilocybin and LSD data," October 15, 2004.

12. Halpern, "Fwd: Psilocybin and LSD data," October 4, 2004.

13. Sewell, "Re: requests for information/records," November 5, 2004.

14. At MAPS's 2017 Psychedelic Science Conference, Erowid's booth had been set up across the way from Clusterbusters' display. When I introduced myself to Earth and explained my research, he gestured toward Clusterbusters' table and described his irritation about having volunteered for research that the organization would later fund at Harvard. Earth seemed to feel better about the experience when I asked him about it at the 2023 Psychedelic Science Conference. We only spoke briefly, but he made sure to express a "great fondness" for Andrew Sewell. I can see this fondness in Erowid's Andrew Sewell "character vault," where the site stores information related to his work. Erowid's biography of Sewell includes a quote attributed to an email he sent in 2008 that captures why he was so beloved by the underground community. "You can either be a serious academic researcher and promote legitimate study of psychedelic drugs, or else run your unauthorized psychedelic clinic, give LSD to patients, grow pot in your back yard and so on, but you can't mix the two; you have to make a choice." Earth, "Confusion over case numbers," October 26, 2004.

15. Erowid and Erowid, "The State of the Stone."

16. Sewell, "LSD and Psilocybin in the Treatment of Cluster Headaches."

17. Sewell, "Clarification of case report," July 19, 2005.

18. Sewell, "Clarification of case report," August 15, 2005.

19. Sewell, "New developments in case series," August 22, 2005.

20. Sewell, Halpern, and Pope, "Response of Cluster Headache to Psilocybin and LSD," 1920.

21. Ibid.

22. Sewell, "re: status of submission," December 28, 2005.

23. Sewell et al., "Treatment of Cluster Headaches with Indole-Ring Psychedelics."

24. Pope told me that he had no memory of this. Halpern argued that the collection of medical records made their research distinct from Clusterbusters.

25. Halpern told me that the collection of medical records, which corroborated a cluster headache diagnosis, distinguished this study from Clusterbusters' research. Peer-reviewers did not have this information. Sewell, "Unauthorized Research on Cluster Headache."

26. Sewell, "re: status of submission," December 28, 2005.

27. Ibid.

## Chapter Fourteen

1. Langlitz, *Neuropsychedelia*, 81.

2. WIRED Staff, "LSD."

3. This scene was captured on video and distributed on YouTube. See Nickles, "Mark McCloud Calls Out DEA Snitch & MAPS Researcher John Halpern January 13th, 2006."

4. The content and [word out] of these documents are not clear but may have come from Leonard Pickard's defense team. Hanna, "Halperngate."

5. During a March 23, 2023, Zoom conversation, Nicolas Langlitz documented people warning one another that Halpern might be an informant in his field notes from Hofmann's one hundredth birthday symposium.

6. MacIntosh, "City Jet-Setter's Bizarre LSD Trip"; Rosenfeld, "William Pickard's Long, Strange Trip."

7. Wilkinson, "Acid King."

8. McDougal, *Operation White Rabbit*; Rosenfeld, "William Pickard's Long, Strange Trip."

9. McDougal, *Operation White Rabbit*; Rosenfeld, "William Pickard's Long, Strange Trip."

10. Ibid.

11. Rosenfeld, "William Pickard's Long, Strange Trip."

12. Elliott, "Life Term Given in Torture Case"; Elliott, "Ex-Informant in Tulsa Jail."

13. Elliott, "Life Term Given in Torture Case."

14. During a March 23, 2023, Zoom conversation, Nicolas Langlitz documented people warning one another that Halpern might be an informant in his field notes from Hofmann's one hundredth birthday symposium.

15. Hanna, "Halperngate."

16. MAPS has been the subject of several controversies in recent years, including allegations of sexual assault of a clinical trial participant by a therapist during an MDMA session and of elder abuse, as well as ongoing complaints about a lack of inclusivity. See, for example, Ross and Nickles, "Trials of Rick Doblin"; Goldhill, "Psychedelic Medicine Group Investigating a Board Member Accused of Financial Elder Abuse"; Lindsay, "Corrective Measures Ordered"; Lekhtman, "Why Indigenous Protesters Stopped a Global Psychedelic Conference."

17. Hanna, "Halperngate," 15.

18. Ibid.

19. Ibid., 16.

20. Ibid., 16.

21. Allen, "A Doctor's Downfall, McLean's Fallout."

22. Doblin, "Updates/restricted accounting," June 11, 2006.

23. Ibid.

24. Sewell, Halpern, and Pope, "Response of Cluster Headache to Psilocybin and LSD."

25. Halpern, "just a clear example . . . ," email exchange titled "well so it isn't" between Halpern and R. Andrew Sewell from January 17, 2006, forwarded to Robert Wold, October 30, 2006.

26. Doblin, Halpern, and Sewell, "Psilocybin cluster headache research," June 14, 2006.

27. Ibid.

28. About a week later, Wold wrote a message to Sewell stating that he, personally, did not care where the fellowship was located but insisted that other important stakeholders should be involved in the discussion, including Dr. Harrison Pope, Rick Doblin, and Marsha Weil. Wold, "Re: Cluster headache research fellowship," June 20, 2006.

29. Sewell, "So You Want to Be a Psychedelic Researcher?"

30. Frauenfelder, "Interview with Marc Franklin."

31. Halpern, "a weekend of patience: besides it's only you and rick . . . ," September 9, 2006.

32. Ibid.

33. Halpern, "A CH'ers complaints," September 16, 2008.

34. Sewell, "Cluster headache studies," October 23, 2006.

35. Halpern, "This is for you only," October 29, 2006.

36. Ibid.

37. Wold, "re: visit," October 21, 2006.

38. Ibid.

39. Wold, "re: 6th death this year," October 15, 2006.

40. Sewell, "Re: Sorry to hear," November 28, 2006.

41. Doblin, "re: updates/Restricted accounting," June 11, 2006; Doblin, "re: money," November 27, 2006.

42. Doblin, "[re: albert's prints]," December 8, 2006.

43. Ibid.

44. Bebergal, "Will Harvard Drop Acid Again?"

45. Hanna, "Halperngate."

46. Giffort, *Acid Revival*.

47. Bebergal, "Will Harvard Drop Acid Again?"

48. Davis, "The Bad Shaman Meets the Wayward Doc."

49. Halpern, "a few more points need fixing," December 25, 2006.

## Chapter Fifteen

1. Huxley, *Island*.

2. Shroder, *Acid Test*, 319.

3. Halpern, "John Halpern Forecasts the Future."

4. Ibid.; Gerard, "Pain, Death and LSD"; Kast, "LSD and the Dying Patient"; Kast, "Attenuation of Anticipation"; Kast and Collins, "Study of Lysergic Acid Diethylamide as an Analgesic Agent."

5. Kast, "Measurement of Pain."

6. Kast and Collins, "Study of Lysergic Acid Diethylamide as an Analgesic Agent."

7. Oram, *Trials of Psychedelic Therapy*.

8. Kast and Collins, "Study of Lysergic Acid Diethylamide as an Analgesic Agent"; Kast, "LSD and the Dying Patient"; Kast, "Attenuation of Anticipation."

9. Ibid.

10. Ibid., 291.

11. Cohen, "Complications Associated with Lysergic Acid Diethylamide (LSD-25)"; Novak, "LSD Before Leary."

12. Cohen, "The Anguish of the Dying."

13. Ibid., 72.

14. Oram, *Trials of Psychedelic Therapy*; Richards et al., "LSD-Assisted Psychotherapy and the Human Encounter with Death."

15. Griffiths et al., "Psilocybin Can Occasion Mystical-Type Experiences Having Substantial and Sustained Personal Meaning and Spiritual Significance."

16. Thirty-three percent ranked it as the most meaningful experience in their life (ibid.).

17. Griffiths et al., "Mystical-Type Experiences Occasioned by Psilocybin Mediate the Attribution of Personal Meaning and Spiritual Significance 14 Months Later."

18. Grob et al., "Pilot Study of Psilocybin Treatment for Anxiety in Patients with Advanced-Stage Cancer."

19. Gasser, Kirchner, and Passie, "LSD-Assisted Psychotherapy for Anxiety Associated with a Life-Threatening Disease"; Griffiths et al., "Psilocybin Produces Substantial and Sustained Decreases in Depression and Anxiety in Patients with Life-Threatening Cancer"; Holze et al., "Lysergic Acid Diethylamide–Assisted Therapy in Patients with Anxiety with and Without a Life-Threatening Illness"; Ross et al., "Rapid and Sustained Symptom Reduction Following Psilocybin Treatment for Anxiety and Depression in Patients with Life-Threatening Cancer."

20. Halpern, "Phase II Dose-Response Pilot Study of 3,4-Methylenedioxy-methamphetamine (MDMA)–Assisted Psychotherapy in Subjects with Anxiety Associated with Advanced-Stage Cancer."

21. Halpern, "Letter #2 review," April 1, 2004.

22. Halpern may have been exaggerating since he provided this estimate to Torsten Passie in email asking if they could bring down the cost of the BOL-148 study. "I hope we can keep the estimated costs to the very lowest possible. The foundation Clusterbusters is patient-driven and is new. They are trying to save as much money as possible to pay for the psilocybin study, which we ballpark coming in at the wallet-busting amount of perhaps $500,000." Halpern, "actual costs," January 23, 2007.

23. Halpern, "re: future plans," November 25, 2006.

24. "Erowid Character Vaults: R. Andrew Sewell."

25. Halpern, "re: future plans," November 25, 2006.

26. Halpern, "CB Budget Committee and Passie Discussion," August 8, 2007.

27. Sewell, Halpern, and Pope, "Response of Cluster Headache."

28. Doblin, email to Wold, February 2, 2009.

29. Ibid.

30. Huertas, "Re: ok . . . let's move ahead . . . JHH comments," March 2, 2009.

31. Doblin, "BOL development prospects," March 27, 2009.

32. Halpern, "BOL development prospects," March 27, 2009.

33. Sewell, "Compositions and Methods for Preventing and/or Treating Disorders Associated with Cephalic Pain," Patent 8859579, filed October 14, 2014, and issued March 20, 2009.

## Chapter Sixteen

1. Fadiman, *The Psychedelic Explorer's Guide*.

2. Gunther, "Carey Turnbull Wears Many Hats as a Donor and Investor."

3. Ibid.

4. "Maharishi School Makes Business Gurus."

5. Griffiths et al., "Psilocybin Can Occasion Mystical-Type Experiences Having Substantial and Sustained Personal Meaning and Spiritual Significance."

6. Pollan, Michael. "The Trip Treatment."

7. Greco, "Yale's Pioneering Research on Psychedelics Gives Hope to Headache Disorder Community."

8. Schindler et al., "Indoleamine Hallucinogens in Cluster Headache."

9. Rusanen et al., "Self-Reported Efficacy of Treatments in Cluster Headache."

10. Greco, "Yale's Pioneering Research on Psychedelics Gives Hope to Headache Disorder Community."

11. Madsen et al., "Psilocybin-Induced Reduction on Chronic Cluster Headache Attack Frequency Correlates"; Schindler, "Psychedelics as Preventive Treatment in Headache and Chronic Pain Disorders"; Rusanen et al., "Self-Reported Efficacy of Treatments in Cluster Headache."

12. Schindler et al., "Exploratory Investigation of a Patient-Informed Low-Dose Psilocybin Pulse Regimen in the Suppression of Cluster Headache."

13. Schindler et al., "Exploratory Controlled Study of the Migraine-Suppressing Effects of Psilocybin."

14. Pollan, *How to Change Your Mind*, 60–61.

15. Schindler et al., "Exploratory Controlled Study of the Migraine-Suppressing Effects of Psilocybin."

16. Madsen et al., "Psilocybin-Induced Reduction on Chronic Cluster Headache Attack Frequency Correlates."

## Conclusion

1. Newberry, "MDMA-Assisted Therapy Could Soon Be Approved by the FDA."

2. U.S. Department of Veterans Affairs, Office of Mental Health and Suicide Prevention, "National Veteran Suicide Prevention Annual Report, 2022."

3. Hooyer et al., "Altered States of Combat."

4. In recent years, several new organizations have been founded to promote psychedelic research and/or therapy for veterans and first responders. Some of the most prominent include VETS and No Fallen Heroes.

5. Lubecky, "From the Personal to the Political."

6. As several scholars have documented, psychedelics have never lived up to the utopian fantasy that they'll "change your mind" to embrace progressive, ecofriendly politics. Rebekah Mercer, one of the chief financiers of the Far Right political movement in the United States, has given MAPS at least $1 million in research support. Peter Thiel, a self-described conservative libertarian and a major donor to Republican candidates, has backed two of the biggest publicly traded psychedelic corporations, Atai and Compass Therapeutics. Jordan Peterson, the philosopher best known for defending traditional gender norms, regularly hosts top psychedelic researchers on his podcast. Then there are the ethical horrors committed by Nazi physicians or "turned on" CIA agents under the cover of MKUltra. Ahlman, "House Moves to Expand Psychedelic Therapy Research"; Pace and Devenot, "Right-Wing Psychedelia."

7. Armstrong and Allen, "Behind the Luxury."

8. Lindsay, "As Psychedelic Therapy Goes Mainstream, Former Patient Warns of Danger of Sexual Abuse."

# INDEX

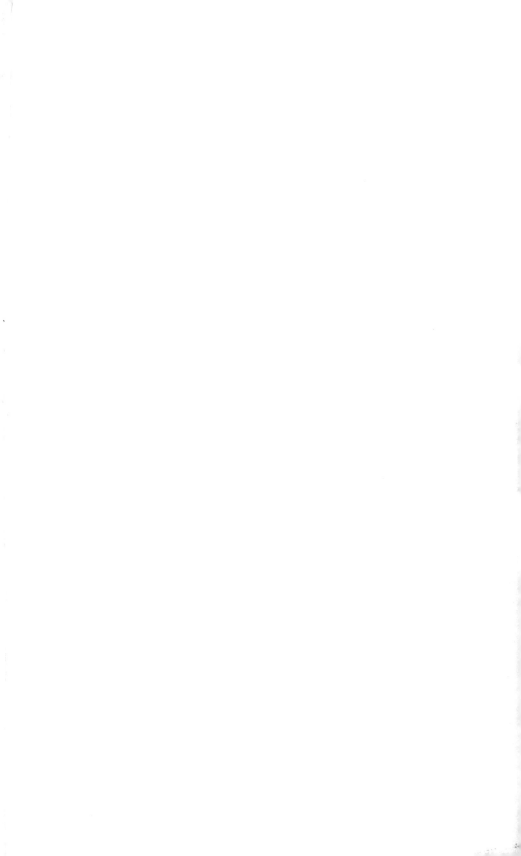